Study Guide

SUZANNE C. BEYEA

Medical
Surgical
Nursing

*Critical Thinking
in Client Care*

SECOND EDITION

LEMONE ■ BURKE

PRENTICE HALL HEALTH
Upper Saddle River, New Jersey 07458

Editor-in-Chief: Cheryl L. Mehalik
Project Editors: Virginia Simione Jutson, Grace Wong
Managing Editor: Wendy Earl
Associate Editor: Stephanie Kellogg
Publishing Assistants: Susan Tehan, Peggy Hammett
Production Supervisor: David Novak
Production Coordinator: Bettina Borer
Director of Manufacturing and Production: Bruce Johnson
Manufacturing Buyer: Ilene Sanford
Cover Designer: Yvo Riezebos Design
Compositor: Marian Hartsough Associates
Printer/Binder: Victor Graphics, Inc.
Cover: The quilt is entitled *Color Blocks #35*,
    ©1993 Nancy Crow. 34 1/2" x 36 1/2";
    Photo by J Kevin Fitzsimons

Previously published by Addison-Wesley Nursing,
A Division of the Benjamin/Cummings Publishing Company, Inc.
Menlo Park, California 94025

Printed in the United States of America.
10 9 8 7 6 5 4 3 2
ISBN 0-8053-8127-9

Prentice-Hall International (UK) Limited, London
Prentice-Hall of Australia Pty. Limited, Sydney
Prentice-Hall Canada Inc., Toronto
Prentice-Hall Hispanoamericana, S.A., Mexico
Prentice-Hall of India Private Limited, New Delhi
Prentice-Hall of Japan, Inc., Tokyo

Preface

Revising and updating this study guide to accompany *Medical-Surgical Nursing, Critical Thinking in Client Care,* Second Edition, by Priscilla LeMone and Karen Burke reinforced my beliefs about the effectiveness of their textbook in presenting and teaching nursing care. As with the first edition of this study guide, the primary goal is to assist students learn and understand what they need to know to provide safe, effective client care. Emphasis has been placed on understanding key concepts as a way to apply critical thinking skills.

Each chapter of the study guide corresponds to the same chapter in the textbook. Assessment chapters focus on a review of anatomy of physiology followed by health assessment. The nursing care chapters are organized by major health problems and the related nursing care. Within the study guide, questions are organized according to the major headings within the textbook, making it easy for students to coordinate the study guide with the textbook.

Questions at the knowledge, comprehension, application, and analysis levels of learning have been included throughout the study guide. Questions are presented in a variety of formats to assist students who have different learning styles. The study guide should be used in conjunction with the textbook and the additional multiple choice questions provided with the textbook. The framework is designed to stimulate learning and thinking and to reinforce knowledge.

▪ ▪ ▪ Acknowledgments

Teamwork was the framework for the first edition of this study guide. Without the efforts of the author group from the first edition, I would not have been able to see this edition through its revisions. Their work and effort lives on in this edition. My sincere thanks are offered to each author and reviewer.

Publication of this study guide, though guided by those at Addison-Wesley Nursing, will occur after many colleagues there move on to new roles within the publishing company. Transition is part of life, but I will forever miss the close relationships of so many at Addison-Wesley Nursing who contributed in such a significant way to my writing. Special and never-ending thanks are extended to:

- Ginnie Simione Jutson, who has believed in my ability to contribute to projects even when I was sometimes unsure.

- Grace Wong, who kept me on schedule and on task and made this revision so much easier than it might have been.

- David Novak and Bettina Borer in production, who made this book a reality.

- Mary Sampel, MSN, BSN; Roger Voekel, RN, MS, Missouri Western State College; and Elizabeth Chandler, MS, RN, Quincy College—the reviewers who contributed their additional perspectives.

- The faculty and students who commented on the first edition and made helpful suggestions for this edition.

- The nursing staff, including many former students, at Catholic Medical Center and the Elliot Hospital, who have kept me grounded in clinical practice and taught me more than they will ever know.

- The Beyea boys (who were men in the last edition), for being there when and where it counts, every day and in my heart.

- BABAMBA, for endless hours of proofreading and editing on this and so many other projects. Words will never fully express my genuine thanks.

Suzanne C. Beyea, PhD, RN, CS
Co-director of Perioperative Nursing Research,
Association of periOperative Registered Nurses (AORN)

Contents

CHAPTER 1

The Medical-Surgical Nurse

▪ ▪ ▪ Focused Study Tips

- Discuss the various roles of the nurse in medical-surgical practice.
- Describe the steps of the nursing process. Keep a record of clinical activities for one day and categorize each activity according to the nursing process.

- Discuss issues and trends regarding nursing care of special populations with experienced nurses.

▪ ▪ ▪ The Medical-Surgical Nurse

1. Medical-surgical nursing practice is designed for the (a) _____ client. Nursing care is planned and implemented for (b) _____ that result in structural and functional changes in the client's body systems. These changes may affect the personal, (c) _____, (d) _____, and (e) _____ life of the client.

▪ ▪ ▪ Roles of the Nurse in Medical-Surgical Practice

2. Identify and describe the six roles that the nurse assumes to promote and maintain health.
   (a) _____
   (b) _____
   (c) _____
   (d) _____
   (e) _____
   (f) _____

3. Which of the following most accurately describes the role of the nurse as caregiver today?
   a. research-based scientist
   b. independent and collaborative professional
   c. highly knowledgeable educator
   d. dependent practitioner

4. Which of the following skills is considered essential to enhancing the teaching/learning process?
   a. effective interpersonal skills
   b. excellent clinical skills
   c. a physician's order
   d. primary nursing practice

5. Discharge planning is a systematic method of preparing the client and family for leaving the health care agency and for maintaining continuity of care after they leave the setting. Teaching is a major part of this process. List three other components of discharge planning.
   (a) _____
   (b) _____
   (c) _____

6. Despite increasing cultural diversity in the population, nursing has been slow to address the need for culturally sensitive care. Two factors that account for this inattention are (a) _____ _____, which is a person's belief that the only acceptable beliefs and values are those of his/her own cultural group, and (b) _____, which is an irrational hostility toward a group or race of people.

7. A client is admitted to the intensive care unit (ICU) with complaints of severe chest pain. During his first night in the ICU, he is extremely anxious and requests that his partner be contacted and asked to stay with him throughout the night, stating, "If he's here, I'll be able to relax." The most appropriate response by the nurse is:
   a. "It's too late tonight. You can call him in the morning."
   b. "Visitors are not allowed in the ICU after 10 PM."
   c. "I'll give him a call now."
   d. "Would you rather call your mother?"

8. A 28-year-old client who is a Jehovah's Witness is refusing a blood transfusion. The nurse knows that a blood transfusion is appropriate therapy for the client's condition. Which of the following nursing interventions is most appropriate?
   a. explain to the client that he must have the transfusion or his condition will worsen
   b. inform the client that the hospital will go to court to make him have the transfusion
   c. explain to the client the benefits of having the transfusion
   d. support the client in his decision even when in disagreement

9. (a) _____ consists of the quality control activities that evaluate, monitor, or regulate the standard of services provided to the consumer. An example of this process is (b) _____.

10. The primary goal of nursing research is to:
    a. improve client care.
    b. support nursing as a profession.
    c. improve the visibility of nursing.
    d. provide accurate information in nursing textbooks.

▪ ▪ ▪ Framework for Practice: The Nursing Process

Identify the step in the nursing process that is best defined by each statement.

11. In this step, the nurse defines the client's health problem based on the nurse's clinical judgment.

_____

12. In this step, the nurse identifies activities that can be used to help a client achieve desired outcomes. _____

13. In this step, the nurse gathers subjective and objective data that may describe the client's health problem. _____

14. During this phase, the nurse examines all other phases of the nursing process. The other phases may be modified based on this examination. _____

15. In this phase, the nurse performs activities to care for the client _____

_____

Match the nursing process step (a–e) that best corresponds to the situations listed in questions 16–28.

_____ 16. the client will have no complaints of chest pain

_____ 17. Anticipatory Grieving secondary to client's end-stage illness

_____ 18. "I am having chest pain."

_____ 19. client's complaints of pain increase following pain medication

_____ 20. client's safety will be maintained at all times

_____ 21. there is a 2 × 2 wound on the client's forearm

_____ 22. turn client q2h

_____ 23. Anxiety related to lack of information about bone marrow aspiration procedure

_____ 24. blood pressure was taken lying down, seated, and standing up

_____ 25. the client's blood pressure is 130/70

_____ 26. following teaching, client cannot correctly describe medication schedule

_____ 27. Fluid Volume Deficit secondary to excessive diaphoresis

_____ 28. client will learn how to self-administer insulin before discharge

a. assessment
b. diagnosis
c. planning
d. implementation
e. evaluation

▪ ▪ ▪ Guidelines for Nursing Practice

29. (a) _____ assessments are ongoing and continuous, occurring whenever the nurse interacts with the client. (b) _____ assessments are conducted through a nursing history and physical assessment and are necessary for facilitation of mutually established goals and outcomes of care.

30. What do the initials in "PES format" represent?

   P _____

   E _____

   S _____

31. Principles of conduct are called _____.

32. A _____ is a statement or criterion that can be used by a profession and by the general public to measure quality of practice.

33. A _____ is a choice between two unpleasant alternatives.

Read the following statement and determine if it is true or false. Correct the statement if it is false.

_____ 34. According to the ANA, the nurse has a moral obligation to provide care for the client with AIDS unless the risk exceeds the responsibility.

35. The purpose of an advance directive is to:
    a. provide the hospital with accurate insurance information about the client.
    b. communicate to all health care professionals the client's complete medical history, including admissions to other hospitals.
    c. communicate to all health care professionals the client's preferences for health care in the event that the client later becomes mentally incapacitated.
    d. detail all of the client's admission orders from the physician.

36. The right to refuse treatment is a client right that may raise nursing dilemmas. During these situations, what is the first intervention the nurse, as client advocate, should complete?

▪ ▪ ▪ Issues and Trends in Medical-Surgical Nursing

Read the following statements and determine if they are true or false. Correct any false statements.

_____ 37. Older adults have more chronic illnesses and recover less rapidly from acute illnesses than young and middle adults, thus requiring a larger number of hospital beds.

_____ 38. Older adults require more long-term care.

_____ 39. The number of older adults in the total population has decreased significantly over the past few years.

_____ 40. Older adults require more community services and home care.

41. Which of the following clients is considered medically indigent?
    a. a 49-year-old disabled U.S. Army veteran
    b. a 28-year-old unemployed actor who is covered by his wife's medical insurance
    c. a 22-year-old nursing student and mother of two who has used student loan money to purchase health insurance
    d. a 40-year-old restaurant cook who is uninsured

42. Which of the following statements about homelessness is false?
    a. Some health problems, such as severe alterations in mental health, may lead to homelessness.
    b. Many homeless individuals have a fixed, regular, and adequate nighttime residence.
    c. Homelessness may lead to illness or to exacerbation of a chronic illness.
    d. Homelessness makes treatment and care of any illness almost impossible.

43. When looking toward the future of health care delivery, hospitals will become centers that focus on two major areas: (a) _____ and (b) _____.

44. Identify at least three goals of critical pathways.
    (a) _____
    (b) _____
    (c) _____

45. Identify at least three uses for computers in health care institutions.

(a) _____

(b) _____

(c) _____

46. In 1991, the ANA published Nursing's Agenda for Health Care Reform, which is a plan focused on (a) _____ rather than (b) _____ .

▪ ▪ ▪ **Critical Thinking Exercises**

47. Compare and contrast the International Council of Nurses Code for Nurses and the American Nurses Association Code for Nurses.

48. The nurse is caring for a homeless woman who is admitted to the hospital with pneumonia. What additional health problems is she at risk of experiencing? How might the nurse approach developing a plan for follow-up care after discharge?

▪ ▪ ▪ **Additional Learning Experiences**

- Volunteer in a soup kitchen or homeless shelter.
- Participate in a hospice as a volunteer.
- Scan the newspaper for health-related articles, and identify any ethical implications.

The Adult Client in Health and Illness

■ ■ ■ **Focused Study Tips**

- Describe the physical changes and healthy behaviors in the young adult years, middle adult years, and older adult years.

- Keep a food diary for a week and classify each item according to food pyramid categories.

- Assess task achievement with a chronically ill person.

■ ■ ■ **The Adult Client**

1. In adult life, changes occur in which three developmental areas?
   (a) _____
   (b) _____
   (c) _____

Match the stages of adult development (a–c) with the related tasks listed in questions 2–8.

_____ 2. identity versus role confusion

_____ 3. integrity versus despair

_____ 4. generativity versus stagnation

_____ 5. taking on civic responsibility

_____ 6. relating to spouse as a person

_____ 7. adjusting to retirement, reduced income, and decreasing health

_____ 8. acquiring a cognitive and an affective faith through questioning one's own faith

a. young adult
b. middle adult
c. older adult

Match the stages of adult development (a–c) with the related risk factors listed in questions 9–15.

_____ 9. In this stage of adult life, weight gain occurs because of continued consumption of calories with a decrease in activities.

_____ 10. Accidents are the leading cause of death in this population.

_____ 11. Ninety percent of this population has at least one chronic illness.

_____ 12. The leading causes of death in this population are cancer, stroke, and heart disease.

_____ 13. Substance abuse occurs most commonly in this stage of adult life.

_____ 14. The number of divorces is highest in this stage of adult life.

_____ 15. Cancer is the third leading cause of death in this population.

a. young adult
b. middle adult
c. older adult

16. Name three community settings for health promotion for young adults.

(a) _____

(b) _____

(c) _____

17. Which gender is most at risk for cardiovascular illness in the middle adult? _____

18. Identify three physical changes that take place in the older adult years.

(a) _____

(b) _____

(c) _____

19. The three major causes of injury in the older adult are (a) _____,
(b) _____, and (c) _____.

20. Which of the following activities might the nurse teach the older adult client when promoting
healthy behaviors?

a. choose a diet high in fat (30% or more of total calories)

b. use sugar, salt, and sodium in moderation

c. have dental checkup and vision exam at least once every 5 years

d. exercise strenuously every day

Match the stages of adulthood (a–d) with the appropriate healthy behaviors listed in questions 21–28.

_____ 21. choose foods from all food groups, and eat a variety of foods   a. young adult

b. middle adult

_____ 22. use sugar, salt, and sodium in moderation   c. older adult

d. all adult groups

_____ 23. have a vision examination every 2 to 4 years

_____ 24. have an annual dental checkup

_____ 25. for females, have a breast examination and a mammogram annually

_____ 26. for females, have Pap tests as recommended by physician

_____ 27. conduct breast or testicular self-examination monthly

_____ 28. consume high-fiber foods

▪ ▪ ▪ The Family of the Adult Client

29. Which one of the following statements is false?

a. The definition of a family stays the same as society changes.

b. Duvall (1977) defined *family* as a unit of people related by marriage, birth, or adoption.

c. In a global society, it may not be realistic for family members to live in close proximity, but
they do remain emotionally involved.

d. Although every family is unique, all families have certain structural and functional features
in common.

30. Identify four risk factors for alterations in health for families with middle adults.

    (a) _____

    (b) _____

    (c) _____

    (d) _____

31. Adjusting to retirement and closing the family home are two possible developmental tasks of which family group?

    a. the family with adolescents

    b. the family with middle adults

    c. the family with older adults

    d. the family with college-age adults

32. Name three health problems associated with the family with school-age children.

    (a) _____

    (b) _____

    (c) _____

▪ ▪ ▪ Health and Illness in the Adult Client

33. _____ is an integrated method of functioning that is oriented toward maximizing an individual's potential within his or her environment.

34. The World Health Organization (WHO) defines _____ as a state of complete physical, mental, and social well-being and not merely the absence of disease or infirmity.

35. List three factors that affect health and give an example of each.

    (a) _____

    (b) _____

    (c) _____

36. Although the emphasis in nursing has been on care of the acutely ill client in the hospital setting, changes in society and health care have shifted the emphasis toward (a) _____ care based in the (b) _____.

Match the levels of preventing illness (a–c) with the correct client activities listed in questions 37–42.

_____ 37. The client performs a breast examination once per month while in the shower.

_____ 38. The client works with a physical therapist after becoming paraplegic from a diving accident.

_____ 39. The client is having a stress test in the cardiac rehabilitation laboratory after having open heart surgery.

_____ 40. The client checks the label on all food products prior to buying them.

_____ 41. Prior to employment at a hospital, the client has a positive purified derivative test (PPD) for TB.

_____ 42. The client uses a filter on the water faucet in her home.

a. primary

b. secondary

c. tertiary

43. The document on national health objectives published by the U.S. Department of Health and Human Services is called _____ .

44. In general, (a) _____ is concerned with illness, while (b) _____ is concerned with disease.

45. Experiencing symptoms, assuming the sick role, seeking medical care, assuming a dependent role, and achieving recovery and rehabilitation are a sequence of behaviors that describe _____ _____.

Match the definitions (a–e) with the correct disease classifications listed in questions 46–50.

_____ 46. communicable

_____ 47. congenital

_____ 48. malignant

_____ 49. psychosomatic

_____ 50. iatrogenic

a. a disease or disorder that exists at or before birth
b. a psychologic disease that is manifested by physiologic symptoms
c. a disease that can spread from one person to another
d. a disease that tends to become worse and cause death
e. a disease that occurs as the result of medical therapy

51. Which of the following is not a task of the chronically ill person?
    a. controlling symptoms
    b. preventing social isolation
    c. preventing and managing a medical crisis
    d. preventing changes in the course of the disease

52. A disturbance in structure or function resulting from physiologic or psychologic abnormalities is called a(n):
    a. disability.   b. chronic illness.   c. handicap.   d. impairment.

53. The process of learning to live to one's maximum potential with a chronic impairment and its resultant functional disability is known as _____.

54. A 75-year-old client has had a stroke and is unable to move her left arm or speak. Identify four nursing interventions that are appropriate for this client.
    (a) _____
    (b) _____
    (c) _____
    (d) _____

55. Before establishing a plan of care, it is critical that the rehabilitation nurse determine the priorities of needs from the perspective of the:
    a. physician.   b. physical therapist.   c. client and family.   d. primary care nurse.

56. Assessment of the client and family includes:
    (a) _____
    (b) _____
    (c) _____
    (d) _____

57. Describe the four general areas of nursing intervention.

    (a) _____

    (b) _____

    (c) _____

    (d) _____

■ ■ ■ Critical Thinking Exercises

58. The nurse is caring for a 14-year-old boy who has been diagnosed with diabetes. Review the tasks of the chronically ill person and develop a teaching plan to assist the client and family in coping with this diagnosis.

59. Discuss nursing strategies to prevent iatrogenic illness.

60. The nurse is caring for a well adult male who is 75 years old. Develop an age-appropriate teaching plan that incorporates primary and secondary levels of prevention.

■ ■ ■ Additional Learning Experiences

- Volunteer at a local nursing home or day care center and work with an age group that is less familiar to you.

- Relate the definitions and functions of *family* to your own family situation.

Community-Based and Home Care of the Adult Client

■ ■ ■ **Focused Study Tips**

- Describe Core Home Health Problems and the various types of home health agencies.
- Describe the roles of the home health nurse.
- Explain the Home Health Agency's Bill of Rights and the ANA Standards for Home Health Nursing Practice to another student.
- Perform a safety assessment in your own home.

■ ■ ■ **The Home Health Care System**

1. Community-based nursing is based on (a) _____ and (b) _____ health care needs.

2. The purposes of home care nursing include (a) _____, (b) _____, (c) _____ health, and (d) _____.

3. _____ are categories for reimbursement of inpatient services, introduced in an effort to control the spiraling cost of health care.

4. Which home care service would Medicare/Medicaid not reimburse?
   a. complex dressing changes
   b. monitoring total parenteral nutrition
   c. adaptive equipment for safety
   d. respiratory assessment for the homebound client

5. When clients are cared for in the home, the coordination of care is the responsibility of the:
   a. home care nurse.
   b. physician.
   c. social worker.
   d. director of the home health agency.

6. Treatments for clients who are cared for in the home are approved by a(n):
   a. registered nurse.
   b. licensed practical nurse.
   c. physician.
   d. agency director.

7. About half of all home care clients are in which age group?
   a. adolescents and young adults
   b. older adults
   c. middle adults
   d. infants and children

8. The _____ is the person recommending home health services and supplying the home health agency with details about the client's needs.

9. Although there are several different types of home health agencies, all are similar in that they must meet uniform standards for (a) _____, (b) _____, and (c) _____.

10. Home care's largest single reimbursement source is (a) _____, and the second largest source of payment is (b) _____.

▪ ▪ ▪ Roles of the Home Health Nurse

11. The philosophy of home health nursing is to provide:
    a. direct nursing care that encourages client self-care.
    b. medical care similar to that provided by a physician in a hospital setting.
    c. nursing care for the community.
    d. for personal care needs.

12. Many home health nurses feel that their primary activity is:
    a. providing personal care.
    b. evaluating the care given by others.
    c. administering medications.
    d. client-teaching.

13. Place a ✔ by the activities listed below that are reimbursable by a third-party payor such as Medicare:

    _____ a. a visit by an RN for a general checkup after hospitalization

    _____ b. a visit by an RN to evaluate a poorly healing wound

    _____ c. a visit by an RN to give intravenous antibiotics

    _____ d. a visit by an RN to give a flu shot

    _____ e. a visit by an RN to a client who cannot afford transportation to the clinic

    _____ f. a visit to a client who is depressed

14. One of the primary problems with current Medicare reimbursement guidelines is:
    a. the client must be at least partially homebound.
    b. the client must require constant care.
    c. the nursing procedures required must be "skilled."
    d. each home care visit must include every step in the nursing process.

▪ ▪ ▪ Nursing Practice in the Home

15. The ANA Standards for Home Health Nursing Practice address such topics as (a) _____, (b) _____, and (c) _____.

16. Another published source of guidance regarding home care is _____.

17. A client is being discharged today from the hospital. He is chronically anemic and will require injections of Epogen three times a week. He performs all the steps correctly; however, the discharge nurse makes a home health referral. The nurse makes the referral based on what principle?
    a. Research shows that recall of specific instructions is less than 50%.
    b. A nurse must supervise all injections.
    c. If the client forgets a step, the hospital could be sued.
    d. All clients have a follow-up home health visit following discharge.

Read the following statement and determine if it is true or false. Correct the statement if it is false.

_____ 18. One important nursing intervention is to obtain a referral for home care from the attending physician.

19. In 1993, Stulginsky studied the art and science of home health nursing. According to the study, goals of home health visits are to:
    (a) _____
    (b) _____
    (c) _____

20. A home health nurse is assigned to a newly diagnosed client with diabetes mellitus. The home health plan includes teaching the client how to draw up, store, inject, and manage insulin therapy. The client must also be taught how to monitor her glucose level. On the first visit, the nurse should teach the client how to (a) _____,
    (b) _____, and (c) _____ insulin.

21. Identify three teaching strategies a nurse can employ to empower a client to learn.
    (a) _____
    (b) _____
    (c) _____

22. Safety assessment in the home is a nursing responsibility and a legal requirement. Name three potential safety hazards in the home the nurse should address.
    (a) _____
    (b) _____
    (c) _____

23. The most important nursing intervention in controlling infection is _____.

24. Infection control in the home centers around protecting clients, caregivers, and the community from the spread of disease. Identify three safety precautions the home health nurse should practice.
    (a) _____
    (b) _____
    (c) _____

25. List three ancillary roles that the home health nurse may perform that are not treatment oriented, and give examples of activities the nurse might perform in each role.
    (a) _____
    (b) _____
    (c) _____

26. In her initial visit to a 76-year-old client with emphysema, the nurse notices a large supply of expired medications on the client's kitchen counter. The nurse alerts the client that these medications are no longer safe to consume, and she suggests they be discarded. The client refuses to discard the medications, stating that he might need them again and that he is sure they are "still good." What further action should the nurse take?
    a. discard the medications herself
    b. document in the clinical record the client's response to her suggestion
    c. tell the client that she will recommend he be placed in a nursing home since he obviously is incapable of caring for himself
    d. no further action is needed

27. A nurse is paying an initial visit to a 19-year-old paraplegic client. During the visit, the client tells the nurse that he wants to return to college immediately. The nurse recognizes that the client has not yet achieved an adequate level of independence to allow for a return to school, and that he requires additional rehabilitative therapy. In discussing the client's goal, the nurse should:
    a. share her assessment data and suggest a process for setting mutually acceptable goals.
    b. explain to the client that he will be unable to meet this goal and should focus on achieving simpler goals.
    c. explain to the client that he is in denial of his condition and requires psychologic counseling.
    d. go along with the client for fear of upsetting him.

28. Contracting is defined as the continuously renegotiated _____
    _____

29. (a) _____ evaluation is the systematic ongoing comparison of the care plan with the goals actually being achieved. In (b) _____ evaluation, the nurse reviews the total care plan and the client's progress toward goals in order to determine the client's eligibility for discharge.

■ ■ ■ Specialized Home Care Nursing

30. Name two benefits of high-technology home care.
    (a) _____
    (b) _____

31. The chief difference between home health nursing and hospice nursing care is:
    a. the nursing process is not applicable to hospice nursing care.
    b. hospice nursing care does not take place in the client's home.
    c. hospice nursing care is principally concerned with promoting quality of life in dying clients.
    d. hospice nursing care is not paid for by Medicare.

32. The Medicare Hospice Benefit would not be available to an individual who has:
    a. less than 6 months to live.
    b. end-stage respiratory failure.
    c. renal failure and is on hemodialysis.
    d. metastatic brain tumors.

33. Nursing management in the home of the client with AIDS includes (a) _____ care, (b) _____ care, and (c) _____ care.

▪ ▪ ▪ Critical Thinking Exercises

34. Develop a teaching plan for a client who is being discharged with a wound that requires irrigations and sterile dressings. Include the family in the teaching plan. Identify key assessments you would perform before implementing the teaching plan.

35. Design a plan to utilize community resources to assist a family in the care of their 67-year-old grandparent with Alzheimer's disease. Consider that there are school-age children in the home and that both parents work full-time outside of the home. There are no other adults in the home situation.

36. Develop a proposed contract with a homebound individual who needs to decrease her intake of concentrated sweets and "junk" food and to test her blood sugar on a more regular basis.

▪ ▪ ▪ Additional Learning Experiences

- Consult with a home care nurse about that role and related professional responsibilities.
- Look at the yellow pages in the phone book and identify community resources.
- Go to a local pharmacy or medical supply store. Do a price-check on durable medical equipment and medical supplies. Identify resources for these supplies if the client/family does not have the financial resources to purchase the items.

Nursing Care of Clients in Pain

■ ■ ■ Focused Study Tips

- Describe the myths and misconceptions about pain. Remember: Pain is whatever the client says it is, and it exists whenever the client says it does.

- Differentiate between acute and chronic pain and differences in treatment.

- Describe the various classes of medication used to relieve pain as well as its associated nursing responsibilities and client/family teaching.

■ ■ ■ Definitions of Pain

1. When caring for a client in pain, it is important for the nurse to keep in mind that:
   a. most pain experienced by clients is exaggerated.
   b. pain is a subjective, personal experience.
   c. pain can only be totally eliminated pharmacologically.
   d. pain always indicates current or impending tissue damage.

Match the manifestations of pain (a–f) with the causative factors listed in questions 2–7.

_____ 2. inflammation	_____ 5. spasm	a. skin rash
_____ 3. compression	_____ 6. conflict, difficulty in life	b. sore throat
_____ 4. heat	_____ 7. chemicals	c. sunburn
		d. psychogenic pain
		e. colon cramping
		f. carpal tunnel syndrome

■ ■ ■ Neurophysiology of Pain

8. The most abundant and potent pain-producing chemical in the body is:
   a. potassium ions.
   b. prostaglandins.
   c. bradykinin.
   d. histamine.

9. Endorphins in the brain:
   a. act to transmit the pain impulse.
   b. intensify the pain response.
   c. are released in response to efferent impulses.
   d. inhibit the pain response.

10. A noxious impulse becomes pain when it:
    a. passes through the medulla and midbrain and reaches the thalamus.
    b. is perceived by the nociceptors in the periphery of the body.
    c. is transmitted by both A-delta and C nerve fibers.
    d. reaches conscious levels and is perceived and evaluated by the person experiencing the sensation.

▪ ▪ ▪ Theories of Pain

For each of the statements below, identify the theory of pain described.

11. In this theory of pain, the perception of pain is based on the summation of afferent impulses. This summation may occur in the spinal cord or the brain. _____

12. In this theory of pain, free nerve endings in the skin act as pain receptors, accept sensory input, and transmit this input along highly specific nerve fibers. _____

13. In this theory of pain, the perception of pain is controlled by two systems. One regulates impulses entering and leaving the spinal cord. The second system is inhibitory. _____

_____

▪ ▪ ▪ Types of Pain

Match the type of pain (a–c) with the correct subjective client statements regarding acute pain listed in questions 14–16.

_____ 14. "When I had a heart attack, I had severe pain in my right arm."

_____ 15. "I can't tell you where the pain is located, but it's dull and makes me feel like I can't sit still."

_____ 16. "It hurts right here and is very sharp."

a. somatic
b. visceral
c. referred

17. Which of the following statements best distinguishes chronic pain from acute pain?
    a. The client in acute pain usually is unable to localize the pain.
    b. Chronic pain often does not respond to conventional medical treatment.
    c. The duration of chronic pain is usually less than 6 months.
    d. The etiology of acute pain typically cannot be explained.

18. Migraine headaches are one example of:
    a. ongoing time-limited pain.
    b. chronic nonmalignant pain.
    c. recurrent acute pain.
    d. chronic intractable nonmalignant pain syndrome.

19. An extensive work-up reveals no clearly identifiable source for the client's pain. The client reports to the nurse practitioner that the pain is brought on when she is fighting with her husband. It is likely that this client is experiencing:
    a. chronic pain.   b. phantom pain.   c. central pain.   d. psychogenic pain.

20. The most common chronic pain condition is _____.

Match the descriptions (a–d) with the appropriate chronic pain conditions listed in questions 21–24.

_____ 21. reflex sympathetic dystrophies

_____ 22. neuralgias

_____ 23. hyperesthesias

_____ 24. chronic postoperative pain

a. painful conditions that result from damage to a peripheral nerve caused by infection or disease
b. conditions of oversensitivity to tactile and painful stimuli
c. characterized by continuous, severe, burning pain
d. rare, but may occur following incisions in the chest wall

25. An 80-year-old client who recently underwent amputation of his left lower leg due to gangrene continually complains of pain in his left foot. This phenomenon is known as _____ _____.

Read the following statement and determine if it is true or false. Correct the statement if it is false.

_____ 26. Treatment of phantom pain is quite simple and successful if the client is willing to see a psychiatrist.

▪ ▪ ▪ Factors Affecting Client Response to Pain

27. Identify six factors that can influence a client's perception of a painful stimuli and give an example of each.
    (a) _____
    (b) _____
    (c) _____
    (d) _____
    (e) _____
    (f) _____

28. Everyone has the same pain (a) _____; what varies is the person's pain (b) _____, which is the amount of pain a person can endure before outwardly responding to it.

29. One change that occurs with aging is slowed reaction time, which slows the older client's avoidance response. What is one negative outcome of this change? _____ _____

30. In clinically depressed clients, (a) _____ is decreased, leading to an increase in (b) _____.

▪ ▪ ▪ Myths and Misconceptions about Pain

31. Which of the following statements about pain is true?
    a. Narcotic medication is too risky to be used in chronic pain.
    b. Offering pain relief before a pain event is well on its way can lessen the pain.
    c. Postoperative pain is best treated with intramuscular injections.
    d. It is best to wait until a client is in pain before administering medication.

32. The client is a 37-year-old statistical analyst suffering from chronic fatigue and fibromyalgia. She expresses concern that she will lose her disability payments if her company finds out that she has been seeing a psychiatrist for the past 6 months for depression. The appropriate action by the nurse is to tell the client that:
    a. pain and depression are chemically related, not mutually exclusive, and often coexist.
    b. the brain chemical serotonin is the major modulator of depression; therefore, depression is the most likely cause of chronic pain.
    c. antidepressants will reduce her chronic pain.
    d. many clients mistake psychologic pain for physical pain, and it is a good thing that she is seeing a psychiatrist.

▪ ▪ ▪ Collaborative Care

Identify the term associated with each client situation.

33. A client used to obtain relief from 10 mg of morphine. He no longer gets the same relief from the same amount of drug. _____

34. A client uses a drug, not prescribed for her, to obtain a "high." _____

35. A client reports that if he does not have caffeine in the morning he gets migraine headaches.
_____

Case Study

Martha Avery is a 46-year-old dancer whose physician has prescribed Toradol (ketorolac), a nonsteroidal anti-inflammatory agent, for the management of her chronic pain.

36. Which assessment is most important for Ms. Avery's nurse to perform prior to administering Toradol?
    a. determine whether Ms. Avery is actually having pain
    b. determine Ms. Avery's temperature
    c. determine whether Ms. Avery is taking oral hypoglycemic agents
    d. determine Ms. Avery's white blood cell count

37. To diminish side effects, the nurse recommends that Ms. Avery take this drug:
    a. with meals.
    b. right before she goes to bed.
    c. only when she feels the pain.
    d. first thing in the morning.

38. Identify three nursing orders that would be appropriate to include in the care plan for Ms. Avery.
    (a) _____
    (b) _____
    (c) _____

Read the following statements and determine if they are true or false. Correct any false statements.

_____ 39. A common myth among health care professionals is that the use of narcotics for pain treatment poses a real threat of addiction.

_____ 40. Giving analgesics before the pain occurs or increases allows the client to experience a confidence in the certainty of pain relief.

_____ 41. Administering morphine sulfate can result in respiratory depression.

_____ 42. When administering narcotic analgesics, the nurse should monitor vital signs, level of consciousness, pupillary response, nausea, bowel function, urinary function, and effectiveness of pain management.

43. Consulting a(n) _____ helps ensure that dosages of different narcotics administered by different routes to the same client will have the same analgesic effect.

Match the descriptions (a–e) with the correct routes of administration listed in questions 44–48.

_____ 44. rectal

_____ 45. transdermal

_____ 46. intravenous

_____ 47. oral

_____ 48. intraspinal (epidural)

a. provides the most rapid onset

b. simplest route for client and nurse

c. helpful for clients who are unable to swallow

d. used to manage chronic and intractable cancer and severe postoperative pain

e. "patch form" of medication—simple, painless, delivers continuous level of medication

49. The most significant advantage of using patient-controlled analgesia (PCA) over conventional methods of pain medication administration (such as nurse-administered) is:
    a. there is less risk of infection with PCA.
    b. PCA is less costly.
    c. PCA reduces the time the nurse must spend medicating clients.
    d. PCA gives clients more control over their pain.

50. Temporary (local) nerve blocks may give the client enough relief to:
    (a) _____
    (b) _____
    (c) _____

51. A client receiving transcutaneous electrical nerve stimulation (TENS) should be taught that:
    a. a slight burn may occur with this therapy.
    b. the client will not be able to use the affected extremity for several days.
    c. the client will feel a gentle tapping sensation with this therapy.
    d. this therapy is experimental and may not work.

52. The principle underlying biofeedback therapy is:
    a. the client will be able to identify stress-related responses and replace them with relaxation responses.
    b. the client is injected with chemicals that promote relaxation.
    c. small electric stimuli are given to the client to relax the muscles.
    d. during a trance state, the therapist suggests ways for the client to achieve pain relief.

■ ■ ■ Nursing Care of the Client with Pain

53. When working with the client with pain, the goal of nursing care is to: _____
    _____.

54. To accurately assess a client's pain, the nurse can use pain rating scales, physiologic responses, and _____.

55. The most reliable indicator of whether a client is in pain is determined by:
    a. the client's blood pressure.
    b. the client's statement of pain.
    c. the client's nonverbal cues.
    d. the client's heart rate.

56. Noninvasive interventions utilized in the management of pain include
    (a) _____, (b) _____,
    and (c) _____.

57. Define guided imagery.

58. Distraction is defined as (a)_____
    _____.
    An example of distraction is (b) _____.

59. Identify three methods of cutaneous stimulation.
    (a) _____
    (b) _____
    (c) _____

60. Which of the following nursing interventions is contraindicated for the client in pain?
    a. teaching the client and family ways in which to substitute noninvasive methods of pain management for narcotic administration, thus eliminating the possibility of addiction
    b. assessing the characteristics of the pain
    c. providing comfort measures, such as changing positions, back massage, skin care, and oral care
    d. providing client and family teaching, and making referrals if necessary to assist with coping, financial resources, and care

61. Touch and massage are effective methods of cutaneous stimulation. The primary advantage of these techniques is that they:
    a. have only temporary effects.
    b. may initiate gate closure.
    c. do not require specialized equipment.
    d. work best for localized pain.

62. A client discusses his pain experience. He expresses grave concern about possible addiction and how his pain has limited his ability to work and socialize with friends. The nurse suspects that he is:
    a. suffering from acute pain.
    b. a depressed malingerer.
    c. experiencing chronic pain.
    d. demonstrating drug-seeking behavior.

63. Which of the following would the nurse not expect to observe when caring for a client with chronic pain?
    a. normal blood pressure
    b. unexpressive facial appearance
    c. dry skin and relaxed posture
    d. grimacing and guarding

▪ ▪ ▪ Critical Thinking Exercises

64. Compare and contrast acute pain and chronic pain. Develop teaching plans for both experiences.

65. The nurse is caring for a client who has a history of chronic back pain. The client has been out of work for 6 months. He recently fell on the ice and suffered an acute muscle strain. Describe the appropriate nursing assessment related to pain. What nursing interventions would be most appropriate? How would the nurse assess the client's coping style?

66. Develop a teaching plan for a client with chronic pain related to cancer who is taking MS Contin and is experiencing "breakthrough pain."

▪ ▪ ▪ Additional Learning Experiences

▪ Interview a client with chronic pain and learn more about their pain experience.

▪ Compare and contrast pain experiences you may have observed in the clinical setting.

▪ Consult with your nursing faculty about attending a pain clinic or pain support group.

Nursing Care of Clients with Alterations in Fluid, Electrolyte, or Acid-Base Balance

▪ ▪ ▪ Focused Study Tips

- Identify clients at risk for alterations in fluid, electrolyte, or acid-base balance.

- Differentiate the various classes of diuretics.

- Explain why daily weights are one of the most important indicators of fluid balances.

- Describe the primary symptoms for each of the electrolyte alterations.

▪ ▪ ▪ Overview of Fluid Balance in the Body

1. Internal and external processes of the body maintain a state of physiologic balance known as (a) _____. This balance is reflected in the normal (b) _____, (c) _____, (d) _____, and (e) _____ of body fluids.

2. Total body water constitutes about (a) _____% of a person's total body weight. Total body water is divided among compartments. The two principle compartments are the (b) _____ and the (c) _____ compartments.

3. Factors that can influence the amount of a person's total body water are age, gender, and _____ _____.

4. For each pair of clients listed below, circle the client who has a lower proportion of water to total body weight.
   (a) a middle-aged client or an elderly client
   (b) an obese client or a slender client
   (c) a male client or a female client

5. The majority of body fluids are contained in which compartment?
   a. transcellular
   b. interstitial
   c. intracellular
   d. intravascular

6. When extracellular fluid is sequestered abnormally in a body cavity, it may contribute to organ malfunction because it:
   a. has a higher sodium content than normal body fluid.
   b. has a lower pH than normal body fluid.
   c. is unavailable for normal physiologic function.
   d. causes changes in the client's weight.

7. An accumulation of excess interstitial fluid is called:
   a. third spaced fluid.
   b. edema.
   c. inflammation.
   d. water intoxication.

Match the type of membrane transport (a–f) with the correct statements listed in questions 8–14.

_____ 8. The movement of fluid across a semipermeable membrane to an area of lower concentration.

_____ 9. The process by which non–lipid-soluble molecules, such as glucose and amino acids, are assisted by substances such as proteins to move across cell membranes.

_____ 10. The movement of molecules across semipermeable membranes.

_____ 11. The force that is primarily responsible for the movement of body fluids between the intracellular and the extracellular fluid compartments.

_____ 12. The process in which hydrostatic pressure is the driving force for fluid to move across cell membranes.

_____ 13. Along with sodium, these particles keep fluid in the intravascular space.

_____ 14. A form of diffusion in which solutes diffuse through a semipermeable membrane by dissolving into a lipid membrane.

a. osmosis
b. facilitated diffusion
c. diffusion
d. filtration
e. plasma protein
f. simple diffusion

15. To determine a client's serum osmolality, the nurse should have available which of the following assessment data?
   a. serum sodium level
   b. urine sodium level
   c. serum potassium level
   d. urine potassium level

16. To estimate the client's serum osmolality, the nurse would:
   a. send the sample to the lab for analysis.
   b. double the serum sodium level.
   c. double the serum potassium level.
   d. add the urine potassium and the serum potassium.

17. Which of the following client data would support the nursing diagnosis of *Fluid Volume Excess?* An osmolarity of:
   a. 275 mOsm/kg
   b. 325 mOsm/kg
   c. 260 mOsm/kg
   d. 300 mOsm/kg

Match the types of solutions (a–c) with the best description listed in questions 18–21.

_____ 18. produces a fluid shift out of the intracellular space into the extracellular space

_____ 19. produces no fluid shift

_____ 20. produces cellular swelling

_____ 21. produces cellular shrinkage

a. isotonic
b. hypotonic
c. hypertonic

Match the types of solution (a–c) with the intravenous fluids listed in questions 22–26.

_____ 22. 5% dextrose in water

_____ 23. 3% sodium chloride

_____ 24. Ringer's solution

_____ 25. 0.45% sodium chloride

_____ 26. 20% dextrose in water

a. isotonic

b. hypotonic

c. hypertonic

▪ ▪ ▪ Fluid Volume Deficit

27. Which of the following nursing assessments would support a nursing diagnosis of *Fluid Volume Deficit?*
    a. bradycardia, poor capillary refill
    b. hypothermia, jugular venous distention
    c. hypertension, wheezing
    d. edema, hypotension

28. For a diagnosis of *Fluid Volume Deficit,* indicate whether the ordered laboratory test results would be low or high.
    (a) serum potassium _____
    (b) hematocrit _____
    (c) urine specific gravity _____

29. A fluid challenge test is ordered for a client. To carry out this order, the nurse administers 300 mL of intravenous fluid over what period of time?
    a. 1 hour   b. 5 minutes   c. 4 hours   d. 24 hours

30. The most likely intravenous solution to be ordered for the client in question 29 would be one that is:
    a. hypotonic.   b. isotonic.   c. hypertonic.   d. hypo-osmolar.

31. In order to measure central venous pressure (CVP) accurately, the nurse places the client in which of the following positions?
    a. side-lying, with the head of the bed 20 degrees
    b. supine, with the head of the bed flat
    c. prone, with the head of the bed 30 degrees
    d. the position of the client does not matter

32. A client's CVP is 12 cm H_2O. This indicates that the client has:
    a. a normal CVP.
    b. fluid volume deficit.
    c. fluid volume overload.
    d. hypovolemia.

Case Study

Twenty-year-old Sharon Meeks is sent to the emergency department (ED). She complains of experiencing nausea and vomiting, diarrhea, thirst, and weakness for 3 days. "I can't hold anything down," she tells the nurse.

33. What assessments should the triage nurse perform?

34. The physician orders the following: CBC, electrolytes, and urinalysis. Interpret the findings below (a–e) as low, normal, or high.

    Results   *Interpretation*

    (a) sodium = 130 mEq/L
    (b) potassium = 3.4 mEq/L
    (c) calcium = 8.4 mEq/L
    (d) hematocrit = 37%
    (e) hemoglobin = 12 g/dL

35. Orthostatic vital signs reveal: 110/60, HR 90 lying; 100/56, HR 100 sitting; 90/50, HR 110 standing. The client complains of weakness and dizziness with position change. What condition do these signs and symptoms indicate?

36. What safety measures should the nurse initiate?

37. Ms. Meeks is prescribed an IV of Ringer's lactate with a bolus of 500 mL, then a decreased IV rate of 250 mL per hour. What are the nurse's responsibilities when administering the IV?

38. Ms. Meeks receives 2 L of fluid and an antiemetic. Following these interventions, her vital signs are within normal limits and she states she feels "much better." What instructions should the nurse include during discharge teaching?

39. How would the treatment change if the client were an 88-year-old woman?

40. To assess a client for orthostatic hypotension, the nurse:
    a. places the client in a Trendelenberg position.
    b. asks the client to bear down when measuring blood pressure.
    c. takes the client's blood pressure in a supine and seated position.
    d. assesses the client's neck veins at a 30-degree angle.

■ ■ ■ **Fluid Volume Excess**

41. Which of the following are signs and symptoms of fluid volume excess?
    a. peripheral edema, weight gain, neck vein distention
    b. decreased skin turgor, sunken eyeballs, decreased blood pressure
    c. full bounding pulses, concentrated urine output, postural hypotension
    d. crackles and wheezes, dry mucous membranes, flattened neck veins

42. The nurse receives the laboratory reports on a client who is being admitted with congestive heart failure (CHF) and a fluid volume excess. Which statement is probably true regarding the client's hematocrit and hemoglobin levels?
    a. The hematocrit and hemoglobin are within normal limits.
    b. The hematocrit and hemoglobin are increased.
    c. The hematocrit is increased and the hemoglobin is decreased.
    d. The hematocrit and hemoglobin are decreased.

43. Which of the following foods would be contraindicated for the client with *Fluid Volume Excess*?
    a. steamed chicken
    b. canned string beans
    c. shredded wheat
    d. fresh broccoli

Case Study

Marina Petroff, RN, is on rounds assessing her clients. She finds that Sue Danowitz, admitted with CHF, has absorbed 600 mL of intravenous fluid over the past 30 minutes. On examination, the client is in distress with a respiratory rate of 32. Auscultation of her lungs reveals crackles and wheezes. Auscultation of her heart reveals a gallop rhythm.

44. Based on the assessment finding, what nursing interventions are indicated?

45. After each physician's order below (a–g), indicate the appropriate rationale.

    Physician's Orders   *Rationale*
    (a) administer Lasix (furosemide) 60 mg IVP
    (b) take portable chest x-ray
    (c) monitor intake and output
    (d) monitor vital signs every hour
    (e) restrict fluid intake
    (f) assess electrolytes in the AM
    (g) monitor daily weight

46. Ms. Danowitz responds well to the medical regimen and will be discharged in 3 days with a prescription for Lasix (furosemide). What discharge teaching should the nurse include about Lasix?

47. The principal intracellular electrolytes are (a) _____ and
    (b) _____.

48. The principal extracellular electrolytes are (a) _____ and
    (b) _____.

■ ■ ■ Hyponatremia

49. Normal serum sodium concentration ranges from (a) _____ to (b) _____ mEq/L.

50. Sodium loss occurs through the (a) _____, (b) _____, and (c) _____.

51. Early indications of hyponatremia include alterations in primarily which system?
    a. nervous system
    b. renal system
    c. gastrointestinal system
    d. peripheral vascular system

52. Late manifestations of hyponatremia include alterations in primarily which system?
    a. nervous system
    b. renal system
    c. gastrointestinal system
    d. peripheral vascular system

53. Identify the manifestations of hyponatremia for each condition below.
    (a) altered gastrointestinal function:

    (b) altered neurologic function:

54. Which of the following most clearly distinguishes the differences between hypovolemic hyponatremia and hypervolemic hyponatremia?
    a. The nurse assesses for neurologic alterations in one and not the other.
    b. The serum sodium level is decreased in one and not the other.
    c. The administration of diuretics is contraindicated in one and not the other.
    d. Slow administration of saline is indicated in one and not the other.

55. Which client statement indicates an understanding about hyponatremia?
    a. "I will drink fluids that contain sodium and other electrolytes when playing basketball this summer."
    b. "I should avoid canned goods, cottage cheese, and cold cuts."
    c. "Doubling my dose of Lasix (furosemide) will aid in preventing an episode of hyponatremia."
    d. "This condition cannot be cured and I will be disabled for life."

■ ■ ■ Hypernatremia

56. When assessing a client for hypernatremia, the nurse would expect to find:
    a. an abnormal EKG and weight loss.
    b. abdominal cramps and possible diarrhea.
    c. dilute urine with a urine specific gravity of 1.001.
    d. altered mental status and lethargy.

57. List three interventions appropriate for the client at *Risk for Injury* related to alterations in neurological function.
    (a) _____
    (b) _____
    (c) _____

Read the statements below and determine if they are true or false. Correct any false statements.

_____ 58. Smoked and cured meats contain more sodium than poultry.

_____ 59. Fruits and vegetables are very low in sodium.

_____ 60. One should use large amounts of salt substitutes to compensate for a low-sodium diet.

_____ 61. Many over-the-counter drugs contain high amounts of sodium.

_____ 62. One's preference for salt can never diminish.

▪ ▪ ▪ **Potassium Disorders**

63. The normal serum potassium level is (a) _____ to (b) _____ mEq/L.

64. Which body systems are affected by potassium deficits or excesses?
    a. neurologic and renal systems
    b. neurologic and cardiac systems
    c. renal and lymphatic systems
    d. cardiac and lymphatic systems

65. Name the potassium imbalance, and describe physiologically how each of the clients is at risk for alterations in potassium imbalance.
    (a) A 55-year-old client receiving large doses of intravenous penicillin for pneumonia

    (b) An 18-year-old client admitted with a diagnosis of anorexia nervosa

    (c) An 87-year-old client who has not urinated in 3 days. His medications include Inderal (propanolol) and Aldactone (spironolactone).

    (d) A 23-year-old client with AIDS-related diarrhea

    (e) A client who has an uncorrected acidosis following a cardiac arrest

▪ ▪ ▪ Hypokalemia

66. Which of the following conditions would not account for a potassium level of 2.2 mEq/L?
    a. severe vomiting and diarrhea
    b. prolonged use of potassium-sparing diuretics
    c. excessive ileostomy drainage
    d. second- and third-degree burns

67. A client is about to receive his morning medications. Prior to administering his Lanoxin (digoxin), a cardiac glycoside, the nurse checks the client's laboratory data. The serum potassium is 3.0 mEq/L. The most appropriate action by the nurse would be to:
    a. withhold the medication, it is contraindicated.
    b. consult with the physician and report the potassium level.
    c. administer one-half of the ordered dose.
    d. double the dose of K-dur and monitor the laboratory data.

68. The nurse would not expect to observe hypokalemia in a client experiencing:
    a. vomiting and diarrhea.
    b. osmotic diuresis.
    c. second- and third-degree burns.
    d. renal failure.

Case Study

Mariko Narita has a serum potassium of 2.7 mEq/L. The medical intern orders potassium chloride 30 mEq IV over 5 minutes.

69. What are the nurse's responsibilities in carrying out this order?

70. The order is rewritten as 30 mEq KCl to 1000 mL of D½NS to run at 150 mL per hour. If the drip factor is 15 drops per mL, how many drops should drip in 1 minute?

71. Ms. Weld complains that she is experiencing burning at the IV site. What should the nurse do?

72. Which of the following is a common nursing diagnosis for a client with hypokalemia?
    a. *Risk for Impaired Skin Integrity*
    b. *Fatigue*
    c. *Decreased Cardiac Output*
    d. *Altered Oral Mucous Membrane*

Case Study

Helen Rice, 77 years old, is being discharged from the hospital after recovering from dehydration and hypokalemia. She expresses reluctance in taking the prescribed potassium medication because of its "terrible taste."

73. What recommendations can the discharge nurse make regarding the "taste" of the medicine?

74. Mrs. Rice's niece asks the nurse how she can recognize if her aunt is becoming ill again. What signs and symptoms of hypokalemia should the nurse teach Mrs. Rice and her niece to monitor?

▪ ▪ ▪ Hyperkalemia

75. The most harmful consequence of hyperkalemia is its effect on the (a) _____ function. This is reflected by changes in the (b)_____ .

76. Which of the following medications is not used to treat hyperkalemia?
    a. insulin
    b. Aldactone (spironolactone)
    c. Kayexalate (sodium polystyrene sulfonate)
    d. sodium bicarbonate

Case Study

Bob Nelson is admitted to the ED with a potassium level of 5.9 mEq/L. Last week, Mr. Nelson's physician placed him on Aldactone for his hypertension. Mr. Nelson started to take the Aldactone, and continued taking K-Lyte/Cl (potassium chloride) as previously prescribed. Also during this period, Mr. Nelson began using a salt substitute.

77. How did each of the above actions contribute to Mr. Nelson's hyperkalemia?

78. The physician orders a Kayexalate enema. Mr. Nelson states that he does not need an enema because he has diarrhea. How should the nurse respond to Mr. Nelson's statement?

79. What food should Mr. Nelson eliminate from his diet?

80. The nurse retrieves her client's laboratory data and finds a serum potassium level of 7.1 mEq/L. After checking the client, the nurse's next appropriate intervention would be to:
    a. move the client next to the nurse's station.
    b. place the client on a cardiac monitor.
    c. increase the rate of the client's intravenous solution.
    d. restrict the client's fluids.

▪ ▪ ▪ Calcium Disorders

81. The normal adult serum calcium is (a) _____ to (b) _____ mg/dl.

■ ■ ■ Hypocalcemia

82. Clients experiencing hypocalcemia have alterations primarily in which one of the following body systems?
    a. cardiovascular system
    b. gastrointestinal system
    c. neuromuscular system
    d. renal system

83. Administration of which of the following substances can potentially contribute to a reduction in a client's serum calcium level?
    a. intravenous fluids
    b. many units of blood
    c. calcium tablets
    d. narcotic analgesia

84. Assessments that may indicate a state of calcium deficiency include:
    a. asking the client to walk while observing his/her gait.
    b. testing the client's intraocular movements.
    c. using tangential lighting to observe the client's neck veins.
    d. stimulating the client's facial nerves and observing for contraction of the facial muscles.

85. To accurately evaluate a client's hypocalcemia, the nurse must also assess the client's:
    a. albumin and magnesium levels.
    b. white blood cell count and hematocrit levels.
    c. 24-hour intake and output.
    d. increased bone density.

■ ■ ■ Hypercalcemia

86. Which of the following clients is at greatest risk for developing hypercalcemia?
    a. a 35-year-old male client with acute pancreatitis
    b. a 20-year-old female multiple trauma victim, in traction, on bed rest
    c. an 85-year-old male abusing laxatives
    d. a 10-year-old female with mitral valve prolapse

87. A client with malignant diseases such as multiple myeloma and lymphoma may develop hypercalcemia. List four signs and symptoms of hypercalcemia.
    (a) _____
    (b) _____
    (c) _____
    (d) _____

88. A client is admitted with a diagnosis of hypercalcemia. He is having profound muscle weakness, vomiting, and bradycardia. Based on these findings, emergency administration of (a) _____ or (b) _____ is indicated. Subsequent to this intervention, the nurse can anticipate that (c) _____ or (d) _____ intravenous solutions will be administered. Other drug therapies can include but are not limited to (e) _____, (f) _____, and/or (g) _____.

89. Which of the following electrolyte disturbances is typical in a client who is hypercalcemic?
    a. hypokalemia
    b. hypophosphatemia
    c. hyperkalemia
    d. hyperphosphatemia

▪ ▪ ▪ Hypophosphatemia

90. Normal serum phosphorus levels in adults range from (a) _____ to (b) _____ mg/dL.

91. An inpatient at a substance abuse treatment center has a serum phosphate level of 1.8 mg/dL. A possible explanation for this finding is _____
_____.

92. Which of the following clients would be at greatest risk for hypophosphatemia?
    a. a client with insulin-dependent diabetes mellitus (IDDM)
    b. a client with iron deficiency anemia
    c. a client receiving total parenteral nutrition
    d. a client with hypertension who is not taking her medication

93. When teaching a client to avoid foods high in phosphorus, the nurse would recommend avoiding:
    a. liver, fish, and poultry.
    b. whole grains, nuts, and oral drug supplements.
    c. milk, milk products, and eggs.
    d. green leafy vegetables and orange juice.

▪ ▪ ▪ Hyperphosphatemia

94. A client with chronic renal insufficiency has a phosphorus level of 5.0 mg/dL. Which clinical signs and symptoms are present in this situation?
    a. dysphagia with absent bowel sounds
    b. shallow respirations and dysrhythmias
    c. complaints of paresthesia and muscle cramping
    d. thirst with altered level of consciousness

95. Explain why neoplastic diseases, such as leukemia, which are treated with a cytotoxic agent, place the client at high risk for hyperphosphatemia.

96. Which of the following interventions is not used to treat hyperphosphatemia?
    a. hemodialysis   b. antacids   c. fluid hydration   d. diuretics

▪ ▪ ▪ Hypomagnesemia

97. The normal serum concentration of magnesium ranges from _____ to _____ mEq/L.

98. Which condition does not place a client at risk for hypomagnesemia?
    a. morbid obesity   c. chronic diarrhea
    b. infection requiring gentamicin   d. chronic alcoholism

99. Assessment of the client with hypomagnesemia is complicated by the fact that:
    a. the manifestations of hypomagnesemia are very subjective.
    b. hypomagnesemia often accompanies multiple electrolyte deficits.
    c. clients with hypomagnesemia are often intoxicated.
    d. the client is often comatose.

100. Clinical manifestations of hypomagnesemia most closely parallel which of the following electrolyte deficits?

    a. hypokalemia   b. hyponatremia   c. hypophosphatemia   d. hypocalcemia

101. Treatment of mild hypomagnesemia would include:

    a. keeping the client npo and administering an IV of D5W.

    b. administering calcium gluconate IV.

    c. omitting all antacids.

    d. encouraging oral intake of green leafy vegetables, seafood, and meat.

▪ ▪ ▪ Hypermagnesemia

102. Which assessment findings would the nurse suspect to be a cause of hypermagnesemia?

    a. anorexia and diarrhea for 3 days

    b. a history of peptic ulcer disease requiring Maalox Plus every 2 hours

    c. hypertension with warm dry skin

    d. hyperactive reflexes and leg cramps

103. Cardiac arrest is associated with which type of hypermagnesemia?

    a. slightly elevated serum magnesium

    b. moderately elevated serum magnesium

    c. markedly elevated serum magnesium

    d. miminally elevated serum magnesium

▪ ▪ ▪ Acid-Base Disorders

104.   The act of breathing is primarily controlled through the concentration of:

    a. ammonia.   b. phosphate.   c. hydrogen ions.   d. plasma proteins.

105. The assessment of $Paco_2$ measures which of the following?

    a. the pressure exerted by carbon dioxide in the blood

    b. the amount of carbon dioxide in the blood

    c. the amount of carbonic acid expired

    d. the level of carbon dioxide in the tissue

106. An elevated $Paco_2$ occurs when:

    a. the kidneys can no longer excrete hydrogen ions.

    b. there is a reduction in ventilation.

    c. there is an increase in ventilation.

    d. the kidneys excrete too many hydrogen ions.

107. The body's normal pH falls between (a) _____ and (b) _____ .

108. The body's normal $Paco_2$ is (a) _____ to (b) _____ mm Hg.

Match the conditions (a–c) with the values listed in questions 109–113.

_____ 109. pH = 7.22

_____ 110. pH = 7.46

_____ 111. Pa_{O_2} = 55

_____ 112. Pa_{CO_2} = 22

_____ 113. Pa_{CO_2} = 57

a. acidosis
b. alkalosis
c. hypoxemia

▪ ▪ ▪ Metabolic Alkalosis/Acidosis

114. Metabolic alkalosis is characterized by (a) _____ pH, a(n)
   (b) _____ in bicarbonate, and (c) _____
   serum potassium.

115. Metabolic acidosis is characterized by (a) _____ pH, a(n)
   (b) _____ in bicarbonate, and (c) _____
   serum potassium.

116. A client is brought to the ED with severe metabolic alkalosis. During assessment, the nurse would observe which objective findings?

117. A nursing diagnosis applicable to the client with metabolic acidosis is *Risk for Injury* related to confusion. Appropriate nursing interventions for this diagnosis include:

▪ ▪ ▪ Respiratory Acidosis/Alkalosis

Case Study

Ann Gardner, age 37, is brought to the ED with complaints of dizziness, dyspnea, and palpitations that started 1 hour ago as she was preparing for a job interview. Arterial blood gases reveal a state of acute respiratory alkalosis.

118. Indicate whether Ms. Gardner's blood gas results would be greater than or less than the stated amount.
   (a) pH _____ 7.35–7.45
   (b) Pa_{CO_2} _____ 35–45

119. What is the most frequent cause of respiratory alkalosis?

120. List four collaborative care/interventions appropriate for Ms. Gardner.

(a) _____

(b) _____

(c) _____

(d) _____

121. A client suffers from chronic respiratory acidosis. Her bicarbonate level is 55. When administering oxygen, the nurse should:

a. increase the flow rate until the bicarbonate level returns to normal.

b. maintain the rate at the ordered level and carefully monitor the client's response.

c. increase the flow rate until the PaO_2 level is >90.

d. withhold oxygen therapy, as it will only increase the bicarbonate level.

Match the conditions (a–b) with the clinical manifestations listed in questions 122–126.

_____ 122. headache

_____ 123. altered mental status

_____ 124. tetany, convulsions

_____ 125. warm, flushed skin

_____ 126. diaphoresis

a. respiratory acidosis

b. respiratory alkalosis

▪ ▪ ▪ Critical Thinking Exercises

127. Develop a teaching plan for a client who must avoid dietary intake of potassium and sodium. Develop a grocery list to assist with shopping.

128. Compare and contrast the metabolic acidosis and respiratory acidosis.

129. The nurse is caring for a client with fluid volume excess. Develop a plan to assist the family in managing the client's fluid and dietary intake at home.

▪ ▪ ▪ Additional Learning Experiences

▪ Review laboratory reports of assigned clients. Determine whether the results are within normal limits. If they are abnormal, try to determine the origin of the imbalance.

▪ Visit a grocery store, and examine food labels for sodium content.

▪ Ask your nursing faculty to arrange a visit to a dialysis center to talk to clients or their family members about their experiences managing dietary restrictions.

CHAPTER 6

Nursing Care of Clients in Shock

■ ■ ■ **Focused Study Tips**

- Describe the stages of shock and the related clinical manifestations.
- Discuss how each body system responds to the process of shock.

- Compare and contrast the types of shock, their cause or precipitating events, as well as associated therapeutic interventions.
- Describe the advantages and disadvantages and rationale for each type of fluid replacement therapy.

■ ■ ■ **The Client in Shock**

1. Shock is characterized by _____.

2. The amount of blood pumped each minute is called:
   a. stroke volume.
   b. mean arterial pressure.
   c. cardiac output.
   d. heart rate.

3. Cardiac output is determined by multiplying which two variables?
   a. stroke volume and mean arterial pressure
   b. stroke volume and heart rate
   c. heart rate and mean arterial pressure
   d. heart rate and systemic vascular resistance

4. When a client is vasoconstricted and has increased sympathetic tone, (a) _____
   _____, (b) _____,
   and (c) _____ increase.

5. A client is given a medication that increases his cardiac output. This action is beneficial in that it increases:
   a. tissue perfusion.
   b. serum potassium level.
   c. heart rate.
   d. respiratory rate.

6. All forms of shock result in:
   a. death.
   b. inadequate tissue perfusion.
   c. bleeding.
   d. hypertension.

7. It is thought that the event that initiates the shock syndrome is: _____
   _____.

8. Which of the following conditions most distinguishes the initial stage of shock from all other stages of shock?
   a. rapid thready pulse
   b. the client may have no symptoms associated with this stage
   c. the client loses consciousness
   d. reduced pulse rate

9. In the compensatory stage of shock, changes may be detected in a client's:
   a. peripheral pulses.
   b. heart sounds.
   c. level of consciousness.
   d. respiratory rate.

10. An increase in heart rate seen in the compensatory stage of shock is the body's attempt to:
    a. increase the stroke volume.
    b. increase the cardiac output.
    c. increase the systemic vascular resistance.
    d. decrease cellular shifts.

11. A beta two response in a client in the compensatory stage of shock would be manifested by:
    a. a decrease in peripheral pulses.
    b. diaphoresis.
    c. a decrease in heart rate and respiratory rate.
    d. an increase in heart rate and respiratory rate.

12. The renin-angiotensin response to decreases in renal blood flow results in:
    a. an increase in respiratory rate.
    b. water and sodium retention.
    c. increased serum potassium.
    d. decrease in systemic vascular resistance (SVR).

13. List three conditions that occur at a cellular level in the progressive stage of shock.
    (a) _____
    (b) _____
    (c) _____

14. In the progressive stage of shock, one would expect to find:
    a. hyperkalemia, acidosis, and oliguria.
    b. hypokalemia, increased urine output, and diaphoresis.
    c. aerobic metabolism, hyperkalemia, and rapid thready pulse.
    d. water and sodium retention.

Match the type of shock (a–e) with the appropriate causes of shock listed in questions 15–24. Questions may have more than one answer.

_____ 15. an acute myocardial infarction (MI)

_____ 16. an incompatible blood transfusion

_____ 17. a client with a burn involving 90% of his body

_____ 18. an acute cervical spine injury

_____ 19. a bowel obstruction

_____ 20. a postpartum hemorrhage

_____ 21. a newly diagnosed diabetic

_____ 22. an immunocompromised client

_____ 23. a bee sting

_____ 24. a client with a laceration to his radial artery

a. hypovolemic
b. neurogenic
c. cardiogenic
d. septic
e. anaphylactic

Case Study

Charley Conor is an 82-year-old client living in an assisted living facility. The nurse's aide reports that Mr. Conor has become very somnolent over the last few hours. Julie, the facility nurse, takes Mr. Conor's vital signs and notes that he is afebrile, his heart rate is 112, and his blood pressure is 98/60. He recently has undergone a cystoscopy and the nurse notices that he has a Foley catheter in place that has drained approximately 200 mL of concentrated urine over the last 8 hours.

25. From her assessment of Mr. Conor, Julie suspects that he is at risk for:
    a. urinary retention
    b. hypovolemic shock
    c. fluid volume excess
    d. septic shock

26. Two factors that place Mr. Conor at risk for this diagnosis are (a) _____
    and (b) _____.

27. What is Julie's first priority in caring for Mr. Conor?
    a. measuring and recording accurate urine output
    b. elevating his legs 20 degrees
    c. continuing to monitor cardiovascular function
    d. administering blood products

28. Julie knows that Mr. Conor's change in mental status is related to:
    a. the effect of endotoxins on the central nervous system.
    b. decreased cerebral perfusion.
    c. low urinary output.
    d. fatigue after a cystoscopy procedure.

29. A client in hypovolemic shock with a blood pressure of 80/50 requires rapid fluid replacement. Which of the following solutions is not appropriate?
    a. lactated Ringer's solution
    b. 25% albumin
    c. 0.9% normal saline
    d. 5% dextrose in water

30. Regardless of the stage or cause, which of the following interventions is always appropriate for the client in shock?
    a. vigorous fluid replacement
    b. elevating the lower extremities 20 degrees
    c. administration of oxygen
    d. application of the MAST (military antishock trousers)

31. A client is admitted in hypovolemic shock. It is suspected that the cause is her abuse of diuretics. Which of the following lab test data would suggest this?
    a. an increase in hemoglobin and hematocrit
    b. a decrease in hemoglobin and hematocrit
    c. no change from the baseline in the client's hemoglobin and hematocrit
    d. the level of hemoglobin and hematocrit cannot provide information to support this diagnosis

32. Antibiotics are essential in the treatment of clients experiencing what type of shock?
    a. anaphylactic   b. cardiogenic   c. septic   d. neurogenic

Case Study

Stan Jacoby, RN, has just received a client from the post-anesthesia care unit (PACU). The transferring RN tells Stan that the client has been very stable in the PACU with a consistent BP of 130/70 and a heart rate of 80. The client, Ron Estes, has undergone a bowel resection for colon cancer. His dressing is dry and intact.

33. While transferring Mr. Estes from the PACU stretcher to his bed, Stan notices that he is extremely pale and diaphoretic. He appears anxious and tremulous and is unable to clearly answer any of Stan's questions. Stan's first priority of care is to:
    a. auscultate his breath sounds.
    b. obtain a BP and pulse rate.
    c. place him in Trendelenberg position.
    d. administer pain medications.

34. Stan notes that Mr. Estes' BP is 90/50 and his heart rate is 118. Stan's next appropriate action is to:
    a. notify the physician.
    b. hang an isotonic intravenous solution wide open.
    c. hang a hypertonic intravenous solution wide open.
    d. none of the above.

35. Stan continues his assessment of Mr. Estes and notes that he has 10 mL of clear yellow urine in his Foley catheter drainage bag. The transferring nurse told Stan that she had emptied the bag approximately 2 hours ago. Stan knows that an adequate urine output is:
    a. 100 mL/hr.   c. 100 mL/shift.
    b. 10 mL/hr.   d. 20–30 mL/hr.

Case Study

Lakshmi Sharma, RN, is visiting a neighbor when the neighbor's daughter falls and lacerates her wrist on an unknown object in the backyard. The child is holding her wrist, which is spurting bright red blood.

36. The most effective way Lakshmi can control the bleeding is to:
    a. find some dressing materials and apply a dressing.
    b. apply a tourniquet above the wound.
    c. apply direct pressure to the bleeding site.
    d. apply pressure to a pressure point above the wound.

37. The child looks pale and is complaining of feeling dizzy. Lakshmi's next priority of care is to:
    a. give her po fluids until an ambulance arrives.
    b. have her lie down with her lower extremities elevated about 20 degrees.
    c. have her lie flat with pillows under her knees.
    d. have her sit up while holding her wrist at a 45-degree angle.

38. The goal for the client in cardiogenic shock is to increase the myocardial oxygen supply. What three interventions can the nurse utilize to support this goal?
    (a) _____
    (b) _____
    (c) _____

39. Nitroprusside is a potent vasodilator. Which of the following statements about the administration of this drug is false?
    a. Vital signs should be monitored every 4 hours when this drug is administered.
    b. The IV solution bag containing the drug needs to be wrapped as this drug is light-sensitive.
    c. This drug must always be administered via an infusion pump.
    d. The IV site should be assessed for infiltration when this drug is administered.

Match the causes of shock (a–d) with the correct type of shock listed in questions 40–43.

_____ 40. the early or warm phase of septic shock

_____ 41. the late or cold phase of septic shock

_____ 42. toxic shock syndrome

_____ 43. DIC (disseminated intravascular clotting)

a. generalized bleeding
b. cool moist skin, oliguria, altered mental status
c. hypotension, headache, and confusion
d. flushed skin, high fevers, and chills

44. The nursing diagnosis that best applies to the client in shock is:
    a. *Fluid Volume Excess.*
    b. *Knowledge Deficit.*
    c. *Altered Tissue Perfusion.*
    d. *Anxiety.*

45. Shock is typically an unanticipated event. Identify four interventions that may help to reduce the anxiety experienced by a client in shock.
    (a) _____
    (b) _____
    (c) _____
    (d) _____

Match the specific type of shock (a–e) with the nursing inverventions listed in questions 46–52.

_____ 46. identifying allergies

_____ 47. monitoring for manifestations of infection

_____ 48. improving myocardial oxygen supply

_____ 49. providing pain relief

_____ 50. assessing fluid status

_____ 51. maintaining immobility

_____ 52. careful aseptic technique

a. hypovolemic shock
b. cardiogenic shock
c. neurogenic shock
d. septic shock
e. anaphylactic shock

Match the specific type of shock (a–e) with the associated pathophysiology listed in questions 53–57.

_____ 53. vasodilation, hypovolemia, and altered cellular metabolism

_____ 54. dramatic reduction in systemic vascular resistance

_____ 55. decrease in cardiac output and mean arterial pressure

_____ 56. complex and not completely understood

_____ 57. decrease in circulating blood volume

a. hypovolemic shock
b. cardiogenic shock
c. neurogenic shock
d. septic shock
e. anaphylactic shock

▪ ▪ ▪ Critical Thinking Exercises

58. Compare and contrast the clinical manifestations that distinguish each stage of shock.

59. An 83-year-old male client just underwent a bowel resection. There is an increasing amount of bloody drainage on his dressing. Identify the key assessments the nurse should make. Design a plan of care to assist the nurse in monitoring for early shock.

60. Develop a teaching plan for the family of a client who suffers from anaphylactic shock following bee stings.

▪ ▪ ▪ Additional Learning Experiences

- Make study cards to help you learn the various types of shock and how to differentiate the clinical manifestations.

- Create abbreviated plans of care for each type of shock.

CHAPTER 7

Nursing Care of Clients Having Surgery

▪ ▪ ▪ Focused Study Tips

- Describe the actions of preoperative medications by category and the related nursing implications.

- Compare and contrast general and regional anesthesia.

- Describe the various stages of wound healing and the related nursing care.

- Identify the various wound drainage devices.

▪ ▪ ▪ The Client Having Surgery

1. Perioperative nursing is:
   a. a specialized area of practice for providing nursing care to the client before, during, and after surgery.
   b. care of the surgical client from entry into the operating room until admittance to the postanesthesia care unit (PACU).
   c. the phase of the surgical experience that begins when the decision for surgery is made and ends when the client is transferred to the operating room (OR).
   d. assisting the surgeon with any medical procedure that is performed to diagnose or treat illness, injury, or deformity.

2. A client has cancer that is considered extensive and incurable. The surgeon decides to remove a portion of the tumor to alleviate her pain. This type of surgery is called:
   a. palliative.
   b. constructive.
   c. ablative.
   d. reconstructive.

3. A client requires surgery to repair his jaw, which was crushed during an automobile accident. This type of surgery is called:
   a. palliative.
   b. constructive.
   c. ablative.
   d. reconstructive.

4. A client is admitted to the emergency department (ED) with the diagnosis of ruptured abdominal aortic aneurysm (AAA). The operating room (OR) is notified of the client's status. The nurse in the OR knows that repairing a ruptured AAA is an example of a(n):
   a. elective procedure.
   b. urgent procedure.
   c. emergency procedure.
   d. reconstructive procedure.

5. A client has a chronic cough. Because her chest x-ray shows a lesion in her right lung field, she must have a biopsy. This type of surgery is called:
   a. ablative.
   b. reconstructive.
   c. diagnostic.
   d. minor.

■ ■ ■ Inpatient Surgery

6. A high school hockey player has been diagnosed with a ruptured spleen. His hemoglobin and hematocrit (H & H) are low. Which procedure must be performed prior to surgery?
   a. type and cross-match for possible transfusion
   b. electrocardiogram (EKG) to detect cardiac arrhythmias
   c. pulmonary function studies to determine the extent of respiratory dysfunction
   d. drug screening to determine the presence of narcotics or other recreational drugs

7. Which of the following descriptions is true of preoperative electrocardiogram (EKG)?
   a. provides an evaluation of the cardiac status of either new or pre-existing cardiac conditions
   b. is prescribed only on clients with a history of cardiac disease
   c. is necessary for all surgical clients over the age of 21
   d. is always prescribed prior to instillation of spinal or epidural anesthesia

8. The major difference between general anesthesia and regional anesthesia is that regional anesthesia does not produce:
   a. analgesia.   b. reflex loss.   c. muscle relaxation.   d. loss of consciousness.

9. During which phase of general anesthesia is surgery performed?
   a. induction phase   b. maintenance phase   c. emergence phase   d. both a and b

10. An important action produced by preoperative atropine sulfate is that it:
    a. increases gastric pH.
    b. decreases anxiety and produces sedation.
    c. reduces oral and respiratory secretions to decrease risk of aspiration.
    d. induces amnesia.

11. A client is scheduled to undergo general anesthesia this morning and has received scopolamine pre-op. She is complaining of a dry mouth. An appropriate intervention by the nurse is to:
    a. offer the client a small glass of water.
    b. tell the client that the dryness is to be expected.
    c. offer the client mouth care to help alleviate the discomfort.
    d. offer the client hard candy to alleviate the discomfort.

12. The rationale for administering Pepcid (famotidine) preoperatively is to:
    a. decrease anxiety.
    b. increase gastric pH and decrease gastric volume.
    c. induce amnesia.
    d. promote drowsiness.

Match the type of regional anesthesia (a–e) with the correct descriptions listed in questions 13–17.

_____ 13. This type of anesthesia, when injected, decreases sensation around a limited area of the body.

_____ 14. This type of anesthesia is applied to skin or mucous membranes. No injection is involved.

_____ 15. This type of anesthesia is injected into a space located outside the dura mater of the spinal cord.

_____ 16. This type of anesthesia is delivered by injecting an agent at the nerve trunk.

_____ 17. This type of anesthesia is injected in the subarachnoid space.

a. nerve block
b. spinal anesthesia
c. topical anesthesia
d. local nerve infiltration
e. epidural blocks

18. A common side effect of spinal anesthesia due to leakage of cerebrospinal fluid (CSF) from the needle insertion site is reduced CSF pressure, resulting in postoperative headache. List three nursing actions that combat this side effect.

(a) _____

(b) _____

(c) _____

19. Pain control postoperatively is best managed when pain medication is administered:

a. regularly.

b. on a PRN basis.

c. when the client complains of pain.

d. only when the client is awake.

20. Contrary to the belief of many health care providers, physical dependence and tolerance to opioid analgesics is (a) _____ in short-term postoperative use. Additionally, opioid analgesics, when used to treat acute pain, (b) _____ lead to psychologic dependence and addiction.

21. Which of the following health care personnel is responsible for obtaining informed consent?

a. the nurse

b. the resident assisting in surgery

c. the surgeon

d. the client's primary care physician

22. What is the priority assessment when caring for a client undergoing conscious sedation?

(a) _____

Name two reversal agents used in conscious sedation.

(b) _____ (c) _____

23. A nurse has just witnessed the physician obtain informed consent from a 73-year-old client. When the physician leaves, the client states, "I don't understand. He said that I could have a stroke. I thought this was a minor procedure." The most appropriate action by the nurse is to:

a. restate what the physician told the client, but in simpler language.

b. reassure the client that a stroke is a rare complication.

c. reassure the client that it is not too late to change her mind about surgery.

d. notify the physician that the client requires further information.

24. Witnessing an informed consent form attests to the fact that the nurse:

a. saw the correct person sign the form, and agrees that the client was alert and aware of what was being signed.

b. verifies that all the client's questions were answered.

c. believes that the client's participation in the decision-making process was voluntary.

d. verifies that the person who gave the client the information is the person who will do the surgery.

25. Regardless of the nature of a surgical procedure, the nurse anticipates that all clients will:

a. require a sedative prior to surgery.

b. receive general anesthesia.

c. have some anxiety.

d. wish all family members to donate blood.

26. Client teaching should be initiated:

a. the morning of surgery.

b. as soon as the client arrives in the postanesthesia care unit (PACU).

c. as soon as the client is made aware of the upcoming surgery.

d. when the surgeon determines the client is ready for discharge from the hospital.

27. If the preoperative client is at risk for developing pulmonary complications, the client is taught coughing exercises. The purpose of coughing is to (a) _____, (b) _____, and (c) _____ pulmonary secretions.

28. Leg exercises are taught to the preoperative client who is at risk for developing _____ _____.

29. Which of the following activities does not occur on the day of elective surgery?
    a. explain the potential risks and benefits of surgery
    b. ensure the client has an identification band
    c. instruct the client to empty the bladder
    d. remove and secure the client's dentures

30. A 50-year-old woman is scheduled to undergo a modified radical mastectomy. She asks the nurse if she should remove her hearing aid and contact lenses before going to the operating room (OR). The most appropriate response by the nurse is:
    a. "I will check with your surgeon."
    b. "What would you be most comfortable doing?"
    c. "You must remove your contact lenses, but you may leave your hearing aid in place."
    d. "You may leave your contact lenses and hearing aid in place."

31. The role the nurse most often assumes on the surgical team is as:
    a. circulating personnel.   c. anesthesia personnel.
    b. scrub personnel.   d. surgical assistant.

32. The surgical scrub is performed to render hands and arms as clean as possible in preparation for a procedure and should last for:
    a. 2 to 3 minutes.
    b. 5 to 10 minutes.
    c. 10 to 15 minutes.
    d. as long as the nurse feels is necessary to adequately clean the skin.

33. Improper positioning of the client on the operating table can lead to:
    (a) _____
    (b) _____
    (c) _____

Match the positions (a–c) with the correct descriptions listed in questions 34–36.

_____ 34. This position is used for gynecologic, perineal, or rectal surgeries.

_____ 35. In this position, the greatest pressure is felt at the bends in the table. The client is supported with pads at the groin, knees, and ankles.

a. lateral chest position
b. jackknife position
c. lithotomy position

_____ 36. In this position, the weight of the upper leg may cause peroneal nerve injury on the downside leg; therefore, both legs must be padded.

37. Nursing interventions for ensuring client safety in the postoperative period include:

   (a) _____

   (b) _____

   (c) _____

38. Which of the following preoperative findings would increase the client's risk postoperatively for deep vein thrombosis (DVT)?

   a. thin, short stature

   b. heart murmur

   c. history of cardiac surgery

   d. varicose veins

39. Once the client is transferred from the PACU to his or her own room, immediate and continuing assessment is essential. After major surgery, the nurse generally assesses the client's vital signs:

   a. every 15 minutes during the first hour, and if stable, every 30 minutes for the next 2 hours, and then every hour during the next 4 hours.

   b. every 4 hours, unless the client's condition changes.

   c. according to the physician's orders.

   d. during routine checks and as indicated.

40. Which of the following nursing interventions is inappropriate for a client with postoperative DVT?

   a. maintaining the client on bed rest

   b. massaging the affected extremity

   c. applying moist heat on the affected area

   d. measuring calf circumference

41. Studies have shown that the client's awareness during the intraoperative period may be greater than once believed. The nurse understands that:

   a. laughing and joking are okay during surgery because the client is unconscious.

   b. nothing should be said while the client is unconscious that would not be said if the client were awake.

   c. the client rarely remembers the intraoperative experience.

   d. there should be complete silence in the OR during surgery.

42. As a result of anesthesia and the cool OR environment, older clients are at higher risk for

   (a) _____, (b) _____,

   and (c) _____.

43. Nursing interventions to prevent postoperative pneumonia include:

   a. maintaining the client on bed rest.

   b. restricting the client's fluids.

   c. encouraging the client to cough and breathe deeply.

   d. maintaining the client in a supine position.

44. Nursing care of the client who is hemorrhaging includes providing care associated with shock as well as (a) _____, (b) _____, or

   (c) _____.

45. Nursing care of the client with atelectasis includes encouraging coughing, turning, and deep breathing every _____ hours.

46. Which of the following interventions may be beneficial for the client who is feeling constipated?
    a. ambulate the client if not contraindicated
    b. offer the client the bedpan frequently
    c. pour warm water over the client's perineum
    d. decrease the client's fluids to 1000 mL per day

Read the following statement and determine if it is true or false. Correct the statement if it is false.

_____ 47. Nursing care of the client with urinary retention includes decreasing the daily oral fluid intake to 500 to 1000 mL.

48. Healing by primary intention describes a surgical wound that:
    a. has large tissue loss.
    b. is well approximated.
    c. is infected.
    d. has an ulcer.

49. Identify the type of wound drainage described:
    (a) This drainage contains serum and red blood cells. It is often reddish in color and thick.

    _____

    (b) This drainage is often clear or slightly yellow. _____
    (c) This drainage is often thick and may be odoriferous. _____

50. A client calls the nurse on the sixth day following abdominal surgery and describes a "giving way" sensation that occurred after coughing. If abdominal wound dehiscence has occurred, assessment of the wound might reveal:
    a. protrusion of a body organ through the surgical incision.
    b. purulent odorous discharge.
    c. drainage that has a thick, reddish appearance.
    d. a separation in the layers of the incisional wound.

51. What primary intervention by the nurse is most appropriate for a client with a wound dehiscence?
    a. prepare the client for emergency surgery
    b. call the surgeon stat and alert the OR team
    c. cover the wound with a sterile dressing moistened with normal saline
    d. cover the wound with a sterile dressing and monitor the amount of drainage from the wound

52. List five key components of discharge teaching for clients following surgery and give an example of each.
    (a) _____
    (b) _____
    (c) _____
    (d) _____
    (e) _____

53. The older surgical client may experience such age-related changes as a decline in vision and hearing ability. Nursing interventions that might compensate for these sensory deficits include:

(a) _____

(b) _____

(c) _____

54. What three interventions can the nurse employ to decrease the chances of intraoperative hypothermia?

(a) _____

(b) _____

(c) _____

▪ ▪ ▪ **Outpatient Surgery**

55. Which of the following is an advantage of outpatient surgery?

a. greater opportunity for the nurse to establish a rapport with the client's family

b. the less formal atmosphere puts the client and family at ease

c. a higher nurse-to-client ratio

d. a reduced risk of hospital-acquired infection

56. Which of the following is a disadvantage of outpatient surgery?

a. decreased revenues for the hospital

b. more surgical complications due to hurried surgical procedures

c. less time for the nurse to spend in client teaching

d. lower nurse-to-client ratio

57. Following outpatient surgery, what criteria must be met by the surgical client prior to discharge?

(a) _____

(b) _____

(c) _____

Case Study

Ken Vu underwent a laparoscopic hernia repair in the ambulatory surgery center. His length of stay is expected to be less than 6 hours. His wife is planning on driving him home.

58. Mr. Vu tells the nurse he cannot void, but states that he is sure he will be able to void at home. The most appropriate action by the nurse is to:

a. discharge him as planned.

b. contact the surgeon.

c. insert a Foley catheter.

d. encourage use of suggestive voiding techniques.

59. Mr. Vu's preoperative BP was 140/88. Prior to discharge the nurse notes that his BP is 110/62 and his P is 98. The most appropriate action by the nurse is to:
    a. discharge him to home and tell him to call with any problems.
    b. assess his wound and monitor his vital signs every 15 minutes.
    c. instruct him about his elevated blood pressure and the importance of follow-up readings.
    d. recognize that this is an expected drop in blood pressure.

60. Which statement by Mr. Vu's wife indicates the need for further teaching?
    a. "He can mow the lawn tomorrow."
    b. "The dressing should be kept dry and clean."
    c. "He should report any fever or chills."
    d. "He should avoid heavy lifting."

■ ■ ■ **Critical Thinking Exercises**

61. Develop a teaching plan for a client undergoing general anesthesia.

62. Design a plan of care for a client receiving conscious sedation.

63. Develop a plan to ensure continuity of care for surgical clients.

64. A 52-year-old woman client just underwent a mastectomy and lymph node dissection in an ambulatory surgical setting. She is discharged 12 hours after surgery. She tells the nurse she is planning to go back to work in 2 days. How might the nurse assess the client's readiness to go back to work? Develop a teaching plan to assist the client in setting realistic goals related to activity and returning to work.

■ ■ ■ **Additional Learning Experiences**

- Ask friends and relatives about any surgical experiences they have had and their perception of the events.
- Ask your nursing faculty about the possibility of observing surgery.
- Interview a perioperative nurse about the role of the nurse in the surgical setting.
- Interview clients about their surgical experiences.

CHAPTER 8

Nursing Care of Clients with Altered Immunity

■ ■ ■ **Focused Study Tips**

- Compare and contrast the three major groups of leukocytes, their percentages, and their functions.

- Describe the five cardinal signs of inflammation.

- Describe the signs associated with transplant rejection. Compare the specific signs and symptoms, causes, presentation, and treatment of rejection episodes for each organ.

- Discuss the clinical presentation, treatment, and related nursing care for the most common opportunistic infections.

- Design a teaching plan for high school students learning the guidelines for safer sex.

■ ■ ■ **Overview of the Immune System**

1. Describe three functions of the immune system.
   (a) _____
   (b) _____
   (c) _____

2. Cells that are involved in both specific and nonspecific immune responses are called:
   a. leukocytes.
   b. T cells.
   c. B cells.
   d. eosinophils.

3. Marginated cells are:
   a. engaged in the digestion of substances.
   b. ineffective for disease fighting.
   c. attached to vascular epithelial cells.
   d. deficient in number.

4. A white blood cell count of 18,000/mm^3 may indicate the client:
   a. is anemic.
   b. has an infection.
   c. is dehydrated.
   d. is experiencing a suppression of bone marrow activity.

5. The purpose of examining a differential in a white blood cell count is to:
   a. determine if the client is anemic.
   b. determine the portion of the total represented by each type of leukocyte.
   c. determine the number of erythrocytes contained in the blood.
   d. tell if the client is experiencing an electrolyte imbalance.

Match the type of cell (a–g) with the correct descriptions listed in questions 6–23. Cell types may be used more than once.

_____ 6. These cells are composed of memory cells.

_____ 7. These cells have a circulating half-life of 30 minutes.

_____ 8. These cells play a role in the destruction of malignant cells.

_____ 9. These cells constitute 55–70% of the total number of circulating leukocytes.

_____ 10. The immature form of these cells are called band cells.

_____ 11. Kupffer cells are a form of this type of cell found in the liver.

_____ 12. These cells account for 1–4% of circulating leukocytes.

_____ 13. These cells are composed of helper cells and suppressor cells.

_____ 14. These cells are the most plentiful of the granulocytes.

_____ 15. These cells are thought to protect the client from parasitic worms.

_____ 16. These cells produce antibodies such as IgA and IgE.

_____ 17. These are the first cells to arrive at the site of an infection.

_____ 18. These cells are granular cells found in the spleen.

_____ 19. The immature form of these cells is called monocytes.

_____ 20. These cells have a circulating half-life of 6–10 hours.

_____ 21. These cells are the largest in size of all the leukocytes.

_____ 22. These cells are involved in the hypersensitivity response.

_____ 23. Microglia is a form of these cells found in the brain.

a. neutrophils
b. eosinophils
c. basophils
d. macrophages
e. B cells
f. T cells
g. natural killer cells

24. The two functions of lymphoid tissue are:
    (a) _____
    (b) _____

25. The predominant cell type found in the white pulp of the spleen is:
    a. macrophages.   b. T cells.   c. B cells.   d. eosinophils.

26. Three days after undergoing a splenectomy, the client tells the nurse, "I know that my spleen is very important in cleansing my blood. How can I live without my spleen?" The most appropriate response by the nurse is:
    a. "You will be on a special machine that will cleanse your blood."
    b. "You will receive another spleen once a donor becomes available."
    c. "Your kidneys and bone marrow will assume the function of your spleen."
    d. "Your liver and bone marrow will assume the function of your spleen."

27. The main purpose of the thymus gland is the:
    a. maturation and differentiation of T cells.
    b. production and proliferation of B cells.
    c. stimulation and dissemination of red blood cells.
    d. stimulation and production of thyroid hormone.

28. Fill in the blanks with the proper terms that describe the events that occur in the nonspecific inflammatory response.

When tissue is damaged, the immediate response by the blood vessels is to (a) _____ _____. Immediately after this, the blood vessels (b) _____. This action releases two inflammatory mediators: (c) _____ and (d) _____. When vasodilatation occurs, the nurse assessing this area will see (e) _____ and will palpate (f) _____, which are two characteristics of inflammation. The inflammatory response also brings fluid to the region to protect and to cleanse the area. This fluid can have various colors. If the mixture is of red blood cells and plasma it is referred to as (g) _____ exudate. Within 1 hour, leukocytes emigrate into the area. They begin their task of engulfing, destroying, and digesting, a process called (h) _____. Inflammation begins wound healing; it is thought of as the first phase. The second phase of wound healing is called (i) _____. When the tissue returns to its original state and sustains no damage, this type of reconstruction is called (j) _____. When regeneration occurs and complete resolution is not possible, healing occurs through the formation of scar tissue. This process is known as (k) _____.

29. A client whose immune system is able to identify antigens and effectively destroy or remove them is said to be:
    a. immunocompromised.
    b. immunocompetent.
    c. immunolatent.
    d. immunopatent.

30. Which of the following statements describing the immune system of the older client is false?
    a. Infections are among the top ten causes of hospitalization in the older client.
    b. Infection is one of the five leading causes of death among persons 65 years or older.
    c. Nonspecific immune defenses and the inflammatory response are reduced in the older client.
    d. Immune defenses are increased twofold in the older client.

31. A frequently occuring symptom of infection in the older adult is:
    a. a low white blood count.
    b. confusion.
    c. fever.
    d. chills.

32. The nurse is teaching an 83-year-old client strategies to prevent infections. Which statement by the client indicates a need for further client teaching?
    a. "I should eat a well-balanced diet."
    b. "I should get a flu shot every year."
    c. "I should limit my fluid intake."
    d. "I should practice thorough hand washing."

33. B cells are activated by contact with:
    a. antibodies.
    b. plasma cells.
    c. antigens.
    d. B lymphocytes.

34. Which immunoglobulin plays an important role in allergic and other hypersensitivity reactions?
    a. IgA
    b. IgE
    c. IgG
    d. IgM

35. T-lymphocytes are the initiators of which type of immune response?
    a. humoral immune response
    b. opsonization
    c. primary immune response
    d. cell-mediated immune response

36. As clients age, thymic hormone levels _____.

▪ ▪ ▪ Assessing the Client's Immune System

37. Which clinical term describes lymph nodes that are swollen and tender upon palpation?

   a. splenomegaly   b. lymphadenopathy   c. hepatomegaly   d. lymphedema

38. Identify the five cardinal signs of inflammation.

   (a) _____   (d) _____

   (b) _____   (e) _____

   (c) _____

39. Identify the four systemic signs of inflammation.

   (a) _____

   (b) _____

   (c) _____

   (d) _____

40. Which of the following statements most accurately describes pus?

   a. Pus is a serous drainage consisting mainly of plasma and digested bacteria.

   b. Pus is a solution consisting of dead neutrophils, digested bacteria, and necrotic tissue.

   c. Pus is a sanguinous drainage consisting chiefly of red blood cells and plasma.

   d. Pus is serosanguineous drainage consisting mainly of plasma and red blood cells.

41. An increase in a client's erythrocyte sedimentation rate (ESR) may indicate that:

   a. the client is anemic.

   b. the client has sickle-cell anemia.

   c. there is some degree of congestive heart failure.

   d. there is an inflammatory process occurring in the client.

42. Which client is at the greatest risk for delayed wound healing?

   a. a 36-year-old client following an appendectomy

   b. a 67-year-old client following a total hip replacement

   c. a 45-year-old client with diabetes mellitus following an exploratory laparotomy

   d. a 56-year-old hypertensive client following a hernia repair

43. Which statement by the client taking corticosteroids indicates a need for further client teaching?

   a. "I should report a weight gain over 5 lbs."

   b. "I should avoid foods high in salt."

   c. "If I gain weight, I should stop taking the corticosteroids immediately."

   d. "I should take the corticosteroids with food."

44. The difference between acetaminophen and acetylsalicylic acid (aspirin) is that acetaminophen is not prescribed as an:

   a. anti-inflammatory.   b. antipyretic.   c. analgesic.   d. antidote.

45. Which statement by the client taking aspirin indicates the need for further client teaching?

   a. "I should take the aspirin on an empty stomach."

   b. "I should report bleeding gums to my health care provider immediately."

   c. "I should not drink alcohol while taking aspirin."

   d. "I should report tinnitus to my health care provider."

46. Identify eight dietary requirements for wound healing.

    (a) _____   (e) _____

    (b) _____   (f) _____

    (c) _____   (g) _____

    (d) _____   (h) _____

47. The most appropriate solution for cleansing an acutely inflamed, noninfected tissue is:

    a. povidone iodine.   b. alcohol.   c. normal saline.   d. hydrogen peroxide.

48. The nurse is teaching a client how to apply heat to an infected wound. Which statement by the client indicates a need for further client teaching?

    a. "The compress should be left on for no longer than 20 minutes at a time."

    b. "The compress should be soaked in boiling water and applied directly to the skin."

    c. "I can use warm compresses several times each day."

    d. "Heat will increase blood flow and relieve pain."

▪ ▪ ▪ **Natural or Acquired Immunity**

49. The occupational health nurse is questioning a client about childhood illnesses. The client had German measles as a child and has a naturally acquired immunity. Her immune status is explained by:

    a. the existence of vaccine which was given to her as a child.

    b. the existence of memory cells which provide long-term immunity.

    c. the administration of antibodies to the chicken pox virus.

    d. the passing of antibodies passed to her in vitro.

50. The purpose of immunizations or vaccinations is to provide:

    a. active immunity.   c. artificial passive immunity.

    b. natural immunity.   d. artificially acquired immunity.

51. A client asks the nurse, "I thought you had to get the measles in order to be immune from catching them again." The correct response by the nurse is that there is a vaccine available that provides:

    a. natural active immunity.   c. active artificial immunity.

    b. natural passive immunity.   d. passive artificial immunity.

52. A laboratory test that breaks down globulin into its specific components is:

    a. serum protein.   c. protein electrophoresis.

    b. antibody testing.   d. skin testing.

53. A 70-year-old grandparent brings his granddaughter to the community clinic for a measles vaccination. He asks the nurse if he should have a measles vaccination, too. An appropriate response by the nurse is:

    a. "Only if you are exposed to the measles."

    b. "Because of your age, you are probably immune."

    c. "Only children need measles vaccine."

    d. "Yes, if you have not been vaccinated before."

54. A 27-year-old woman arrives at the doctor's office for treatment of a wound in her foot caused by a rusty nail. When questioned, she cannot recall when she last received a tetanus injection. The correct action by the nurse is to:
    a. prepare to give a booster injection of 0.5 mL.
    b. prepare to give the initial series of injections.
    c. assume that the client received a tetanus shot as a child and is not at risk.
    d. recognize that there is no risk of tetanus in this situation.

55. The nurse would not recommend hepatitis B vaccine to which of the following clients?
    a. a nursing student
    b. a prison guard
    c. a client on hemodialysis
    d. a client with hepatitis B

56. A client has undergone an anergy panel and the results indicate that he is anergic. This means that:
    a. his immune system is fully functional.
    b. he possesses no antibodies in his blood.
    c. he has normal humoral immunity.
    d. he has a depressed cell-mediated immunity.

57. The purpose of a gamma globulin injection is to:
    a. provide passive immunity to a known antigen.
    b. protect the client from the HIV virus.
    c. stimulate an immune response.
    d. give the client a tetanus booster.

58. Which of the following assessments is important to make prior to the administration of a measles, mumps, and rubella (MMR) vaccine?
    a. ask the client about allergies to shellfish
    b. ask the client about allergies to eggs
    c. ask the client about hypersensitivity to horse serum
    d. ask the client about allergies to beef or pork

59. A client has been diagnosed with AIDS. She asks the nurse if her 1-year-old daughter should receive oral polio vaccine. The daughter has tested negative for HIV. The correct action by the nurse is to:
    a. set up appointments for the series of vaccines.
    b. explain to the client that live vaccine may cause disease in immunosuppressed individuals.
    c. explain to the client that all children must receive the vaccines to attend school.
    d. discuss with the client the research that suggests polio vaccine may cause AIDS.

60. Immediately following administration of an inoculation, the nurse should monitor the client for:
    a. redness around the injection site.
    b. fever, chills, and muscle aches.
    c. irritability and restlessness.
    d. respiratory distress.

▪ ▪ ▪ Infection

61. Fill in the blanks (a–d) with the correct pathogens.

    (a) _____ are obligate intracellular parasites incapable of reproducing outside a living cell.

    (b) _____ are single-celled organisms transmitted via direct or indirect contact or an arthropod vector.

    (c) _____ are single-celled organisms capable of autonomous reproduction.

    (d) _____ are similar to bacteria, but they are smaller and have no cell wall.

62. Fill in the blanks (a–c) with the correct stage of infectious process.

    (a) During the _____ stage of the infectious process, the host begins to show signs and symptoms associated with the infection. These signs are often nonspecific such as fever, malaise, and myalgias.

    (b) During the _____ period of the infectious process, the organism has infected the host; it replicates, but does not cause any symptoms.

    (c) During the _____ state of the infectious process, the host defense mechanisms have been successful in eliminating the disease state but the organism is still present and continues to multiply on certain sites.

63. Early in septic shock, the nurse would expect to observe:

    a. hypertension.   b. bradycardia.   c. restlessness.   d. decreased urine output.

64. Which of the following nursing interventions would be the most effective in reducing a client's risk for nosocomial infections?

    a. ambulating the client twice per day

    b. performing passive range-of-motion exercises

    c. changing the intravenous tubing every day

    d. removing Foley catheters as soon as possible

65. When monitoring for infection with the older client, the nurse would expect to observe:

    a. more dramatic signs of infection.

    b. shaking chills, but no fever.

    c. changes in mental status.

    d. fever, shivering, and restlessness.

66. A student nurse tells his clinical instructor that his client has an infection because the client has a "shift to the left" in his differential. This means that:

    a. there are more immature neutrophils than normal in circulation.

    b. there are more eosinophils than normal in circulation.

    c. the client's temperature is increasing to the left side of the temperature scale.

    d. both leukocytosis and leukopenia are present.

67. A client is taking gentamicin IV piggyback every 8 hours at 12 AM, 8 AM, and 4 PM. The physician prescribes daily peaks and trough levels. The nurse would order blood levels at:

    a. 11:45 PM and 12:30 AM.   c. 7:45 AM and 9 AM.

    b. 7 AM and 9 AM.   d. 3:45 PM and 4:30 PM.

68. A drug that inhibits bacterial growth but does not necessarily kill organisms is classified as:
    a. antiviral.　　　　　b. bacteriostatic.　　　　c. antibiotic.　　　　d. bactericidal.

69. List six factors of the host that affect the choice of an antimicrobial agent and give an example of each.
    (a) _____
    (b) _____
    (c) _____
    (d) _____
    (e) _____
    (f) _____

70. When a client is taking an antibiotic, the chances of resistance can be lessened by:
    (a) using a broad-spectrum antibiotic.
    (b) taking all the prescribed doses.
    (c) taking the medication on an empty stomach.
    (d) taking the highest dose that is safe.

71. During the administration of parenteral penicillin, the nurse monitors for:
    (a) _____
    (b) _____
    (c) _____

72. A client is allergic to penicillin. She has no other known allergies. Her doctor prescibes Ancef (cefazolin) IV. An appropriate intervention by the nurse is to:
    a. administer the medication as ordered; there is no known allergy.
    b. confer with the physician regarding possible cross-sensitivity.
    c. refuse to administer the medication due to a possible allergy.
    d. obtain a prescription for Benadryl (diphenhydramine) to minimize a histamine response.

73. A client is receiving gentamicin. The nurse should monitor the client's:
    a. electrolytes and CBC.　　　　　　　c. white blood count and electrolytes.
    b. BUN and creatinine.　　　　　　　　d. urinalysis and CBC.

74. A client is taking Bactrim (trimethroprim-sulfamethoxazole) BID. Which statement by the client indicates the need for further client teaching?
    a. "If this medicine upsets my stomach, I should stop taking it."
    b. "I should drink 2 quarts of fluid each day."
    c. "I should avoid excessive sun exposure."
    d. "I should report rashes or itching and any easy bruising and bleeding gums."

75. In which of the following clinical situations is the nurse not required to wear gloves?
    a. when administering an injection of subcutaneous insulin
    b. when performing peritoneal dialysis on a patient in renal failure
    c. when changing the linen on a client who is diaphoretic
    d. when assisting with a pelvic exam and Pap smear

76. The most important aspect in the prevention of infection is:
    a. identification of clients at risk.　　　　c. monitoring of vital signs.
    b. aseptic technique with all procedures.　　d. vigorous hand washing.

▪ ▪ ▪ Hypersensitivity Reactions

77. An example of an immediate hypersensitivity reaction is:
    a. hay fever allergy. b. rhinorrhea. c. anaphylaxis. d. contact dermatitis.

78. A client is to have an intradermal skin test to determine the cause of his hypersensitivity response. His nurse must record the results of this test. If this test is positive, what local response will the nurse observe?
    a. cyanosis and shortness of breath
    b. a wheal initially and then erythema
    c. no observable change
    d. crusting, peeling, and irritation

79. To prevent a client from having a hypersensitivity reaction, which of the following nursing activities is a priority?
    a. a thorough physical examination
    b. a carefully performed health history interview
    c. a proper nursing care plan
    d. excellent nursing resources

80. A client just received an "allergy shot." The nurse observes that immediately after the shot, the client starts to wheeze and break out in hives. Within seconds he begins to have increasing difficulty breathing. The nurse should anticipate that the physician will prescribe the following medication:
    a. oral diphenhydramine hydrochloride
    b. epinephrine 1:1000 subcutaneous
    c. cromolyn sodium
    d. epinephrine 1:100,000 intravenous

81. When a client experiences anaphylaxis, the nurse's priority assessment is:
    a. rate and quality of respirations.
    b. blood pressure and pulse.
    c. patency of airway.
    d. neurovital signs.

82. While a client is receiving a blood transfusion, his nurse suspects a blood transfusion reaction. The correct intervention by the nurse is to:
    a. stop the blood and IV and monitor for further signs of reaction.
    b. contact the physician and report the symptoms.
    c. stop the blood, maintain the IV with normal saline, and contact the physician.
    d. contact the blood bank, as they may want to check the crossmatch.

83. The most likely time for a blood transfusion reaction to occur is:
    a. after the client has received about half of the transfusion.
    b. after the client has received the entire transfusion.
    c. during the first 15 minutes of the transfusion.
    d. after the first 15 minutes of the transfusion.

84. A client is taking hydroxyzine for allergy symptoms. Which statement by the client indicates a need for further client teaching?
    a. "I should report chest tightness or wheezing to my physician immediately."
    b. "I can have a couple glasses of wine daily while I'm taking hydroxyzine."
    c. "I should not drive my car or operate hazardous machinery while I'm taking hydroxyzine."
    d. "Hard candy and gum may relieve the mouth dryness I'll experience from the medicine."

■ ■ ■ The Client with a Tissue Transplant

Match the grafts (a–c) with the correct descriptions listed in questions 85–87.

_____ 85. This type of graft comes from living donors.

_____ 86. This type of graft is transplanted from animal to human.

_____ 87. This type of graft occurs between identical twins.

a. xenograft
b. isograft
c. allograft

88. The most common and treatable type of tissue rejection occurs:
   a. 2 to 3 days after transplant.
   b. between 4 days and 3 months after the transplant.
   c. between 4 months and 1 year after the transplant.
   d. during the first 100 days following the transplant.

89. A client underwent a kidney transplant 3 days ago. His brother wants to visit him, but he is just getting over a cold. The most appropriate action by the nurse is to:
   a. allow the client's brother to visit, but only if he wears a mask.
   b. tell the client's brother that it is best to wait until his cold is completely gone.
   c. allow the client's brother to visit since it is unlikely that he is contagious.
   d. tell the client's family that he could die if he caught a cold, and that everyone must stay away for now.

90. A nurse who works in a transplant unit notices that her client, 2 weeks following a liver transplant, has a maculopapular rash on the palms of her hands and the soles of her feet. She asks the client if the rash itches. This finding is characteristic of:
   a. graft-versus-host disease.
   b. hyperacute rejection.
   c. acute tissue rejection.
   d. chronic tissue rejection.

91. A client taking immunosuppressive drugs is at higher risk for infection due to the fact that _____
   _____
   _____.

92. Identify six topics the nurse should address when performing client teaching following transplant.
   (a) _____
   (b) _____
   (c) _____
   (d) _____
   (e) _____
   (f) _____

■ ■ ■ The Client with HIV Infection

93. AIDS is the leading cause of death in which of the following groups?
   a. adults over 65
   b. females 35–44
   c. males 35–44
   d. males 45–65

94. The primary mode of HIV transmission is thought to be through:
   a. sexual contact.
   b. kissing.
   c. breast milk.
   d. needlestick injuries.

95. Risk factors associated with HIV transmission are thought to be:
    a. associated with groups of people such as homosexuals or drug abusers.
    b. highest in the prison population.
    c. of no concern to the heterosexual population.
    d. associated with other negative health behaviors.

96. A student is seen by the nurse in his campus health clinic. He reports that he had unprotected sex the previous night and wants to have an HIV antibody test. The appropriate action by the campus nurse is to inform the client that:
    a. there is no antibody test for the HIV virus.
    b. an antibody test taken today will not indicate if the previous night's encounter exposed him to the HIV virus.
    c. he should have the antibody test right away.
    d. he should begin taking AZT right away as a cautionary measure.

97. The primary cell infected by the HIV virus is the:
    a. RBC.   b. CD8.   c. helper T.   d. macrophage.

98. A CD4 cell count of less than 200/μL is significant in the HIV client in that:
    a. it coincides with the appearance of opportunistic infections.
    b. it indicates the client's immune status is improving.
    c. it indicates death is imminent.
    d. it is an indicator of nutritional status.

99. The most common opportunistic infection seen in the HIV client is:
    a. tuberculosis.   c. lymphoma.
    b. esophageal candidiasis.   d. pneumocystis pneumonia.

100. The most common cancer seen in the HIV client is:
    a. Kaposi's sarcoma.   b. lymphoma.   c. cervical cancer.   d. oat cell cancer.

101. A nurse is teaching high school juniors about safe sex. One of the students asks about using natural skin condoms. What would be the correct response by the nurse to this question?

102. In screening for HIV, a positive enzyme-linked immunosorbent assay (ELISA) test is always followed by:
    a. a CD4 cell count.   c. a Western blot.
    b. a blood culture for HIV.   d. a polymerase chain reaction (PCR).

103. A client is currently taking antiretrovirals for an HIV infection. While providing her health history, she reports that every month she takes a different antiretroviral drug. The rationale for this therapy is:
    a. to diminish viral resistance to one drug.
    b. because some of the drugs she is taking are ineffective.
    c. to diminish the toxic effects of some of the drugs.
    d. due to the short supply of these medications.

104. Which of the following findings is not seen in the client with HIV-wasting syndrome?
    a. weight loss of 10–15% of baseline weight
    b. fever
    c. constipation
    d. fatigue

▪ ▪ ▪ Critical Thinking Exercises

105. Develop a plan of care to promote an older adult's immune function.

106. Design a teaching plan that will enhance healing to assist a family who is providing home care for a 65-year-old woman with HIV and a non-healing decubitus ulcer.

107. The school nurse is developing a program to teach parents about immunizations. Develop a plan to evaluate the success of the teaching program.

▪ ▪ ▪ Additional Learning Experiences

- Ask your faculty member about participating in an immunization clinic.

- Review your own immunization records. Consider the reasons you may or may not have kept your immunizations up-to-date.

- Interview an infection control nurse about the various aspects of that role.

- Review the laboratory reports of your assigned clients. Determine whether they indicate an altered immunity or infection.

- Consider volunteering at a facility that provides services and care to clients with HIV/AIDS.

CHAPTER 9

Nursing Care of Clients with Cancer

▪ ▪ ▪ Focused Study Tips

- Describe the incidence, prevalence, and mortality rates of the four most prevalent cancers.

- Discuss the risk factors for cancer.

- Compare and contrast benign and malignant neoplasms.

- Describe the system for classifying, grading, and staging cancers.

- Discuss the nursing implications for clients undergoing tests to diagnose cancer.

- Compare and contrast the different classes of chemotherapy drugs, their side effects, and nursing implications.

- Describe the different types of radiation therapy used in the treatment of clients with cancer and the nursing implications for client care.

- State the American Cancer Society guidelines for early detection and guidelines for cancer prevention.

▪ ▪ ▪ The Client with Cancer

1. Cancer kills _____ percent of its victims over time.

2. Cancer occurs when:
   a. normal cells multiple abnormally.
   b. normal cells mutate into abnormal cells.
   c. abnormal cells become tumor cells.
   d. abnormal cells are exposed to toxins.

3. The primary focus of nursing care for the client with cancer is to _____
   _____.

4. Cancer ranks as the number _____ cause of death in the United States.

5. _____ is the type of cancer with the highest mortality rate.

6. The cancer mortality rate is declining. Which two groups have not demonstrated equal gains in surviving cancer?
   (a) _____
   (b) _____

7. List the top four most frequently occurring cancers in the United States.
   (a) _____
   (b) _____
   (c) _____
   (d) _____

8. Cancer deaths are most likely to occur in which age group?
   a. children and adolescents
   b. young adults
   c. middle adults
   d. older adults

For questions 9–11, indicate which phase of the cell cycle is described.

9. This phase is referred to as the "resting" phase. _____

10. The cell is actively reproducing its interior components in preparation for cell division in this phase. _____

11. The parent cell divides into daughter cells in this phase. _____

12. The three subphases are the (a) _____, (b) _____, and (c) _____.

13. In mitosis each daughter cell has _____.

14. The normal process that allows cells to specialize in a certain task is called:
    a. mitosis.　　　　　b. differentiation.　　　c. hyperplasia.　　　　d. anaplasia.

Match the unproductive cellular alterations (a–d) with the correct descriptions listed in questions 15–18.

_____ 15. the regression of a cell to an immature or undifferentiated cell type

_____ 16. change in the normal pattern of differentiation

_____ 17. increase in the number or density of normal cells

_____ 18. cells show an abnormal degree of variation in size, shape, and appearance, and a disturbance in the usual arrangement

a. hyperplasia
b. metaplasia
c. dysplasia
d. anaplasia

19. Which of the following statements applies to all of the present theories about the etiology of cancer?
    a. Cancer occurs mostly in young people.
    b. There is impairment of the immune system with cancer.
    c. In cancer, proteins inhibit the growth of cells.
    d. In cancer, the actions of oncogenes are repressed.

20. A client has cervical cancer. She asks the nurse if it is possible that the cancer was caused by a virus. The correct response by the nurse is:
    a. "Probably not—that is only one of many theories."
    b. "All cancers have a viral etiology."
    c. "I am not sure—you will have to ask your doctor."
    d. "Some cancers such as yours have a strong association to viruses."

21. In which of the following cancers is heredity not recognized as a risk factor?
    a. breast cancer
    b. colon cancer
    c. malignant melanoma
    d. brain cancer

22. Which of the following clients probably has the lowest occupational risk of developing cancer?
    a. a coal miner
    b. a carpenter
    c. an oncology nurse
    d. an English teacher

23. List the nine controllable risk factors for cancer.

    (a) _____   (f) _____
    (b) _____   (g) _____
    (c) _____   (h) _____
    (d) _____   (i) _____
    (e) _____

24. Identify three concerns regarding the older client with cancer.

    (a) _____
    (b) _____
    (c) _____

25. Which of the following is characteristic of a benign neoplasm?

    a. rapid growth   b. invasive   c. noncohesive   d. well-defined borders

26. *For each of the terms listed below (a–g), place a* ✔ *by those that are characteristic of malignant cells.*

    _____ a. rapid growth

    _____ b. contact inhibition is present

    _____ c. local

    _____ d. transplantable

    _____ e. can recur

    _____ f. encapsulated

    _____ g. cell specialization is present

27. Metastasis occurs through (a) _____,
    (b) _____ and
    (c) _____.

28. A major factor in the establishment of metastatic lesions is the _____
    _____.

29. A client was recently diagnosed with breast cancer. She asks the nurse what steps she can take to boost her immune system. The best response by the nurse is:
    a. "Refuse chemotherapy; it weakens the immune system."
    b. "Learn techniques to relieve or manage stress more effectively."
    c. "Ask your doctor to prescribe an antidepressant."
    d. "Research herbal remedies."

30. A client's breast cancer has metastasized to the lymph nodes. Which statement is correct regarding this condition?
    a. Metastasis means that the client will eventually die from cancer.
    b. The cancer has spread only to the lymph nodes.
    c. Chemotherapy and radiation will be only palliative in this situation.
    d. Aggressive treatment may reduce risks of further spread of the cancer.

Match the manifestations (a–h) with the appropriate physiologic or psychologic effects listed in questions 31–38.

_____ 31. anemia and clotting disorders

_____ 32. ascites syndromes

_____ 33. septicemia

_____ 34. rapid weight loss

_____ 35. severe hypercalcemia

_____ 36. lung cancer and deep vein thrombosis

_____ 37. fatigue and altered chemistries

_____ 38. grief and fear

a. creation of ectopic sites

b. paraneoplastic syndrome

c. anorexia-cachexia syndrome

d. infection

e. disruption of function

f. hematologic alteration

g. pyschologic stress

h. physical stress

39. Which lab test is it most important to monitor for a client with lung cancer that has ectopic sites?
   a. T_3 b. T_4 c. serum glucose   d. blood culture

40. The pain associated with cancer can be classified as (a) _____ and
   (b) _____.

41. Which statement about cancer pain is false?
   a. Chronic cancer pain may be treatment-related.
   b. Fear and hopelessness may contribute to suffering of the client with cancer.
   c. Chronic cancer pain may affect objective manifestations.
   d. Pain relief is not a goal of cancer care.

42. For each test listed below (a–c), identify the type of cancer the test helps diagnose.
   a. PSA _____
   b. Papanicolaou smear _____
   c. alkaline phosphatase _____

43. For each of the statements below (a–c), fill in the appropriate diagnostic term.
   (a) This system is used to describe the amount of cell differentiation. _____.
   (b) This system describes the size of the tumor. _____.
   (c) This system describes tumors by the tissue or cell of origin. _____.

44. The physician has told a client that the results of the biopsy reveal a papilloma. This statement means that the client has:
   a. a cancer.   b. metastatic disease.   c. a malignancy.   d. a benign tumor.

45. In the TNM classification system, the N stands for:
   a. no metastasis.   b. node involvement.   c. numerical grade.   d. name.

46. Which of the following explanations should the nurse utilize regarding the magnetic resonance imaging test used to diagnose a suspected brain tumor?
   a. "This test uses sound waves."
   b. "Before this test, the physician will inject you with a radiopaque dye and then films will be taken."
   c. "The machine for this test is like a tube, and you will lie inside. It may make thumping noises."
   d. "You must drink a radioactive substance before this test."

47. A client says, "The doctor explained so many things to me that I forgot what she said about the gastroscopy test I'm having tomorrow." The nurse should explain that in this test there is direct visualization of the:
    a. sigmoid colon.
    b. upper gastrointestinal tract.
    c. urethra.
    d. tracheobronchial tree.

48. For each of the laboratory tests below (a–e), state at least one type of cancer the test helps diagnose.
    (a) increased alpha-fetoprotein (AFP): _____.
    (b) prolonged bleeding time: _____.
    (c) elevated calcitonin: _____.
    (d) increased CEA: _____.
    (e) increased aspartate aminotransferase (AST): _____.

49. A client is undergoing diagnostic testing as part of the staging process. She tells the nurse, "I am so worried they will find cancer everywhere; what will happen if I die before my children are grown up?" The most appropriate response by the nurse is:
    a. "There is no way of knowing what the future holds."
    b. "No matter what happens, your children will be fine."
    c. "You sound like you are afraid."
    d. "Don't worry until you know the results."

50. Which of the following client statements indicates the need for further client teaching about chemotherapy?
    a. "Chemotherapy is a local treatment."
    b. "I may experience nausea, vomiting, diarrhea, and hair loss during the treatments."
    c. "I may receive both oral and IV medications."
    d. "I may receive a combination of drugs over different periods of time."

51. Which of the following statements is true about the cell-kill hypothesis?
    a. It explains the body's mechanism of protection from carcinogens.
    b. It forms the basis for selecting specific classes of chemotherapeutic drugs.
    c. It accounts for the severity of side effects.
    d. It is the reason why several courses of chemotherapy are given.

52. For each of the following statements (a–g), indicate the class of chemotherapeutic drugs that is described.
    (a) These drugs are phase-specific, acting during mitosis. _____
    (b) These non–phase-specific drugs work on both proliferating and nonproliferating cells.

    _____
    (c) These phase-specific drugs work best in the S phase. _____
    (d) The main example of a drug in this category is cisplatin. _____
    (e) These non–phase-specific drugs are derived from streptomyces. _____
    (f) An example of this class of phase-specific drugs is prednisone. _____
    (g) Tamoxifen, an example of this class of drugs, competes with estradiol receptors in breast tumors. _____

53. An example of a chemotherapy catheter that is tunneled under the skin on the chest into the subclavian vein is:
    a. Hickman.
    b. peripherally inserted central catheter (PICC).
    c. Mediport.
    d. Port-a-Cath.

54. Which of the following nursing interventions is contraindicated for a client receiving Cytoxan (cyclophosphamide)?
    a. monitoring the client's WBC, BUN, and liver enzyme lab data
    b. teaching the client about ways to manage hair loss
    c. restricting daily fluid intake to 1 L during treatment
    d. enouraging the client to use relaxation techniques

55. Assessing for arrhythmias, gallops, and congestive heart failure is an especially important nursing intervention for a client receiving:
    a. vinblastin (Velban).
    b. doxorubican (Adriamycin).
    c. 5-Fluorouracil (5-FU).
    d. vincristine (Oncovin).

56. When preparing and administering chemotherapy and disposing of the equipment, the nurse should:
    a. use universal precautions.
    b. wear gloves.
    c. wear gloves, a mask, and a gown.
    d. wear gloves and a mask.

57. A client is scheduled to start chemotherapy. Which statement by the client indicates a need for further teaching?
    a. "I will have to drink plenty of fluids each day."
    b. "Visits from my school-aged grandchildren will help my spirits."
    c. "I will need extra rest during this period of time."
    d. "I may need extra help at home to clean and prepare meals."

58. A client is scheduled for surgery to remove a cancerous tumor. She remarks to the nurse, "Why have surgery? I am going to have to have chemotherapy just the same." The most appropriate response by the nurse is to:
    a. tell the client that surgery must be performed.
    b. encourage her to confer with the surgeon and the oncologist about the surgery.
    c. tell her that the combination of surgery and radiation may lead to a cure.
    d. document her concerns and give her reassurance.

59. Which of the following statements best describes brachytherapy?
    a. Brachytherapy involves placing radioactive materials at some distance from the tumor.
    b. Brachytherapy involves placing radioactive material directly into the tumor site.
    c. Brachytherapy is a holistic, nontraditional cancer treatment.
    d. Brachytherapy is also referred to as teletherapy.

60. Which of the following nursing actions is most appropriate when caring for a client with an unsealed, implanted radioisotope?
    a. wearing an abdominal apron
    b. having the other client in the room wear a monitoring device to measure exposure
    c. picking up any dislodged implants found in the bed linen with a sterile gloved hand
    d. disposing of the client's body fluids in specially marked containers

61. Which of the following statements indicates that the client teaching prior to an external radiation was successful?
    a. "If I have pain at my treatment site, I will apply an ice pack."
    b. "I will not have any intimate sexual contact while I am receiving treatments."
    c. "I should protect my skin from sun exposure during treatments."
    d. "I will wash the skin in the treatment area daily using soap and hot water."

62. List two newer types of therapies that are being used to treat clients with cancer.
    (a) _____
    (b) _____

63. A male client is receiving a combination therapy of alpha-interferon with another chemotherapeutic agent. Which statement indicates that the client and family require further teaching from the nurse?
    a. "I will observe my husband for any changes in his mental status."
    b. "I understand how to give the drug subcutaneously."
    c. "I can have severe flulike symptoms while taking these drugs."
    d. "I will limit my fluid intake."

Read the statements below (64–68) regarding pain management for clients with cancer and determine if they are true or false. Correct any false statements.

_____ 64. Terminally ill individuals should die pain-free.

_____ 65. Narcotic doses must be limited.

_____ 66. Gradually increasing narcotic doses means there is no limit on the amount a client can receive.

_____ 67. Most clients can tolerate the level of medication needed to control pain.

_____ 68. Morphine is the drug of last resort.

69. Place a ✔ by the statements below (a–f) that describe proper adherence to the American Cancer Society guidelines for cancer checkups.

    _____ (a) a 47-year-old female who has a breast examination by her physician every 2 years

    _____ (b) a 56-year-old female who has an annual mammogram

    _____ (c) a 21-year-old female who performs a monthly breast self-exam

    _____ (d) a 58-year-old male who has an annual digital rectal exam

    _____ (e) a 68-year-old male who has an annual flexible sigmoidoscopy

    _____ (f) a 57-year-old male who has an annual PSA test

70. A nurse using the Karnofsky scale to assess a client with cancer is evaluating the client's:
    a. amount of pain.
    b. stress level.
    c. performance status.
    d. nutritional intake.

71. Which finding would support a diagnosis of poor nutrition?
    a. oral mucous membranes pink-red and moist
    b. tongue bright to dark red and swollen
    c. slight hair loss
    d. acne

72. A client with prostate cancer is trembling and is pacing in his room. His blood pressure and pulse are slightly elevated. The client may be experiencing:
    a. some type of drug reaction.
    b. anxiety.
    c. body image disturbance.
    d. fear of the unknown.

73. Which of the following statements indicates that the client has misunderstood client teaching about alopecia from chemotherapy?
    a. "I can wear a colorful scarf or turban."
    b. "I have already bought a wig."
    c. "My neighbor will be driving me to the 'Look Good, Feel Better' program."
    d. "After the chemotherapy is finished, my hair will grow back the same as it was before the treatments."

74. Which finding indicates a possible infection in the client with cancer who is immunosuppressed?
    a. a decreased respiratory rate
    b. a decreased pulse rate
    c. a normal temperature
    d. an increased blood pressure

75. The partner of a client with cancer has been provided with guidelines regarding when to call for help. Which of the following statements by the client's partner indicates that further teaching about the guidelines is needed?
    a. "I'll contact the physician if I see any new bleeding from her rectum."
    b. "If her oral temperature is 100F, I'll notify the physician."
    c. "If she becomes withdrawn and cries frequently, I'll notify the physician."
    d. "I'll contact the physician if I notice a change in her eating patterns."

76. Which of the following nursing assessments would indicate an improvement in a cancer client with the nursing diagnosis *Altered Nutrition: Less than Body Requirements*?
    a. serum albumin less than 3.0 g/dL
    b. a PPD response of more than 5 mm of induration
    c. a decrease in urinary creatinine level
    d. an anthropometric measurement of 75% of the standard

77. Which of the following nursing interventions would be most helpful in managing the nausea and vomiting of a client with cancer?
    a. instructing the client to drink plenty of fluids with each meal
    b. instructing the client to lie down for an hour after eating
    c. encouraging the client to eat dry foods
    d. instructing the client to follow a high-fat food plan

78. Which of the following nursing actions is contraindicated for the client with leukemia?
    a. assessing the client's oral mucous membranes daily
    b. instructing the client to brush and floss the teeth three times per day
    c. preventing dry mouth by using moisturizing agents such as Blistex
    d. teaching the client to use smooth rather than sharp utensils for eating

79. A 48-year-old client has just undergone a mastectomy. When the nurse is performing the first dressing change, the client states, "I just do not want to look at it." The most appropriate response by the nurse is:
    a. "You are going to have to look at it some time."
    b. "You do not have to look at your incision."
    c. "You will eventually be able to look at it."
    d. "Every woman with this kind of surgery feels that way."

80. The doctor has told Martin Rodriguez and his family that he has about 6 to 9 months to live. The family asks the nurse about making funeral arrangements ahead of time. The most appropriate response by the nurse is:
    a. "Many people do make arrangements ahead, but it might upset Mr. Rodriguez if you tell him about the plans."
    b. "If you would like to do this, you should try to include Mr. Rodriguez in the planning."
    c. "Don't give up hope; he may still respond to therapy."
    d. "You should wait until Mr. Rodriquez dies before making funeral plans."

81. Which strategy would not be recommended to a cancer client with problems eating? Eating:
    a. icy-cold foods
    b. frequent, small meals
    c. semisoft and liquid foods
    d. spicy, warm foods

82. Which of the following statements indicates that the teaching about the American Cancer Society's dietary guidelines to prevent cancer was understood by the client?
    a. "I should take vitamin supplements every day."
    b. "My food pattern should include a serving of salt-cured foods four times a week."
    c. "I will include high-fat foods in my meal plan."
    d. "Eating more high-fiber foods will be better for me."

83. A client with lung cancer is experiencing facial and arm edema. The nurse should suspect that the client has:
    a. allergic drug reaction.
    b. pericardial effusion.
    c. sepsis.
    d. superior vena cava syndrome.

84. A client has metastatic breast cancer and is admitted to the hospital for pain management. During the night she becomes incontinent, which has never occurred before. The appropriate action by the nurse is to:
    a. recognize that the incontinence occurred as a result of oversedation.
    b. notify the physician that spinal cord compression is suspected.
    c. realize that incontinence can occur in metastatic bone disease.
    d. wait until the morning to see if the incontinence recurs.

85. Describe the signs and symptoms and the two phases of septic shock observed in individuals with cancer.
    (a) hyperdynamic (warm) shock:

    (b) hypodynamic (cold) shock:

■ ■ ■ Critical Thinking Exercises

86. A 42-year-old mother of 3-year-old twins was just diagnosed with metastatic breast cancer. She is planning to undergo surgery, chemotherapy, and radiation. She is considering a bone marrow transplant. Develop a plan of care that focuses on her physiologic needs. Design a teaching plan regarding her upcoming therapies.

87. Design a plan of care to assist the client in question 86 in coping with the body image disturbance she may experience.

88. The client in question 86 develops impaired tissue integrity in the oral-pharyngeal mucous membranes. Develop a teaching plan that will promote comfort and prevent recurrent tissue trauma and injury.

■ ■ ■ Additional Learning Experiences

- Attend a cancer screening clinic.
- Volunteer for the local American Cancer Society or for your local hospice.
- Attend a cancer support group.
- Identify and evaluate Internet resources for clients with cancer.

CHAPTER 10

Nursing Care of Clients Experiencing Trauma

▪ ▪ ▪ Focused Study Tips

- Describe all aspects of the primary assessment and secondary assessment of the trauma client.

- Discuss how the mechanism of injury may result in hidden, life-threatening injuries.

- Define minor trauma, major trauma, multiple trauma, blunt trauma, acceleration injuries, deceleration injuries, and penetrating trauma. Provide examples of these types of trauma.

- Describe the priority and ongoing assessments when caring for a trauma client.

▪ ▪ ▪ Components of Trauma

1. Which of the following injuries is commonly seen in adult clients of all ages?
   a. ultraviolet radiation injuries
   b. drug-related injuries
   c. motor vehicle accidents
   d. fire-related injuries

2. Which person is at highest risk for traumatic injuries?
   a. a 19-year-old unemployed male who abuses alcohol
   b. a 2-year-old toddler in day care
   c. a 32-year-old pregnant woman working 40 hours a week
   d. a 59-year-old overweight male executive who smokes

3. Which of the following injuries is commonly seen in clients over the age of 65?
   a. motor vehicle accidents
   b. falls
   c. fire-related injuries
   d. poisons

4. List three principles of physics that influence the amount of injury that a host may sustain.
   (a) _____
   (b) _____
   (c) _____

5. List the energy sources that cause physical injury.
   (a) _____
   (b) _____
   (c) _____
   (d) _____
   (e) _____
   (f) _____

6. Classify the following injuries as either blunt, penatrating, inhalation, or thermal.

   Injury   *Classification*

   (a) impalement

   (b) sunburn

   (c) flying shrapnel

   (d) gas fumes

   (e) gunshot wound

   (f) head hitting windshield

   (g) radiator steam to face

7. For each of the following emergencies (a–c), list the appropriate assessments and anticipated interventions.

   (a) airway obstruction
      assessment

      interventions

   (b) tension pneumothorax
      assessment

      interventions

   (c) shock due to external or internal hemorrhage
      assessment

      interventions

8. Diagnostic measures to determine the presence and location of internal hemorrage include:

   a. complete blood count with differential.

   b. blood pressure and apical pulse every 15 minutes.

   c. diagnostic peritoneal lavage with CT scan.

   d. chest x-ray with arterial blood gases.

9. List three nursing responsibilities to prepare a client for diagnostic peritoneal lavage.

   (a) _____

   (b) _____

   (c) _____

10. Needle thoracostomy may be used in the emergency treatment of which traumatic disorder?
    a. internal hemorrhage
    b. airway obstruction
    c. tension pneumothorax
    d. spinal cord injury

11. A client is admitted to the emergency department in severe hypovolemic shock. The client is hypotensive and requires immediate fluid resuscitation. The blood type and crossmatch is unavailable. The most appropriate blood type to transfuse at this time is:
    a. A.   b. B.   c. AB.   d. O.

12. Which of the following clients would be able to donate his/her organs upon death?
    a. a client who has breast cancer
    b. a client who is HIV positive
    c. a client with a brain tumor
    d. a client with tuberculosis

13. Which of the following is the most common nursing diagnosis for the family of a client who has just expired from a traumatic injury?
    a. *Anticipatory Grieving*
    b. *Anxiety*
    c. *Spiritual Distress*
    d. *Ineffective Family Coping: Compromised*

▪ ▪ ▪ Effects of Traumatic Injury

Match the integument injuries (a–d) with the correct descriptions in questions 14–17.

_____ 14. partial thickness denudations

_____ 15. open wounds that result from sharp cutting or tearing

_____ 16. occur when the skin is penetrated by a sharp object

_____ 17. superficial injuries that cause breakage of small blood vessels

a. lacerations
b. contusions
c. abrasions
d. puncture wounds

Case Study

Alex Schiano, 36 years old and father of two young children, sustains a pelvic fracture in a motor vehicle accident.

18. Explain why this musculoskeletal injury is considered a high priority.

19. Identify several necessary nursing interventions for Mr. Schiano during the first 2 hours after the accident.

20. What long-term results from the accident could alter the lives of this client and his family?

21. The cardinal signs of neurologic injury are:
    (a) _____
    (b) _____
    (c) _____

▪ ▪ ▪ Trauma Care

22. List the steps involved in the primary assessment of a trauma client and the rationale for each step.
    (a) _____
    (b) _____
    (c) _____
    (d) _____
    (e) _____
    (f) _____
    (g) _____

23. Secondary assessment is (a) _____.
    It is performed following (b) _____
    and after (c) _____
    by either the (d) _____,
    (e) _____, or (f) _____.

24. Provide the rationales for the following nursing interventions.
    (a) administering a tetanus immunization to a client who comes to the emergency department (ED) with a fish hook in her hand

    (b) checking distal pulses after splinting an extremity of a client who has suffered a fracture

    (c) instructing a client who has sustained a head injury and has clear drainage from the nose not to blow the nose

    (d) requesting that members of the Social Service Department be present in the ED for family and friends during trauma resuscitation

25. Identify the actions the nurse should take if, after the first 30 minutes of a blood transfusion in the ED, a client complains of lumbar pain, headache, and chills.

26. What assessments are included in a psychosocial assessment of a trauma client following a serious accident?

27. What are the appropriate interventions for a client who is experiencing a post-traumatic response to a disastrous event?

28. When organ donation is being considered, the donor's care must be carefully managed by the nurse in order to (a) _____. This is done by maintaining

(b) _____,
(c) _____,
and (d) _____.

29. Define brain death and list the clinical signs associated with this state.

Case Study

A frantic young male arrives in the emergency department (ED) shouting, "My brother has been shot! Help him!" The emergency staff follow him out to the car at the ambulance entrance. The 22-year-old male gunshot victim is slumped over in the front seat. Blood is splattered everywhere. On examination, the client is hypotensive and tachycardic and has a wound to the upper left portion of his chest.

30. What type of injuries might be expected with this history?

After the primary examination, the client is intubated and intravenous lines are put in place. However, the client suffers a cardiac arrest, and efforts to revive him are unsuccessful.

31. What factors make this death reportable?

32. What are the forensic considerations in managing a client with a gunshot wound?

33. What are the nurse's responsibilities with regard to documenting this case?

34. Explain the term "chain of custody" with regard to evidence.

Case Study

Mike Adams, 32 years old, arrives in the emergency department (ED) by ambulance after sustaining multiple facial wounds when his snowmobile flipped, and he hit a tree. He does not remember whether he lost consciousness.

35. The triage nurse wrote *Risk for Ineffective Airway Clearance* as a nursing diagnosis for Mr. Adams. How will the nurse assuming care for this client monitor for this potential problem?

36. What other nursing diagnoses would be appropriate for Mr. Adams?

37. Several of Mr. Adams' lacerations require suturing. Identify the nursing interventions necessary when caring for these wounds.

38. After extensive evaluation, Mr. Adams is discharged home. What information should the nurse include in the discharge teaching plan?

39. Develop a teaching plan to assist Mr. Adams in preventing further trauma.

40. Mr. Adams experiences posttrauma response. Identify key nursing interventions.

▪ ▪ ▪ **Critical Thinking Exercises**

41. Discuss how the nurse might approach a family whose loved one is brain dead and is a candidate for donating organs.

42. Debate the ethical issues related to stopping life support once brain death is determined.

43. Develop a community teaching plan aimed at reducing trauma-related injury. How would the success of such a program be measured?

▪ ▪ ▪ **Additional Learning Experiences**

- Determine which hospitals in your city or town are designated trauma centers.
- Assess the system of prehospital care in your community.
- Consider volunteering at a center that provides chronic care to adults who suffer from traumatic brain injury.

Nursing Care of Clients Experiencing Loss, Grief, and Death

■ ■ ■ Focused Study Tips

- Describe the processes and theories of loss and grief.

- Compare and contrast age-related and cultural responses to loss and grief.

- Identify nursing interventions appropriate for clients and families experiencing loss.

- Differentiate anticipatory grieving and dysfunctional grieving.

- Explain the concepts of euthanasia and advanced directives.

■ ■ ■ Loss, Grief, and Death

1. Complete the following statements with the term they define.
   (a) The actions of a bereaved person are called _____.
   (b) An actual situation in which a valued object, person, or body part is changed and can no longer be experienced is called _____.
   (c) The emotional response to a loss is called _____.

■ ■ ■ Theories of Loss, Grief, and Dying

For questions 2–7, fill in the name of the theorist identified with the theories of the grief process described below.

2. Name the theorist who observed in *Mourning and Melancholia* that normal mourning entails a gradual withdrawal of attachment. _____

3. Name the theorist who identified ways in which personal history affects the quality and meaning of the loss. _____

4. Name the theorist who described stages of the grief process during the first year following a loss as shock and disbelief, developing awareness, and restitution. _____

5. Name the theorist who identified a response to loss consisting of five stages: denial, anger, bargaining, depression, and acceptance. _____

6. Name the theorist who stated that grief involves finding meaning with what was lost in relation to what was, what is, and what is yet to be. _____

7. Name the theorist who described the five categories of symptoms characteristic of normal grief. _____

8. The three phases of loss as described by Bowlby are (a) _____,
   (b) _____, and (c) _____.

9. List the three factors that, according to Caplan, influence a person's ability to deal with a loss.

   (a) _____

   (b) _____

   (c) _____

▪ ▪ ▪ **Relationship of Age to Loss**

10. At which developmental stage is a client most likely to view death as a spiritual reunion with deceased loved ones?

    a. childhood   b. adolescence   c. middle adulthood   d. older adulthood

11. At which developmental stage is a client most likely to experience waves of death anxiety?

    a. childhood   b. adolescence   c. middle adulthood   d. older adulthood

12. At which age do children understand the finality of death?

    a. 3–5 years   b. 6–10 years   c. 11–12 years   d. 13 years or older

13. During adolescence, the concept of death is:

    a. thought about only when confronted with it.
    b. experienced in waves of death anxiety.
    c. accompanied by thoughts of an afterlife.
    d. viewed as distant or a challenge.

14. List at least four symptoms that are not characteristic of a "normal" grief reaction.

    (a) _____

    (b) _____

    (c) _____

    (d) _____

15. A client's husband died 2 months ago. She tells the visiting nurse, "I just wish I could go to sleep and not wake up. I wish I had done more for my husband before he died, he suffered so." The nurse observes overfilled trash bags and a smell of rotting food in the kitchen. The appropriate intervention by the nurse is to:

    a. acknowledge the client's loss and offer support.
    b. accept this as a cultural norm and clean up the kitchen.
    c. refer her for a depression evaluation.
    d. recognize these as signs of uncomplicated bereavement.

▪ ▪ ▪ **Nursing Care**

16. What is the rationale for nurses promoting self-awareness about loss and grief?

17. A client has always been healthy, but in the 16 months since her sister's death she has begun to develop patterns of increased illness which have not been attributed to a physical cause. The client may be experiencing:

    a. phantom pain.   c. referred pain.
    b. dysfunctional grieving.   d. normal bereavement.

18. Explain why a spiritual assessment is important when caring for a grieving client.

19. A client has been diagnosed with a malignant brain tumor and she and her husband have just been told that she has about 6 months to live. When conducting a psychosocial assessment, the nurse should:
    a. determine the phase of grief they each are experiencing.
    b. focus on the meaning of the loss.
    c. primarily address the client's needs.
    d. refer the client's husband to a hospice organization.

Match the phase in the grief process (a–e) with the client statements listed in questions 20–29.

_____ 20. "If I hadn't insisted we go on vacation, this wouldn't have happened."   a. anger

_____ 21. "Why me?"   b. guilt

_____ 22. "What's the use?"   c. depression

_____ 23. "Nothing is wrong."   d. awareness

_____ 24. "My mother had suffered a long time; it's for the best."   e. denial

_____ 25. "Chemotherapy is simply hopeless."

_____ 26. "I can see he had a good life."

_____ 27. "If I had only quit smoking."

_____ 28. "This just should not happen to someone so young."

_____ 29. "I cannot possibly have cancer."

30. Identify four factors that can interfere with successful grieving.
    (a) _____
    (b) _____
    (c) _____
    (d) _____

31. Identify one purpose of ceremonies at the time of death.

32. A 58-year-old client is terminally ill and is staying in a hospice. His children have accused the hospice staff of not doing enough for their father. They are also missing work and having heated verbal discussions when they visit the hospice. An appropriate explanation for their behavior is that the family is:
    a. dysfunctional.
    b. experiencing a normal stress response.
    c. in denial regarding their father's condition.
    d. experiencing dysfunctional grief.

33. The state in which an individual responds to a perceived loss before the loss occurs is called _____
    _____.

34. The state in which an individual has an exaggerated response to a perceived loss is called _____
    _____.

35. A client's wife has just died of cardiac arrest. Which nursing intervention is most appropriate for him?
    a. encouraging him to stop crying and verbalize his feelings
    b. leaving him alone to gather his thoughts
    c. sitting with him and letting him cry
    d. explaining that he needs to be strong for his children

36. A client has recently experienced the death of her newborn son. The nurse caring for her has determined that the nursing diagnosis of *Ineffective Individual Coping* related to her son's death as evidenced by altered sleep patterns, altered communication patterns, and feelings of worthlessness is appropriate for the client. The nurse knows that:
    a. the client is clinically depressed.
    b. the client's condition is chronic.
    c. there is a basis for nursing intervention.
    d. the client cannot be responsible for treatment goals.

37. Which of the following techniques is an appropriate nursing intervention for the grieving client?
    a. asking the client direct questions about the loved one who died
    b. discouraging the client's anger
    c. encouraging the client to talk about the loss
    d. avoiding talking about the loved one who died

38. A client has pancreatic cancer. He asks the nurse, "How long do I have to live?" The most appropriate response by the nurse is:
    a. "You will have to ask your doctor."   c. "Do you think you are dying?"
    b. "No one can know for sure."   d. "You shouldn't give up hope."

39. A client has been diagnosed with lung cancer. He is verbally abusive to the nursing staff and his family. He angrily tells nurses and visitors, "Just leave me alone." The most appropriate response by the nurse would be to:
    a. allow him time alone to grieve.
    b. tell him his behavior is unacceptable and set limits.
    c. acknowledge his anger and encourage him to verbalize.
    d. accept this as a normal part of the grief process.

40. Following a mastectomy, the client tells the nurse, "I just hate the way I look." The most appropriate response by the nurse is:
    a. "You are so lucky—you lost your breast, not your life."
    b. "In time you will accept this loss and feel better about yourself."
    c. "This must be a difficult time for you."
    d. "A breast prosthesis will make you look just like before."

▪ ▪ ▪ **Special Interventions for Dying Clients**

41. An intervention the nurse uses to encourage the client and family to talk about past accomplishments, pleasures, and hardships is called _____.

42. An intervention in which the nurse encourages the client to give significant others meaningful information to pass on to future generations is called _____.

43. According to Kübler-Ross, the greatest fear expressed by dying clients is:
    a. dying in pain.
    c. not going to heaven.
    b. dying alone.
    d. dying in a hospital.

44. A client tells the nurse that her mother has been dead for 6 months and that her father should be ready to get on with his life. The most appropriate response by the nurse is:
    a. "Six months is really a very short time to grieve a death."
    b. "He probably needs additional support from you."
    c. "You could suggest that he join a singles club."
    d. "A death usually affects all family members—how has your mother's death affected you?"

45. A hospice nurse is caring for a client who is terminally ill with pancreatic cancer. As she concludes her visit, which statement by the nurse would best reflect therapeutic reassurance for the client?
    a. "It will be great for you to go fishing again in the spring."
    b. "I hope that you have a comfortable night. I'll see you in the morning."
    c. "Don't worry, your wife is here; nothing will happen."
    d. "Just take your medication, and you'll sleep right through the night."

46. The best way to predict whether an individual might develop dysfunctional grieving is by determining:
    a. degree of closeness with the deceased.
    b. length of illness prior to the occurrence of death.
    c. previous methods of coping with loss.
    d. belief in an afterlife.

47. Two weeks after the death of her 70-year-old husband, a client tells the nurse she needs something for her "nerves." She asks for Valium (diazepam). The primary reason that the client should refrain from using antianxiety agents is that they tend to:
    a. interfere with the normal grieving process.
    b. be addictive.
    c. be metabolized slowly in the elderly.
    d. decrease muscular tension.

48. In an effort to comfort a bereaved client, an appropriate statement by the nurse would be:
    a. "At least your loved one didn't suffer much."
    b. "Your loved one lived a long life."
    c. "You'll get over the shock with the help of your family."
    d. "The loss of your loved one is very intense right now."

49. Two years after the death of her partner, which action would best indicate that an individual has grieved successfully?
    a. She sets her partner's dinner plate every evening.
    b. She cries readily at the mention of her partner's name.
    c. She has yet to cry or experience feelings of loss.
    d. She recalls their relationship with positive and negative memories.

50. Which behavior would indicate that a person is not progressing through the normal grieving process?
    a. experiencing waves of intense pain
    b. keeping overly busy with work or activities
    c. discussing unfinished business associated with the deceased
    d. discussing feelings of guilt

51. List two resources that may assist clients and families cope with loss.
    (a) _____
    (b) _____

52. Family members are standing around a client's bed. Death is imminent and the client seems unresponsive. The most appropriate advice the nurse can give the family is:
    a. "Whisper so you will not disturb this rest period."
    b. "Why not go for coffee; he doesn't even know you are here."
    c. "He can't hear you or possibly understand what you are saying."
    d. "Do not whisper or say things you would not want him to hear."

53. For a nurse to resolve losses, the nurse must first: _____.

54. List three broad goals for grieving clients.
    (a) _____
    (b) _____
    (c) _____

▪ ▪ ▪ Legal and Ethical Issues Related to Loss, Grief, and Dying

55. Define euthanasia.

56. What distinguishes involuntary euthanasia from voluntary euthanasia?

57. An advance directive allows the client to:
    a. plan for the management of his/her health care in the event of incapacitation.
    b. assign a financial provider in the event of his/her death.
    c. specify which caregivers are allowed to handle him/her.
    d. direct his/her care for the duration of his/her hospitalization.

58. The purpose of the Patient Self-Determination Act (PSDA) is to:
    a. require the client to sign an advance directive to be treated at any facility.
    b. require facilities to report which clients they will or will not treat.
    c. require that facilities provide written materials to all clients about advance directive.
    d. ensure that all clients will be cared for by a registered nurse.

59. Participating in a "slow code" is considered:
    a. an ethical response with terminally ill clients.
    b. a response for which, currently, there are no legal or ethical guidelines.
    c. an ethical response with clients who do not have a DNR order.
    d. malpractice.

60. A client is undergoing surgery for colon cancer. He asks about a durable power of attorney for health care. The nurse's responsibilities do not include:
    a. assisting with determination of the client's competence.
    b. telling the client to make decisions before surgery.
    c. providing education to the client and family.
    d. ensuring that decisions are strictly voluntary.

61. Differentiate a living will from a durable power of attorney for health care.

62. A client is suffering from *Dysfunctional Grieving* related to stress 1½ years after the death of her mother. Which nursing intervention would not be appropriate?
    a. demonstrating empathy, caring, and respect
    b. helping the client see the importance of "letting go"
    c. exploring the client's past experiences with losses
    d. encouraging client participation in a grief support group

63. Describe clients who may experience *Dysfunctional Grieving*.

64. Which of the following is not a sign of grief resolution?
    a. frequently talking about the loss and past experiences
    b. experiencing recurrent painful "waves" of grief and loss
    c. breaking ties with the lost object or person
    d. making plans for the future and engaging in activities

▪ ▪ ▪ Critical Thinking Exercises

65. Think about losses you have experienced. Examine those losses using the major theories of loss, grief, and dying. Identify the theory that best represents your loss experiences.

66. Develop arguments for and against euthanasia. Discuss these perspectives with another student.

▪ ▪ ▪ Additional Learning Experiences.

- Ask hospice nurses and volunteers about their views on loss and grief.
- Consider volunteering for a local hospice.
- Obtain the appropriate documents for a durable power of attorney for health care. Review them and consider signing them, if you haven't already.

Assessing Clients with Nutritional Disorders

▪ ▪ ▪ Focused Study Tips

- Describe the processes involved in the digestion, absorption, and metabolism of foods and fluids.

- Compare and contrast the purposes, effects, and sources of each of the major nutrient groups.

- Practice the skills of inspection, auscultation, palpation, and percussion.

- Evaluate your dietary intake and compare it to dietary recommendations.

▪ ▪ ▪ Anatomy and Physiology

1. The main purposes of the gastrointestinal tract are to (a) _____ foods and to break them down into end products for (b) _____ into the (c) _____ and (d) _____.

2. Which of the following is not a function of the gastrointestinal tract?
    a. to secrete enzymes   b. to move wastes   c. to absorb acids   d. to secrete mucus

3. Food moves through the gastrointestinal tract from the mouth to the (a) _____
    to the (b) _____ to the (c) _____
    to the (d) _____ to the (e) _____
    to the (f) _____ to the anus.

4. Identify the three purposes of saliva.
    (a) _____
    (b) _____
    (c) _____

5. Peristalsis is defined as _____.

6. Which of the following gastric cells is responsible for secreting hydrochloric acid in the stomach?
    a. mucous cells   b. zymogenic cells   c. parietal cells   d. enteroendocrine cells

7. After an adult consumes a normal, well-balanced meal, the stomach empties completely within approximately:
    a. 1 hour.   b. 1–2 hours.   c. 2–4 hours.   d. 4–6 hours.

8. The phase of secretory activity in which preparation for digestion is triggered by the sight, odor, taste, or thought of food is called the:
    a. cephalic phase.   b. gastric phase.   c. intestinal phase.   d. excretory phase.

9. Which statement about the small intestine is false?
   a. Nutrients are absorbed through the mucosa of the intestinal villi.
   b. The small intestine begins at the pyloric sphincter and jejunum.
   c. Ten liters of fluids, foods, and secretions enter the small intestine each day.
   d. The small intestine is about 20 feet long and about 1 inch in diameter.

10. The digestive function of the liver is to:
    a. release glucose during times of hypoglycemia.
    b. produce bile.
    c. synthesize plasma proteins to maintain plasma oncotic pressure.
    d. convert amino acids to carbohydrates (ketoacids) through deamination.

Match the descriptions (a–h) with the correct terms listed in questions 11–18.

_____ 11. metabolism

_____ 12. mastication

_____ 13. bile

_____ 14. anabolism

_____ 15. positive nitrogen balance

_____ 16. adenosine triphosphate

_____ 17. bolus

_____ 18. catabolism

a. a greenish, watery substance used to burn fats
b. breakdown of complex structures into simpler ones
c. mass of food, and saliva formed during chewing
d. energy molecule that fuels cellular activity
e. process of building complex structures from simpler ones
f. complex biochemical reactions occurring in cells
g. condition when protein intake exceeds protein breakdown
h. process of grinding food with teeth to break it down

19. The primary source of carbohydrates is _____.

20. Carbohydrates supply (a) _____ kcal per gram. The recommended daily intake is (b) _____ to (c) _____ grams.

21. The nurse is helping a client to select a menu high in complex carbohydrates. Which diet selection would be best?
    a. grilled cheese and tomato sandwich on white bread with tomato soup
    b. grilled chicken, baked potato, milk, and a whole-grain roll
    c. sliced turkey sandwich on whole-grain bread with lettuce and cranberry juice
    d. tuna fish sandwich with celery on whole wheat bread, an apple, and grape juice

22. Proteins are either (a) _____ or (b) _____.

23. The healthy adult requires a daily intake of protein equal to _____ g/kg of body weight.

24. The nurse is assisting a client to select a lowfat diet. Which diet selection would be the most appropriate snack?
    a. coconut milk and cookies
    b. lean roast beef and crackers
    c. carrot sticks, celery, and an apple
    d. milk and toast with peanut butter

25. The nurse is assisting a client to further reduce his intake of foods with cholesterol. Which diet selection would be most appropriate?
    a. liver, carrots, and rice and milk
    b. chicken, green beans, and potatoes
    c. lean roast beef, beets, and pasta
    d. cheese and vegetable omelet and toast

26. The intake of fats should be less than (a) _____ % of the total daily caloric intake, and saturated fats should account for no more than (b) _____ % of the total daily caloric intake. Cholesterol intake should not exceed (c) _____ mg/day.

Match the food sources (a–h) with the vitamins listed in questions 27–34.

_____ 27. vitamin A

_____ 28. vitamin E

_____ 29. vitamin K

_____ 30. thiamine

_____ 31. riboflavin

_____ 32. pyridoxine

_____ 33. niacin

_____ 34. folic acid

a. vegetable oils, margarine, whole grains, and dark green leafy vegetables
b. liver, dark green vegetables, lean beef, eggs, whole grains
c. green leafy vegetables, cabbage, cauliflower, pork
d. meat, poultry, fish, liver, peanuts, green leafy vegetables
e. lean meats, liver, eggs, green leafy vegetables, legumes
f. meat, poultry, fish, potatoes, tomatoes, spinach
g. fish liver oils, egg yolk, liver, fortified milk, margarine
h. liver, egg whites, whole grains, meat, poultry, fish, milk

▪ ▪ ▪ **Assessment of Digestion and Nutritional Status**

35. Identify the six assessment categories the nurse analyzes in the client with a health problem involving digestion or nutrition.
    (a) _____
    (b) _____
    (c) _____
    (d) _____
    (e) _____
    (f) _____

36. Anthropometric measurements consist of data gathered by:
    a. inspecting, auscultating, and palpating the client's four abdominal quadrants.
    b. interviewing the client and family members.
    c. determining the client's height, weight, triceps skinfold, and midarm circumference.
    d. evaluating the nutritional value of all foods/fluids ingested by the client in 24 hours.

37. Which of the following assessment findings should the nurse recognize as a sign of malnutrition?
    a. pale conjunctiva
    b. normotension
    c. lustrous hair
    d. rough papillae on tongue

Perform the calculations listed in questions 38–40 using the following data: ideal weight = 142 lb; current weight = 167 lb; usual weight = 160 lb; triceps skinfold = 16.5 mm; midarm circumference = 12 inches

38. percentage of ideal body weight:

39. percentage of usual body weight:

40. midarm muscle circumference:

Match the descriptions (a–j) with the appropriate assessment findings listed in questions 41–50.

_____ 41. cheilosis

_____ 42. borborygmus

_____ 43. gingivitis

_____ 44. candidiasis

_____ 45. bruits

_____ 46. venous hum

_____ 47. leukoplakia

_____ 48. atrophic smooth glossitis

_____ 49. striae

_____ 50. Cullen's sign

a. continuous medium-pitched sound that may be heard over a cirrhotic liver
b. small white patches on the buccal mucosa
c. bluish umbilicus (intra-abdominal hemorrhage)
d. hyperactive and high-pitched tinkling, rushing, or growling bowel sounds
e. swollen, red gums that bleed easily
f. painful lesions at corners of the mouth
g. white, cheesy patches on buccal surface that bleed when scraped
h. blowing sounds due to restricted blood flow in a vessel
i. whitish-silver stretch marks
j. bright red tongue in vitamin and iron deficiencies

51. The size of the liver may be determined by (a) _____ and (b) _____.

52. Normal assessment findings during palpation of the abdomen include:
    a. tympany over stomach and bowel.
    b. rough, grating sounds over the liver or spleen.
    c. presence of the aorta, rectus abdominus muscle, and colonic feces.
    d. rigid, boardlike abdomen.

53. The second step in the examination of the abdomen is:
    a. inspection.　　　b. palpation.　　　c. percussion.　　　d. auscultation.

54. When examining the abdomen, the nurse should position the client:
    a. prone with arms in a comfortable position.
    b. in a reclining position that is comfortable for the client.
    c. supine with a pillow under the knees and arms at the sides.
    d. supine with a pillow at the head and hands behind the head.

55. Older adults are at increased risk for alterations in nutrition. Which of the following statements is not true? Older adults:
    a. have slower processes related to digestion.
    b. may experience malabsorption of B_{12} and calcium.
    c. may have limited access to food and cooking facilities.
    d. have decreased nutritional requirements.

Case Study

Irene Rousseau is a 63-year-old client who arrives at the nurse practitioner's office complaining of abdominal pain for the last 5 days. Mrs. Rousseau is retired and has recently moved to Florida. She is a widow and not currently sexually active. She tells the nurse practitioner she would like to find a boyfriend, but has not had any luck. On examination, the abdomen is soft and nondistended with quiet bowel sounds in all four quadrants. Mrs. Rousseau complains of tenderness in the right lower quandrant. There is a well-healed surgical scar in the right upper quadrant. She tells the nurse practitioner that her last bowel movement was 4 days ago, and it was dark brown and hard.

56. List the subjective and objective data, and identify any abnormal assessment findings and their possible etiologies.

    subjective findings:

    objective findings:

    abnormal findings and etiologies:

57. Physical examination of the abdomen starts with _____.

58. To check for rebound tenderness, the nurse _____
    _____.

59. If a nurse practitioner palpates a mass on exam, the client should be instructed to _____
    _____
    _____.

60. The rationale for this instruction is that _____
    _____
    _____.

61. On auscultation, the nurse practitioner hears borborygmus. What does this mean? _____
    _____
    _____

62. What might borborygmus indicate? _____
    _____

■ ■ ■ Critical Thinking Exercises

63. A 23-year-old married woman is admitted to the hospital with complaints of abdominal pain. How would the evaluation of her abdominal pain differ from a 23-year-old male with the same complaint?

64. Develop a teaching plan for an 83-year-old woman with weight loss and malnutrition who needs to increase her intake of calories and nutrients. Her major complaint is a lack of appetite.

■ ■ ■ Additional Learning Experiences

- Assess your nutritional intake and evaluate whether your diet is adequate.
- Visit a local health food store or pharmacy. Explore the vitamin and supplement sections. Read the labels on various supplements.
- Visit your school cafeteria and assess whether the selections are consistent with dietary recommendations.

CHAPTER 13

Nursing Care of Clients with Nutritional, Oral, and Esophageal Disorders

▪ ▪ ▪ Focused Study Tips

- Compare the physical and psychosocial issues that contribute to obesity and undernutrition.

- Describe preventive measures and management of clients with oral disorders.

- Compare and contrast symptoms and collaborative management for clients with esophageal disorders.

▪ ▪ ▪ Obesity

1. Identity the term that describes the following clients whose energy consumption exceeds their energy expenditure.
   a. This client's body weight is more than 20% above ideal body weight. _____
   b. This client weighs no more than 20% over ideal body weight. _____
   c. This client weighs more than 100% over ideal body weight. _____

2. List five health-related problems in obese clients.
   (a) _____   (d) _____
   (b) _____   (e) _____
   (c) _____

3. The two standard measurements used to assess for obesity are the (a) _____ _____ and the (b) _____.

4. The percentage of lean body mass and body fat which is measured by body density is called body _____.

5. Which gender has a higher percentage of body fat at ideal body weight? _____

6. For each of the following diagnostic tests, indicate what the rationale would be for performing the test on a client with obesity.
   (a) serum glucose:

   (b) serum cholesterol:

   (c) lipid profile:

   (d) electrocardiogram (EKG):

Case Study

Erin Greene, an 18-year-old high school student, confides to the school nurse that she no longer wants to be fat. She is 5' 4" tall and weighs 190 pounds. "I have always been overweight," she states. "I think obesity is in my genes." Ms. Green currently leads a sedentary lifestyle.

7. List four environmental factors that influence a teenager's increased food intake.

   (a) _____   (c) _____

   (b) _____   (d) _____

8. After Ms. Green receives medical clearance, what type of exercise program should the nurse recommend ?

9. Which of the following is not an effective behavioral change strategy for the obese client?
   a. reducing the frequency of eating out at restaurants, parties, and picnics
   b. eating a salad or drinking a beverage before all meals
   c. eating a "forbidden" food as a reward for meeting a goal
   d. using small plates and cups

10. Identify three surgical interventions used to treat obesity.

    (a) _____

    (b) _____

    (c) _____

11. Identify three nursing diagnoses that are common in the client who is obese.

    (a) _____

    (b) _____

    (c) _____

■ ■ ■ Undernutrition

12. List five conditions associated with undernutrition.

    (a) _____   (d) _____

    (b) _____   (e) _____

    (c) _____

Match the following calorie and nutrient deficiencies (a–e) with proper clinical findings listed in questions 13–17.

_____ 13. confusion, apathy, ataxia, muscle cramping, neuropathy, cardiomegaly

_____ 14. listlessness, fatigue, smooth tongue

_____ 15. thin/sparse hair, hepatomegaly, flaking skin

_____ 16. easy bruising, delayed wound healing, weakness, depression, swollen gums

_____ 17. altered taste and smell; dry, scaling, rough skin; night blindness

a. iron deficiency
b. vitamin C deficiency
c. thiamine deficiency
d. vitamin A deficiency
e. protein deficiency

18. An undernourished hospitalized client is at risk for:
    a. diabetes mellitus.
    c. poor wound healing.
    b. low back pain.
    d. high LDL levels.

19. An 81-year-old client is brought to a walk-in clinic by her neighbor who is worried because "she doesn't eat right, she's lost weight, and she always has a cold." List the physiologic data and psychologic issues that place this client and all older clients at risk for undernutrition.
    (a) Physiologic data:

    (b) Psychologic issues:

20. Explain the difference between kwashiorkor and marasmus.

21. Which of the following serum albumin laboratory data results would support a diagnosis of malnutrition?
    a. 6.0 mg/dL
    c. 4.0 mg/dL
    b. 5.0 mg/dL
    d. 3.0 mg/dL

22. What are the most common side effects of enteral tube feedings?
    a. obesity and GI bleeding
    c. diarrhea and gastric distress
    b. fluid and electrolyte imbalance
    d. aspiration and pneumonia

23. An example of an enteral feeding formula that provides 1.5 kcal/mL is:
    a. Ensure.
    c. Pulmocare
    b. Isocal.
    d. Sustacal.

24. To avoid aspiration of an enteral tube feeding, the nurse should:
    a. instill 250 mL of saline before and after each feeding.
    b. elevate the client at least 30 degrees during and for 1 hour after feeding.
    c. never administer more than 150 mL of feeding every 2 to 4 hours.
    d. hold the feedings for 24 hours if vomiting occurs.

25. Which nursing action is essential prior to beginning the infusion of a client's initial bag of total parenteral nutrition (TPN) solution?
    a. record the amount of intake and output
    b. check for x-ray verification of the catheter tip placement
    c. assess the client's temperature
    d. add the client's medications to the TPN solution

26. List three complications of TPN.
    (a) _____
    (b) _____
    (c) _____

27. Which of the following is not an appropriate nursing diagnosis for the client with undernutrition?
    a. *Risk for Infection*
    b. *Risk for Fluid Volume Imbalance*
    c. *Risk for Impaired Skin Integrity*
    d. *Feeding Self-Care Deficit*

28. Provide the rationale for each of the following nursing interventions for the undernourished client.
    (a) eliminate foul odors; provide oral hygiene before and after meals; offer frequent, small meals
    (b) monitor oral mucous membranes, specific gravity of urine, level of consciousness, laboratory data
    (c) maintain medical asepsis when providing care or surgical asepsis when carrying out procedures

Match the vitamins (a–f) with the correct descriptions listed in questions 29–33. Vitamins can be used more than once, and some descriptions may have more than one correct answer.

_____ 29. This vitamin should be administered with food.

_____ 30. This is an example of a water-soluble vitamin.

_____ 31. This vitamin should never be administered intravenously.

_____ 32. This vitamin is stored in the liver.

_____ 33. This is an example of a fat-soluble vitamin.

a. vitamin A
b. vitamin D complex
c. vitamin C (ascorbic acid)
d. vitamin D (cholecalciferol, ergocalciferol)
e. vitamin E (alpha-tocopherol)
f. vitamin K (menadione)

■ ■ ■ Stomatitis

34. List three causes of oral lesions.
    (a) _____
    (b) _____
    (c) _____

35. Clients with inflammations, infections, and neoplastic lesions of the mouth often complain of
    (a) _____, (b) _____,
    and (c) _____.

36. The nurse assessing a client's mouth notices white, slightly raised patches in the mucous membranes. Based on this finding, the client probably has:
    a. an aphthous ulcer (canker sores).
    b. thrush (candidiasis).
    c. a viral infection (herpes simplex).
    d. oral cancer.

37. A client is being treated with Mycostatin (nystatin) for an oral fungal infection. When administering the medication for the first time, the nurse should instruct the client to:
    a. refrain from swallowing because of danger of impairing the gag reflex.
    b. take with meals for maximum absorption.
    c. apply to lips qid for 3 days only.
    d. swish and swallow the solution.

38. The medication usually prescribed to reduce the severity and frequency of oral fungal infections is:
    a. Orajel.
    b. triamcinolone acetonide.
    c. acyclovir.
    d. clotrimazole.

39. Which of the following interventions is contraindicated in the client with stomatitis?
    a. providing mouth care q2–4h while awake
    b. assisting with alcohol-based mouthwashes after every meal
    c. assessing client's oral mucous membranes q4h while awake
    d. suggesting gauze toothettes if client is unable to tolerate a toothbrush

▪ ▪ ▪ **Neoplasms of the Mouth**

40. Risk factors for oral cancers include:
    a. smoking, drinking alcohol, and chewing tobacco.
    b. obesity, high fat intake, and sedentary lifestyle.
    c. diabetes, high carbohydrate intake, and undernutrition.
    d. family history, poor dental care, and alcohol intake.

41. The earliest symptom of oral cancer is:
    a. difficulty chewing.   c. painless oral lesions.
    b. blood-tinged sputum.   d. swollen lymph nodes.

42. The client with an oral cancer is at risk for *Ineffective Airway Clearance*. For each of the rationales of care below (a–e), identify the appropriate nursing intervention:
    (a) helps to thin and loosen secretions _____

    _____

    (b) necessary for cell life _____

    _____

    (c) promotes lung expansion _____

    _____

    (d) understanding promotes client participation in care _____

    _____

    (e) maintains a patent airway by preventing pooling of secretions _____

    _____

    _____

43. A client has been diagnosed with oral cancer that will require extensive oral surgery. During preoperative teaching, the client confides to the nurse that after surgery, he is afraid that he will need help and will not be able to call out. What can the nurse tell the client to reassure him?

▪ ▪ ▪ **Gastroesophageal Reflux**

44. List three controllable factors that contribute to gastroesophageal reflux disease (GERD).
    (a) _____
    (b) _____
    (c) _____

45. Which of the following statements by a client with GERD indicates that the client is managing his/her care correctly?
    a. "I have a snack right before I go to sleep."
    b. "Instead of coffee, I now am drinking 6 cups of orange juice a day."
    c. "I still am 40 pounds over my ideal weight."
    d. "I sit upright for 2 hours after my meals."

46. Discuss how each of the following drugs aid in the treatment of GERD.
    (a) antacids:
    (b) H$_2$-receptor antagonists:
    (c) omeprazole (Prilosec):

47. Which of the following nursing interventions is appropriate for a client who has just returned to the nursing unit following an esophagogastroduodenoscopy (EGD)?
    a. administering an enema to remove the barium
    b. assessing the ostomy pouch for drainage q2h
    c. collecting the 24-hour sputum specimen
    d. withholding fluids until the swallowing response returns

48. A client has been diagnosed with achalasia.
    (a) What symptoms would the client experience?

    (b) What would be included in initial treatment for the client?

    (c) Explain how calcium channel blockers and nitrates decrease the symptoms of dysphasia.

■ ■ ■ **Esophageal Cancer**

49. The most common symptom of esophageal carcinoma is:
    a. regurgitation.
    b. persistent coughing.
    c. weight loss.
    d. pain on swallowing.

50. The most common postoperative problems following an esophagogastrectomy are:
    a. dysfunctional gastric emptying and cardiovascular complications.
    b. esophageal perforation and hemorrhage.
    c. weight gain and dysphagia.
    d. body image disturbance and inability to communicate.

51. The nursing diagnoses of a client admitted with esophageal cancer following thoracic and eso-phageal surgery are *Risk for Aspiration* and *Ineffective Airway Clearance.* On the second post-operative day, the client who is receiving a tube feeding states, "I feel so full and bloated." Which intervention by the nurse is appropriate at this time?
    a. assuring the client that this feeling is normal
    b. adding 200 mL of water bolus to clear the feeding tube
    c. stopping the feeding solution
    d. changing the client's position to high Fowler's

52. Following an esophagogastrectomy, which statement by the client indicates a need for further teaching?
    a. "I should take my protein supplements as ordered."
    b. "I should ingest excessive calories."
    c. "I should report any redness or drainage from my wound."
    d. "I should report difficulty swallowing or vomiting."

■ ■ ■ **Critical Thinking Exercises**

53. Design a contract for a client desiring a weight loss program.

54. Develop a teaching plan for a client who is going to be discharged with total parenteral nutrition.

55. Design a diet for a client with oral stomatitis.

■ ■ ■ **Additional Learning Experiences**

■ Review warning signs of cancer. Develop a community health program to identify individuals with early oral or esophageal cancer.

■ Consider attending a weight-loss support group in your community.

■ Identify resources in your community for adults with undernutrition.

CHAPTER 14

Nursing Care of Clients with Gastric Disorders

■ ■ ■ Focused Study Tips

- Describe differences between acute and chronic gastritis and their clinical manifestations.

- Discuss the pharmacology related to antiemetics, antacids, and H_2-receptor antagonists.

- Describe the risk factors, pathophysiology, and clinical presentations for the different types of ulcers.

- Discuss the various types of gastric surgery and the related postoperative care.

■ ■ ■ Gastritis

1. To prevent attacks of acute gastritis, the nurse should teach the client to avoid which of the following foods?
   a. broccoli   b. alcohol   c. lemonade   d. pastas

2. The difference between acute gastritis and chronic gastritis is that in acute gastritis:
   a. there are changes in the glandular tissue of the stomach.
   b. autoimmune dysfunction is a causative factor.
   c. Helicobacter pylori has been associated with this form of gastritis.
   d. there is destruction of the mucosal barrier.

3. One hundred percent of all people over the age of 70 experience:
   a. acute gastritis.   c. type A gastritis.
   b. stress-induced gastritis.   d. type B gastritis.

4. Vitamin B_{12} levels are measured to evaluate the client with chronic gastritis for _____ _____.

5. Which of the following is not a preoperative nursing care intervention for a client having a gastroscopy?
   a. explaining the procedure to the client
   b. inserting a nasogastric tube the morning of the procedure
   c. checking the client's mouth for loose teeth
   d. maintaining the client NPO for 6 to 12 hours

6. A client returns to the medical unit after a gastroscopy. He complains of feeling hungry and requests the breakfast that he missed. Before feeding the client, the nurse should:
   a. take his vital signs every 30 minutes for 1 hour.
   b. offer him clear liquids in small amounts.
   c. check for a gag and swallow reflex.
   d. provide him with warm saline gargles.

Case Study

Ali Nekourouh, a 21-year-old college student, arrives in the emergency department (ED) complaining of hematemesis, nausea, and abdominal pain during the previous 12 hours. Mr. Nekourouh states that he had "a little too much to drink" at a party the previous night. He also took 3 aspirins to prevent a hangover. A diagnosis of acute gastritis is made. The physician orders Compazine (prochlorperazine) 10 mg IM now, and writes a prescription for compazine suppository every 6 hours .

7. Identify the actions that put Mr. Nekourouh at risk for acute gastritis.

8. What are the nursing responsibilities when administering this drug?

9. Dietary management is one aspect of treatment for the client who has acute gastritis. The reintroduction of food occurs in stages. After being npo for 6–12 hours, the diet progresses to
   (a) _____. Examples of foods allowed on this diet are
   (b) _____. The diet then progresses to
   (c) _____. Examples of food allowed on this diet are
   (d) _____. The diet then progresses to solid food.

10. Which of the following medications does not inhibit gastric acid secretion?
    a. Carafate (sucralfate)   c. Tagamet (cimetadine)
    b. Pepcid (famotadine)   d. Zantac (ranitidine)

11. For which type of gastritis would H$_2$ antagonist be of no benefit?
    a. acute gastritis   c. type A gastritis
    b. stress-induced gastritis   d. type B gastritis

12. The primary symptoms seen in the client with acute gastritis are (a) _____,
    (b) _____, (c) _____. Because of nausea, the client may have a(n) (d) _____ po intake. Vomiting may lead
    to (e) _____ and (f) _____ abnormalities.

▪ ▪ ▪ Ulcers of the Stomach and Duodenum

13. A client is admitted to the hospital for a below-the-knee amputation. His physician prescribes an H$_2$ antagonist for him even though he has no history of ulcerative disease. The rationale for this therapy is that:
    a. the client may develop stress ulcers due to his current illness.
    b. H$_2$ antagonists are prescribed preoperatively to dry up secretions.
    c. H$_2$ antagonists are used to decrease the vascularity of the leg to receive the amputation.
    d. H$_2$ antagonists are prescribed preoperatively to increase blood flow.

14. One key feature that distinguishes peptic and gastric ulcers from stress-induced ulcers is that stress ulcers:
    a. occur only in the young adult.
    b. occur only in the older adult.
    c. are painless.
    d. are often related to gastric irritants.

15. Peptic ulcer disease is thought to be due to:
    a. major trauma.
    b. a bacteria that colonizes the stomach.
    c. sodium bicarbonate.
    d. incompatible blood transfusions.

16. The name of the gram-negative bacteria thought to cause peptic ulcer disease is _____ _____.

17. The most common site of peptic ulcers is:
    a. esophagus.
    b. stomach.
    c. duodenum.
    d. colon.

18. Nursing assessment of the client with a peptic ulcer would reveal pain that occurs:
    a. on an empty stomach.
    b. with eating.
    c. immediately after eating.
    d. continuously.

19. A client is admitted with melanotic stools. This finding indicates that the stool is:
    a. hard and not easily passed.
    b. filled with blood.
    c. filled with bile.
    d. pale in color.

20. A 47-year-old client is suspected to have perforated his peptic ulcer. He has severe upper abdominal pain radiating throughout the abdomen and shoulder. Which of the following findings would also indicate the presence of a perforation?
    a. numbness in the legs
    b. abdominal pain that is intermittent
    c. a soft abdomen on palpation
    d. absent bowel sounds

21. Signs and symptoms of shock that may follow the perforation of a peptic ulcer include (a) _____ _____, (b) _____, and (c) _____.

22. An 88-year-old client has an ulcer perforation. Signs and symptoms of ulcer perforation differ in the older client because the older client may not experience (a) _____ and may present with (b) _____.

23. Unlike peptic ulcers, gastric ulcers are considered to be:
    a. a problem of young adults.
    b. premalignant lesions.
    c. a problem of older adults.
    d. undetectable by physical exam.

24. Stress ulcers that occur as a result of burns are called _____.

25. Stress ulcers that occur as a sequela of head injury are called _____.

26. The majority of stress ulcers occur in which portion of the stomach?
    a. antrum
    b. duodenum
    c. pylorus
    d. fundus

27. Which of the following clinical manifestations most clearly distinguishes the peptic ulcer caused by Zollinger-Ellison syndrome when compared to other peptic ulcers?
    a. the presence of steatorrhea
    b. the presence of melena
    c. the presence of diarrhea
    d. the presence of hematchezia

28. When performing client teaching about the proper use of antacids, the nurse should instruct the client to:
    a. stagger the administration of the antacids with other medications.
    b. take the antacids with all other medications.
    c. take other medications in the daytime and antacids only at night.
    d. drink a glass of water immediately after taking the antacids.

29. A client complains to the advice nurse that the antacid he has been taking for 1 week makes him constipated. He wants to discontinue taking it because he "feels fine." Identify three recommendations the advice nurse can give to the client.
    (a) _____
    (b) _____
    (c) _____

30. Identify two reasons why a nasogastric tube is inserted into a client with a gastric bleed.
    (a) _____
    (b) _____

Fill in the blanks with the correct term concerning gastric lavage.

31. The nurse uses a # _____ to _____ gauge French nasogastric tube for lavage.

32. The solution used to irrigate a nasogastric tube is _____.

33. The irrigating solution should be at _____ temperature.

34. If the irrigating solution is too cold or iced, the client is at risk for _____ _____ of the gastric mucosa.

35. Explain how the nurse would verify placement of a nasogastric tube.

36. The nurse monitoring a client receiving a continuous infusion of vasopressin should be aware that this drug can also cause:
    a. nosebleeds.
    b. fluid imbalances.
    c. impaired drug absorption.
    d. fatigue.

37. When a client is being treated for active bleeding, it is best to recommend which of the following diets?
    a. a clear liquid diet
    b. a full liquid diet
    c. a low-fat diet
    d. the client should be kept npo

38. A Billroth II is most clearly distinguished from a Billroth I in that in a Billroth II:
    a. the duodenum is removed.
    b. the distal half of the stomach is removed.
    c. a portion of the jejunum is anastamosed to the stomach.
    d. the duodenum is anastamosed to the stomach.

39. The most common symptom seen in clients who have surgical procedures for the treatment of peptic ulcer disease is:
    a. tachycardia.　　　b. dumping syndrome.　　　c. achlorhydria.　　　d. hypertension.

40. Early symptoms of dumping syndrome occur within _____ to_____ minutes after eating.

41. Identify three early symptoms related to increased peristalsis.
    (a) _____
    (b) _____
    (c) _____

42. Identify four early symptoms related to decreased blood volume.
    (a) _____
    (b) _____
    (c) _____
    (d) _____

43. The rationale for performing a vagotomy with most gastric surgery is that:
    a. the distal third of the stomach is almost always diseased.
    b. the vagus nerve is responsible for the contraction of the stomach.
    c. the vagus nerve stimulates gastric acid production.
    d. it is always necessary to control bleeding postoperatively.

44. The nurse caring for a client following a truncal vagotomy would be sure to monitor the client for which of the following adverse effects of this procedure?
    a. hypotension　　　　　　　c. tachycardia
    b. fatigue　　　　　　　　　d. diarrhea

45. A client returns to the surgical unit following a Billroth procedure. She complains of nausea, and her abdomen is firm and distended. An appropriate intervention by the nurse is to:
    a. medicate her with a narcotic analgesic.
    b. reposition or replace the nasogastric tube.
    c. gently irrigate the nasogastric tube with normal saline.
    d. give the client sips of water.

46. Identify three major complications related to fluid, electrolyte, and acid-base balance a client is at risk for immediately following surgery for peptic ulcer disease.
    (a) _____
    (b) _____
    (c) _____

47. A client has been diagnosed with dumping syndrome. To prevent the symptoms associated with this syndrome, the nurse should:
    a. provide him with antacids with his meals.
    b. encourage him to drink large amounts of water before, during, and after his meal.
    c. instruct him to drink all liquids one-half hour before eating.
    d. instruct him to chew his food more than usual and then ambulate immediately after eating.

48. The nurse should place the client in question 47 in which of the following positions 30–60 minutes after he completes a meal?
    a. high Fowler's
    b. prone
    c. ambulatory
    d. supine

49. What is the rationale for using saline as opposed to water when irrigating a nasogastric tube?

50. A client who has an active gastrointestinal bleed is likely to have an elevation in which of the following lab data?
    a. sodium
    b. hemoglobin
    c. hematocrit
    d. blood urea nitrogen (BUN)

■ ■ ■ Cancer of the Stomach

51. Identify four factors that the nurse would assess for risk of gastric cancer.
    (a) _____
    (b) _____
    (c) _____
    (d) _____

Match the statements (52–55) with the correct terms (a–d).

_____ 52. lack of hydrochloric acid secretion

_____ 53. most common form of gastric cancer

_____ 54. state of very poor health and malnourishment

_____ 55. one-half of gastric cancers are located here

a. antrum or pyloric region
b. achlorhydria
c. adenocarcinoma
d. cachectic

56. A client's partner is being taught to care for the client's gastrostomy tube. Which statement by the partner indicates a need for further teaching?
    a. "I check the placement of the tube by checking its length and checking for stomach contents."
    b. "I should only give him the ordered tube feedings."
    c. "I should keep the dressing dry and clean."
    d. "I should report any redness, swelling, or drainage."

57. A major concern with a gastrostomy tube is that:
    a. it will easily become displaced.
    b. sterile technique must always be used for dressing changes.
    c. self-care, independence, and self-image must be encouraged.
    d. mouth care will result in stomatitis.

58. A client's gastrostomy tube insertion site is covered with a dressing. List the steps in the procedure for changing the dressing.

Case Study

Josh Ivan is seen at the physician's office. He is complaining of early satiety, anorexia, and indigestion. The physician wants to rule out gastric cancer.

59. What diagnostic and laboratory tests should the nurse expect to be ordered?

60. If the diagnosis is gastric cancer, what laboratory and diagnostic findings are consistent with this diagnosis?

■ ■ ■ Critical Thinking Exercises

61. Develop a teaching plan for a client who will be discharged with a gastrostomy tube.

62. Design a diet program for a client who is experiencing dumping syndrome.

63. The nurse is caring for a 38-year-old European American male client who underwent a total gastrectomy. His nasogastric tube was removed 2 days ago and discharge is anticipated for tomorrow. He complains of nausea and vomits 500 cc of bright red blood. What are the priority nursing interventions at this time?

■ ■ ■ Additional Learning Experiences

- Ask your clinical faculty about observing the role of the nurse in an endoscopy procedure.
- Observe a dietician providing diet teaching to a client with ulcer disease.
- Visit your local pharmacy, become more familiar with over-the-counter products for heartburn, indigestion, and gastric distress.

CHAPTER 15

Nursing Care of Clients with Gallbladder, Liver, and Pancreatic Disorders

■ ■ ■ **Focused Study Tips**

- Discuss the care for a postoperative client having undergone gallbladder, liver, or pancratic surgery, particularly the purposes of and the care for all drains and tubes.

- Describe the four broad categories of liver dysfunction.

- Compare and contrast the pathophysiology, clinical manifestations, and nursing care of clients with portal hypertension, ascites, esophageal varices, and hepatic encephalopathy.

- Compare normal and abnormal levels of serum lipase and serum amylase.

■ ■ ■ **Cholelithiasis and Cholecystitis**

1. The most common form of obstruction of the biliary tract is due to:

   a. tumors.   b. fluid.   c. gallstones.   d. abscesses.

2. Two factors that contribute to stone formation are:

   (a) _____

   (b) _____

3. Which gender is more prone to gallstone formation? _____

Match the conditions (a–d) with the correct clinical terms listed in questions 4–7.

_____ 4. The clinical term for gallstone formation.

_____ 5. The clinical term for inflammation of the gallbladder.

_____ 6. The clinical term that describes stones in the common bile duct.

_____ 7. The clinical term used to describe duct inflammation.

   a. cholecystitis
   b. cholangitis
   c. cholelithiasis
   d. choledocholithiasis

8. The pain associated with acute cholecystitis is often located:

   a. in the precordial area.
   b. diffusely in the abdominal area.
   c. in the right upper quadrant of the abdomen.
   d. posteriorly with radiation to the legs.

9. When palpating the abdomen of a client with cholelithiasis, the nurse obtains a positive Murphy's sign. This indicates that pain occurred:

   a. with inspiration.
   b. with expiration.
   c. in the prone position.
   d. in the left lateral decubitus position.

10. A client with cholelithiasis may have pain when consuming which of the following foods?

   a. raspberry sorbet
   b. salad with blue cheese dressing
   c. pasta with fresh tomato sauce
   d. steamed chicken, rice, and vegetables

11. All of the following tests can be used to visualize gallstones. Which one is the least beneficial in detecting stones in the biliary duct system?
    a. HIDA scan   b. ultrasound   c. x-ray study   d. cholecystogram

12. The major disadvantage of using dissolvers (such as UDCA and chenodiol) in the treatment of gallstones is that:
    a. dissolvers cannot be used in the elderly client.
    b. these drugs may cause diarrhea.
    c. dissolvers must be given intravenously.
    d. there is the possibility of recurrence of gallstones.

13. A nurse is caring for a client from the postanesthesia care unit following gallbladder surgery. The client has a peripheral intravenous line and no abdominal dressing or tubes. Which type of gall-bladder surgery did this client have?
    a. choledochostomy
    b. simple cholecystectomy
    c. laparoscopic cholecystectomy
    d. the client probably did not have the surgery

14. The client having a laparoscopic cholecystectomy, without complications, typically is discharged:
    a. the day after the procedure.   c. two weeks after the procedure.
    b. the week following the procedure.   d. immediately following the procedure.

15. If a client has had a common bile duct exploration, the nurse should expect that the client will:
    a. require an ICU stay.   c. not have pain.
    b. return with a T-tube in place.   d. have a portion of the liver removed.

16. The rationale for inserting a T-tube into a client who had a common bile duct exploration is:
    a. because the common bile duct has been removed.
    b. to provide an outlet for urine to flow.
    c. to prevent edema from stopping the flow of bile.
    d. to decrease the client's feeling of nausea.

17. Four days after a common bile duct exploration, the nurse should expect the bile in the drainage bag to be what color?
    a. sanguinous
    b. serosanguineous
    c. green-brown
    d. there should be no drainage after four days

18. Removal of the T-tube may be indicated when nursing assessments show a decreasing amount of drainage and:
    a. drainage that is blood-tinged.   c. leakage around the tube.
    b. increased complaints of pain.   d. stools of normal brown color.

19. It is important to teach the client having extracorporeal shock wave lithotripsy that:
    a. there will be some discomfort following the procedure.
    b. there is intense pain associated with the procedure.
    c. sedatives cannot be given for the procedure.
    d. there are relatively few symptoms postprocedure.

20. A client is having severe pain due to an attack of acute cholecystitis. The physician prescribes analgesia. Which medication prescription is contraindicated in this situation?
   a. Demerol (meperidine) 75 mg IM
   b. Tylenol (acetominophen) 625 mg PO
   c. codeine 15 mg PO
   d. morphine sulfate 10 mg SQ

21. A 59-year-old client, who is 5' 8" and 250 lbs, has just returned from the PACU following an open cholecystectomy. He has been medicated for incisional pain. The nurse observes that the client's respirations are a bit shallow and that he is guarding when he is encouraged to breathe deeply. The most appropriate intervention by the nurse would be to:
   a. allow him to rest and get some relief with his pain medication.
   b. encourage him to use his incentive spirometer when he is more comfortable.
   c. assist him out of bed and encourage him to ambulate and fully expand his lungs.
   d. splint his incision and encourage him to cough and deep breathe.

22. A client has been home for a week following a cholecystectomy. She complains to the visiting nurse that she has fever and chills. The most appropriate intervention by the nurse would be to:
   a. schedule an appointment for the client to see her surgeon.
   b. encourage the client to increase her fluid intake.
   c. tell the client to monitor her symptoms and report any vomiting or diarrhea.
   d. recognize that fever and chills may occur following any surgery.

▪ ▪ ▪ Hepatitis

Match each of the laboratory tests for the detection of the hepatitis B virus (a–e) with the appropriate descriptions in questions 23–27.

_____ 23. This antibody test is useful in determining if a client is a chronic carrier of the virus.

_____ 24. This antibody test is used to detetermine if the client has a current infection.

a. anti-HBs
b. anti-HBe
c. HBsAg
d. HBeAg
e. anti-HBc-IgM

_____ 25. This antigen test identifies when the virus is actively replicating.

_____ 26. This antigen test is used to determine if the client has active disease.

_____ 27. Elevations in this antibody test suggest the client has mounted an immune response to the hepatitis virus.

28. The transmission of hepatitis A virus occurs primarily through:
   a. blood transfusions.
   b. fecal contamination.
   c. needlestick injuries.
   d. environmental pollutants.

29. A client in the preicteric phase of viral hepatitis would typically present with:
   a. anorexia.
   b. brown urine.
   c. jaundice.
   d. fever and chills.

30. Assessment of the abdomen of a client with hepatitis will reveal:
   a. pain without palpation.
   b. pain with palpation in the LUQ.
   c. pain with palpation in the RUQ.
   d. diffuse abdominal pain.

31. The icteric phase of hepatitis begins:
    a. exactly 2 weeks after the prodromal phase.
    b. when RUQ pain diminishes.
    c. when jaundice appears.
    d. when serum bilirubin begins to decline.

32. The posticteric phase lasts for:
    a. several days.   b. 2 weeks.   c. several weeks.   d. several months.

33. Which of the following tests is the most appropriate for determining liver dysfunction?
    a. alkaline phosphatase (ALP)
    b. gamma-glutamyl transferase (GGT)
    c. prothrombin time
    d. lactic dehydrogenase isoenzymes 4 and 5

34. Identify three conditions that cause chronic active hepatitis.
    (a) _____
    (b) _____
    (c) _____

35. A student nurse asks her clinical instructor about hepatitis B protection. The most appropriate response by the instructor is:
    a. "You should have received a vaccine when you were a baby."
    b. "All health care workers should receive protection."
    c. "Wearing gloves will protect you from exposure."
    d. "If exposed, immune globulin will provide you enough protection."

36. A client has hepatitis A. It is believed he ingested contaminated seafood. His wife calls and asks the nurse if the family needs protection. The most appropriate response by the nurse is:
    a. "Everyone who ate the seafood should come in for an IG injection."
    b. "Hepatitis A is transmitted through blood and body fluids only."
    c. "All of the client's household contacts and sexual partners should receive an IG injection."
    d. "Only household memebers who have not been immunized should receive an IG injection."

37. A certified nurse assistant has been inadvertently exposed to blood contaminated with hepatitis B. The nurse assistant has never received a hepatitis immunization. The hospital nurse should recommend that the nurse assistant:
    a. begin immunizations at her next medical appointment.
    b. wait for the results of her hepatitis test before beginning immunizations.
    c. do nothing, since hepatitis B is not transmitted through contact with blood.
    d. receive HBIG and start the HBV protection right away.

38. A client is being admitted with hepatitis E and has had fecal incontinence. He should be placed in a _____ room.

39. A client is recuperating from hepatitis E. His oral intake of food and fluids has been limited. The nurse should encourage him to eat a:
    a. small breakfast and increase intake throughout the day.
    b. large breakfast and eat less later in the day.
    c. high-fat diet to ensure adequate intake of calories.
    d. low-calorie diet that is low in roughage and fiber.

▪ ▪ ▪ Cirrhosis

40 The clinical manifestations associated with cirrhosis of the liver are the result of the liver's inability to perform which four essential functions?

(a) _____

(b) _____

(c) _____

(d) _____

41. A complication not associated with portal hypertension is:

a. edema.
b. formation of ascites.
c. bleeding varices.
d. an elevated blood pressure.

42. In the client with cirrhosis of the liver, which of the following problems does not contribute to fluid volume excess?

a. portal hypertension
b. thrombocytopenia
c. hypoalbuminemia
d. hyperaldosteronism

43. Which of the following foods should the nurse teach a client with cirrhosis of the liver to avoid?

a. almonds
b. smoked ham
c. apple pie
d. red and green peppers

44. Three early clinical manifestations of hepatic encephalopathy are:

(a) _____

(b) _____

(c) _____

45. Assessment for hepatic encephalopathy can be made through the observation of which of the following signs?

a. asterixis
b. Chvostek's sign
c. Trousseau's sign
d. Homan's sign

46. The clinical manifestations of hepatic encephalopathy can be controlled through the reduction of dietary:

a. nitrates.
b. fats.
c. protein.
d. carbohydrates.

47. Anasarca in the client with cirrhosis can best be explained by the presence of:

a. hyponatremia.
b. thrombocytopenia.
c. hypokalemia.
d. hypoalbuminemia.

48. Aldactone (spironolactone) is the preferred drug for a client with cirrhosis because it performs two pharmacologic actions: it acts as a (a) _____, and it competes with (b) _____, which reduces sodium reabsorption.

49. The physician has prescribed neomycin for a client who has cirrhosis and is taking digoxin for chronic atrial fibrillation. When administering these two medications, the nurse should:

a. refuse to administer the neomycin because it is contraindicated.
b. monitor the client for diarrhea, as it is a common side effect.
c. monitor the client's digoxin level and heart rate.
d. check with the physician about increasing the dose of digoxin.

Case Study

Ira Therwell is admitted with cirrhosis. A number of laboratory tests are obtained. The nurse is notified of the results at 10 pm. For each of the following laboratory test results, state whether it is normal or abnormal and whether the nurse should notify the physician of the findings at this time. Also indicate any related nursing interventions.

50. Sodium 127 mEq/L

51. Potassium 3.6 mEq/L

52. GGT = 230 U/L

53. Glucose = 250 mg/dL

54. Serum albumin 3.0 mg/dL

55. Prothrombin time = 24 seconds

56. A client is taking lactulose. He complains to the nurse that he is having two to three soft stools each day. The most appropriate response by the nurse is:
    a. "I will contact the doctor and get something to slow down your bowels."
    b. "Don't worry unless you have loose, watery stools."
    c. "It is a temporary effect of medication; it will wear off in time."
    d. "This medication acts as a laxative and helps remove ammonia through the stool."

57. A paracentesis is done when:
    a. the client's abdominal girth is greater than 45 cm.
    b. fluid leaks from the client's umbilicus.
    c. the client gains more than 3 lb in 1 day.
    d. the client's respirations are labored.

58. A client is scheduled for a liver biopsy at 7 AM. Which statement by the client indicates a need for further client teaching?
    a. "I can have nothing to eat or drink after midnight."
    b. "When the needle goes in, I will experience severe pain for a short time."
    c. "I must avoid lifting, coughing, or straining for about 10 to 14 days."
    d. "During the biopsy, I will have to hold my breath after expiration."

59. A client with cirrhosis is experiencing some gastritis. She tells the visiting nurse that the doctor recommended an antacid. The nurse would expect the client to be taking:
    a. Riopan.   b. Amphogel.   c. Tums.   d. Maalox.

60. A client is admitted to the hospital with cirrhosis. Her laboratory studies indicate anemia, a low platelet count, and delayed prothrombin time. List four nursing interventions appropriate for the client that will help prevent bleeding.
    (a) _____
    (b) _____
    (c) _____
    (d) _____

61. A client is admitted with esophageal varices. Emergency department personnel inserted a Minnesota nasogastric tube. List four nursing interventions appropriate for the client.

    (a) _____

    (b) _____

    (c) _____

    (d) _____

62. A client has severe jaundice. When teaching the client about skin care, which statement by the client indicates a need for further client teaching?

    a. "I should use warm water for bathing."

    b. "I can take antihistamines whenever my skin itches."

    c. "I should avoid soap and lotions with alcohol."

    d. "I should change my position at least every 2 hours."

▪ ▪ ▪ Liver Cancer

63. A woman's father has just died from primary liver cancer. The woman asks the nurse if liver cancer is an inherited disease. The most appropriate response by the nurse is:

    a. "Many cancers are inherited and there may be a genetic connection."

    b. "The causes of liver cancer appear to be chronic infections, chronic cirrhosis, and environmental toxins."

    c. "Anyone can get cancer; we never know what causes it."

    d. "Your father's liver cancer was the result of metastasis from another site."

64. List at least four key early symptoms of hepatic cancer.

    (a) _____

    (b) _____

    (c) _____

    (d) _____

▪ ▪ ▪ Liver Trauma

65. A client is admitted to the emergency room after a blunt traumatic injury. The injury occurred in the RUQ of his abdomen. The most immediate concern of the trauma team is that:

    a. the client may develop acute hepatitis as a result of his injury.

    b. trauma to the RUQ of the abdomen almost always progresses to the development of ascites.

    c. because of his injury, the client is at high risk for hemorrhage.

    d. because of his injury, the client is at high risk for the development of hepatic encephalopathy.

66. A client had emergency surgery to control bleeding that occurred from liver trauma as a result of a car accident. In the immediate postoperative period, his nurse should:

    a. encourage coughing, deep breathing, and early mobility.

    b. expect a moderate amount of postoperative bleeding.

    c. encourage fluids and food to tolerance.

    d. encourage ambulation.

▪ ▪ ▪ Hepatic Abscess

67. In terms of onset, how do pyrogenic and amebic abscesses of the liver differ?

68. Identify two drugs that are used to treat amebic hepatic abscesses.

(a) _____

(b) _____

69. Identify two interventions that help individuals prevent the spread of amebic infection:

(a) _____

(b) _____

▪ ▪ ▪ Pancreatitis

70. The pancreas is:

a. both an exocrine and an endocrine gland.

b. an exocrine gland.

c. an endocrine gland.

d. not truly a gland.

71. The key pathophysiologic feature of acute pancreatitis is:

a. autodigestion of the pancreas.

b. hemorrhage within the pancreas.

c. insufficient pancreatic enzymes.

d. overproduction of pancreatic enzymes.

72. In acute pancreatitis, which of the following laboratory data will remain elevated for at least 1 week after the acute event?

a. serum amylase   b. serum lipase   c. serum calcium   d. serum magnesium

73. In acute pancreatitis, the presence of bruising in the flanks is called _____
_____.

74. In acute pancreatitis, bruising or discoloration around the client's umbilicus is called _____
_____.

75. A client is being treated for acute pancreatitis. Her nurse finds her tearful. The client states, "I am hungry, and I want to know when I can eat again." The nurse should tell the client that she can eat:

a. after 24 hours.

b. after her pancreas has been removed.

c. when her serum amylase level returns to normal.

d. after her chemotherapy treatment.

76. The nurse may observe that the client with pancreatitis has stools that:

a. are watery.

b. have occult blood.

c. are pale in color.

d. contain a large amount of fat.

77. The physician has prescribed cotazym for a client. Which statement by the client indicates a need for further client teaching?
    a. "I should eat a lowfat diet."
    b. "I should not chew or crush the tablets."
    c. "I should take the medication with food."
    d. "I should take the medication when I notice pain or discomfort."

78. A client is admitted with acute pancreatitis. A Foley catheter is inserted. In the last 4 hours, her urine output was 75 mL. An appropriate nursing intervention is to:
    a. recognize that dehydration may co-occur with pancreatitis.
    b. increase the IV rate and monitor output.
    c. report this finding to the physician.
    d. continue to monitor output and obtain a urine specific gravity.

79. When caring for a client with acute pancreatitis, the nurse should:
    a. allow the client to take the position of comfort.
    b. position the client in high Fowler's.
    c. position the client on his side, with knees flexed and HOB up 45 degrees.
    d. encourage activity as tolerated.

80. The client with pancreatitis should follow a diet that is:
    a. high in fat, high in protein, and high in calories.
    b. low in fat, high in carbohydrates, and low in protein.
    c. low in fluids.
    d. low in fat, high in carbohydrates, and high in protein.

81. The client with pancreatitis is having frequent stools. What assessments should the nurse record on a stool chart?
    (a) _____
    (b) _____
    (c) _____
    (d) _____

Case Study

Theodore Salvitori is admitted to the hospital with abdominal pain, nonspecific complaints of nausea, weight loss, dark-colored urine, and pruritis. He is a two-pack per day smoker and has a history of pancreatitis. He works for a cheddar cheese factory and tells the nurse that he no longer can eat cheese at work every day because of nausea.

82. What are Mr. Salvitori's major risk factors for pancreatic cancer?

83. The nurse should assess Mr. Salvitori for the purpose of obtaining objective data. What assessments should be made?

84. Once the diagnosis of pancreatic cancer is made, Mrs. Salvitori confides in the nurse. She tells the nurse, "I am just sure he is going to die; everyone with pancreatic cancer does." What is the most appropriate response by the nurse?

85. Mr. Salvitori undergoes surgery. He has a Salem tube. The nurse notes that the tube is not draining. The most appropriate intervention by the nurse is to:
    a. vigorously irrigate the tube until it is patent and draining fluid.
    b. recognize that this is a normal finding during the postoperative period.
    c. advance the tube to ensure that it is in the correct position.
    d. obtain an order to irrigate and do so with minimal pressure.

86. Specify the major complications following a Whipple's procedure.

87. What are the key nursing assessments to assist in early detection of major complications?

■ ■ ■ **Critical Thinking Exercises**

88. Develop a teaching plan for a client who will be discharged from the hospital with a T-tube.

89. A 23-year-old client is admitted with acute viral hepatitis. He is a college student and hoping to return to school. Develop a discharge plan for him that addresses his health needs.

90. Review laboratory results related to liver function tests. Decide whether they are within normal limits. If the results are abnormal, try to determine why.

■ ■ ■ **Additional Learning Experiences**

■ Ask your instructor if you can observe a laparoscopic cholecystectomy or watch a videotape of the procedure.

■ Design a community health intervention to increase awareness of strategies to protect oneself from viral hepatitis.

CHAPTER 16

Assessing Clients with Skin Disorders

▪ ▪ ▪ Focused Study Tips

- Assess the skin of clients, family members, and friends for both normal and abnormal findings.

- Categorize skin abnormalities and work on perfecting your skill in one category at a time.

- Practice palpating for clubbing of the fingers, degree of edema, skin temperature, and scalp contours.

- Examine the skin of clients of various cultural groups as often as possible.

▪ ▪ ▪ Anatomy and Physiology

1. Name four components of the integumentary system.
   (a) _____   (c) _____
   (b) _____   (d) _____

Match the descriptions (a–g) with the terms related to the structure of skin in questions 2–8.

_____ 2. epidermis

_____ 3. ceruminous glands

_____ 4. stratum basale

_____ 5. melanocytes

_____ 6. stratum spinosum

_____ 7. superficial fascia

_____ 8. dermis

a. the deepest layer of the epidermis
b. a layer of subcutaneous tissue underlying the skin
c. modified apocrine sweat glands that secrete a yellow-brown, sticky substance
d. the second layer of skin
e. epidermal cells that produce pigment responsible for skin color
f. outermost part of skin composed of epithelial cells
g. second most common site of epidermal mitosis

9. Which of the following statements is true?
   a. Eccrine glands produce sweat.
   b. Eccrine glands are found in axillary, anal, and genital regions.
   c. Apocrine glands are sebaceous glands.
   d. Ceruminous glands are modified eccrine glands.

Match the descriptions of skin color (a–d) with questions 10–13.

_____ 10. erythema

_____ 11. cyanosis

_____ 12. pallor

_____ 13. jaundice

a. yellow-to-orange color visible in skin and mucous membranes
b. a reddening of the skin
c. a paleness of the skin
d. a bluish discoloration of the skin and mucous membranes

14. A nail consists mainly of (a) _____ and has an active growing part called the (b) _____ and a white crescent at the proximal end called the (c) _____.

▪ ▪ ▪ Assessment of Integumentary Function

15. If a client presents with a skin problem, the nurse analyzes what five elements?

(a) _____

(b) _____ and _____

(c) _____

(d) _____ and _____ factors

(e) any _____

16. Explain the reason for investigating the medical history of clients with skin disorders.

17. Identify the equipment necessary for assessment of the skin.

(a) _____

(b) _____

(c) _____

Case Study

Jason Williams is a 35-year-old African American male who has been admitted to the same-day surgery unit for revision of an old surgical scar. During the interview, Mr. Williams reveals he has no known allergies, heals well when injured, seldom spends time in the sun, and hasn't noticed any itching, burning, numbness, or tenderness of his skin. A physical assessment of his skin shows warm, moist skin with good turgor overall; a small, white patch of skin on his right hand; spooning of his nails; and an elevated, irregular, darkened area of excess scar tissue over his right forearm. Mr. Williams has no family history of skin cancer or melanoma.

18. The small, white patch of skin on Mr. Williams' hand may be _____.

19. Spooning of the nails often indicates _____.

20. The elevated, irregular, darkened area is probably a(n) _____.

21. The clinical term used to describe patches of pale, itchy wheals in an erythematous area is:

a. psoriasis.   c. paronychia.

b. tinea dapitis.   d. urticaria.

22. Port wine stains, strawberry marks, spider angioma, petechiae, and venous stars are all examples of _____ skin lesions.

Match the descriptions (a–h) with the assessment findings in questions 23–30.

_____ 23. clubbing

_____ 24. basal cell carcinoma

_____ 25. hirsutism

_____ 26. papule

_____ 27. fissure

_____ 28. lichenification

_____ 29. actinic keratoses

_____ 30. furuncles

a. rough, thickened epidermis resulting from chronic irritation
b. pearly-edged nodules with a central ulceration
c. red, swollen pustules around infected hair follicles
d. angle of the nail base is greater than 180 degrees
e. increased growth of coarse hair, usually on face and trunk
f. linear skin crack with sharp edges extending into the dermis
g. elevated, solid, palpable mass with a circumscribed border
h. raised, reddish plaques on areas of high sun exposure

31. The condition in which the nail plate separates from the nail bed in trauma, psoriasis, and *Pseudomonas* and *Candida* infections is known as:
    a. paronychia.   b. vitiligo.   c. alopecia.   d. oncolysis.

32. Thinning of the nails is often seen in _____.

33. The common name for senile lentigines, the normal variation in the skin in the older adult characterized by localized hyperpigmentation, is _____.

Match the nutrient (a–g) with the resulting deficiency in questions 34–40.

_____ 34. dark, round spots in the areas of skin exposed to the sun

_____ 35. bleeding gums, delayed wound healing

_____ 36. dry skin, loss of skin color

_____ 37. oily skin, sores in the mouth, cheilosis

_____ 38. patches of baldness, eczema

_____ 39. thickened skin that is rough or dry

_____ 40. flaky skin, sores in the mouth

a. vitamin A
b. protein
c. niacin
d. riboflavin
e. vitamin B_6
f. essential fats
g. vitamin C

Match the lesion (a–e) with the correct description in questions 41–45.

_____ 41. bright red dot with radiating blood vessels

_____ 42. raised, irregularly shaped, elevated swelling

_____ 43. flat red or purple rounded "freckles"

_____ 44. flat, reddish-blue, irregularly shaped patches

_____ 45. flat, irregularly shaped lesions of varying color

a. purpura
b. ecchymosis
c. hematoma
d. spider angioma
e. petchiae

▪ ▪ ▪ Critical Thinking Exercises

46. A client has dry skin, bleeding gums, cracks at the corners of his mouth, and sores in his mouth. Develop a diet program to assist him in resolving his nutritional deficits.

47. Design a teaching program for fifth grade students to assist them in understanding the function of skin and how they can promote "healthy" skin.

▪ ▪ ▪ Additional Learning Experiences

- ▪ Observe and assess the skin of your assigned clients. Note any lesions and try to identify them.
- ▪ Make flash cards of the various skin lesions.

Nursing Care of Clients with Common Skin Disorders

▪ ▪ ▪ Focused Study Tips

- Give an example of the most commonly seen infections within each group (bacterial, fungal, parasitic, and viral).

- Describe a psoriatic lesion and discuss the treatments for psoriasis.

- Teach self-examination of benign and malignant skin lesions to clients and friends.

- Compare and contrast the characteristics of commonly seen malignant skin lesions.

- Compare and contrast the care of skin grafts and flaps.

- Describe the various stages of pressure ulcers and their treatment.

▪ ▪ ▪ Pruritus

1. A diagnosis of pruritus would be supported by which of the following objective data?
   a. hyperpigmentation
   b. edema
   c. wheals
   d. maceration

2. To limit possible causative factors for a widespread pruritus, the physician may recommend that the client:
   a. rub the skin vigorously with a dry towel.
   b. discontinue all unnecessary medications.
   c. eliminate all citrus fruits from the diet.
   d. take hot baths three times each day.

3. A pharmacologic agent used to suppress the immune response and to help a client who itches is:
   a. Vaseline.   b. Xylocaine.   c. hydrocortisone.   d. Lubriderm.

4. A client has recently experienced an episode of widespread pruritus. The nurse has taught her how to care for her skin. Which statement by the client indicates a need for further teaching?
   a. "I should trim my nails short and wear gloves at night."
   b. "Some creams with alcohol may provide relief from itching."
   c. "I should not use fabric softeners, and I should rinse my clothes twice."
   d. "I can use Vaseline on my skin after my bath to prevent dryness."

5. An ideal temperature for a therapeutic bath is:
   a. between 110F and 115F.
   b. hot enough to bring relief.
   c. between 105F and 125F.
   d. between 37C and 47C.

▪ ▪ ▪ Dry Skin

6. Elderly clients are at high risk for developing dry skin because they:
   a. take fewer baths.
   b. stay indoors more.
   c. have less subcutaneous tissue.
   d. have decreased sebaceous activity.

7. Planned nursing care to reduce the effects of drying of the skin should include:
   a. using hot water and deodorant soap for the daily bath.
   b. entering a nursing order to bathe the client every other day.
   c. decreasing oral intake of fluids.
   d. limiting the use of bath oils.

8. A client is experiencing dry skin. The advise nurse has provided instructions on how to prevent dry skin. Which statement by the client would indicate a need for further teaching?
   a. "I should increase my intake of fluids."
   b. "I should use creams and lotions when the skin is still damp."
   c. "I should bathe less frequently but use extra soap to stay clean."
   d. "A humidifier will humidify the air and my skin."

▪ ▪ ▪ Psoriasis

Match the components of care (a–f) with the correct treatment of psoriasis listed in questions 9–14.

_____ 9. topical steroids

_____ 10. tar preparations

_____ 11. topical anthralin (dithranol)

_____ 12. tretinoin (Retin-A)

_____ 13. photochemotherapy

_____ 14. UVB

a. This agent should be applied during the evening shift. The nurse should thoroughly assess the client's skin prior to its application and should not apply it to any areas of broken skin.

b. This treatment is given daily. The nurse should inform the client that he will develop a mild erythema with this treatment.

c. When applied, this drug inhibits keratinization. The nurse should inform the client that effects of the medication may not be seen for a few weeks.

d. These agents decrease inflammation and are well absorbed through the skin. The nurse should use an occlusive dressing to increase absorption.

e. This medication should be stopped if the client exhibits erythema. The client who receives this treatment should be informed to stay out of direct sunlight for at least 12 hours.

f. When applying these preparations, the nurse should wear gloves and inform the client that the medication may have an unpleasant odor.

Case Study

Hannah Prichard is a 15-year-old with psoriasis on her arms, legs, and scalp. Hannah tells the nurse, "I look awful. How can I wear a swimsuit?"

15. Which of the following is the most appropriate response by the nurse?
    a. "All teenagers feel that way."
    b. "Your psoriasis will improve over time."
    c. "You have a great figure; you'll look fine."
    d. "Tell me more about how you feel."

16. The nurse teaches Hannah how to apply her topical medications. Which statement by Hannah indicates a need for further teaching?
    a. "I should use a plastic wrap as a covering for 12 hours each day."
    b. "I should avoid getting the medication in my eyes or mucous membranes."
    c. "I should apply the lotion in a thick layer on a regular basis."
    d. "I can use gloves, a wooden tongue depressor, or gauze pad to apply the medication."

17. Hannah calls the nurse a few days after starting a new topical medication for her psoriasis. She tells the nurse that she has swelling, redness, and pain in the lesions on her arm. The nurse should suspect that this is:
    a. an allergic reaction to the medication.
    b. a therapeutic reaction to the new medication.
    c. evidence of infection.
    d. an exacerbation of the psoriasis.

▪ ▪ ▪ Bacterial Infections of the Skin

18. To prevent bacterial infections of the skin, the nurse should teach the client the importance of:
    a. keeping the skin clean.
    b. squeezing lesions to keep them clear of pus.
    c. discontinuing antibiotics once the lesions disappear.
    d. allowing draining lesions to remain uncovered.

19. A 45-year-old male who weighs 280 pounds visits the employee health nurse with a large, tender cystic nodule that appears to be draining purulent material. The nurse suspects that this lesion is:
    a. cellulitis.   b. impetigo.   c. erysipelas.   d. a furuncle.

20. The skin condition of the client in question 19 is often associated with:
    a. hypertension.   b. diabetes.   c. poor hygiene.   d. fever and chills.

21. The primary treatment for skin infections is:
    a. topical antibiotics.   c. systemic antibiotics.
    b. hydrogen peroxide.   d. pHisohex baths.

22. One of the most effective ways to prevent the spread of infection is:
    a. daily showers with antibacterial soaps. c. careful hand washing.
    b. avoiding exposure to skin infections.   d. hand washing with antibacterial agents.

▪ ▪ ▪ Fungal Infections of the Skin

23. The most important factor in the development of fungal infections is:
    a. age.   b. moisture.   c. pregnancy.   d. cold weather.

24. A client complains of a white, cheesy, foul-smelling vaginal discharge with itching and burning. The nurse should suspect that the client has:
    a. a sexually transmitted disease.   c. a candidiasis infection.
    b. tinea cruris.   d. diabetes mellitus.

25. A 28-year-old client has a fungal skin infection. The nurse is teaching the client about home care. Which statement by the client indicates the need for further teaching?
    a. "All skin folds should be dried carefully."
    b. "I should use a clean towel and washcloth each day."
    c. "My condition is not usually contagious."
    d. "I should not share linens or personal items with others."

26. Which of the following clients is not at high risk for candidiasis infections?
    a. 46-year-old with diabetes
    b. 27-year-old who is HIV-positive
    c. 33-year-old pregnant woman
    d. 22-year-old following an appendectomy

▪ ▪ ▪ Parasitic Infections of the Skin

27. When caring for a client who has a parasitic infection, which of the following is essential?
    a. ensuring the client has no visible eggs
    b. evaluating the client's knowledge of universal precautions
    c. evaluating the family members' knowledge of body fluid precautions
    d. ensuring that all family members are treated for the same infection

28. Which statement is true about pediculosis?
    a. Only individuals with poor hygiene are prone to these infections.
    b. It is a sexually transmitted disease.
    c. It is spread by contact with an infested person or item.
    d. It is a parasitic infection caused by mites.

Case Study

Anissa LaFerme is sent home from the third grade with head lice. Her mother asks the school nurse, "What should I do?"

29. Develop a teaching plan for the mother to help her cope with this infestation.

30. What are some appropriate nursing diagnoses for Anissa and her mother?

31. Her mother tells the nurse, "Oh, this is so disgusting. I feel so dirty."
    What is the most appropriate response by the nurse?

■ ■ ■ Viral Infections of the Skin

32. When providing care for the client with herpes zoster lesions, it is important for the nurse to know that:
    a. contact isolation should be practiced.
    b. strict isolation is required.
    c. a mask will prevent exposure.
    d. pregnant women have adequate immunity.

33. A 75-year-old client suffers from herpes zoster. The nurse would expect the physician to prescribe:
    a. antibiotics.
    b. topical steroids.
    c. acyclovir (Zovirax).
    d. salicylic acid.

34. A client visits the nurse with vesicular lesions that have an erythematous base. The lesions appear to have started on a dermatome, but have now extended over the entire trunk, face, and thorax. The nurse should recognize that this is:
    a. a typical presentation of shingles.
    b. probably herpes simplex.
    c. disseminated herpes zoster.
    d. postherpetic neuralgia.

35. A client has herpes zoster across her thorax. The nurse instructs her on pain-reducing strategies. Which statement by the client indicates a need for further teaching?
    a. "I should take my pain medication on a regular basis."
    b. "Calamine lotion or cool compresses may relieve the burning."
    c. "Warm compresses will be most effective in relieving the itch."
    d. "Distraction or relaxation techniques may reduce pain."

36. Which statement about herpes zoster is true?
    a. There is a high risk of secondary bacterial infection.
    b. Only immunocompromised individuals are at risk for secondary infections.
    c. The client is contagious to individuals who have had chickenpox.
    d. Contact isolation is appropriate for immunocompromised clients.

■ ■ ■ Dermatitis

37. An essential part of the teaching plan for a client who has been prescribed medications for a skin condition caused by dermatitis is:
    a. the medications must be taken for life to prevent recurrence.
    b. the medications will cure the disease if taken properly.
    c. factors that contributed to the dermatitis must be identified.
    d. oral steroids should be stopped as soon as improvement occurs.

Match the descriptions (a–d) with the correct type of dermatitis listed in questions 38–41.

_____ 38. contact dermatitis

_____ 39. atopic dermatitis

_____ 40. seborrheic dermatitis

_____ 41. exfoliative dermatitis

a. involves the scalp, eyebrows, eyelids, ear canals, axillae, and trunk
b. a hypersensitivity response or chemical reaction
c. also called eczema; characterized by chronic lichenification, erythema, and scaling
d. characterized by excessive peeling or shedding

▪ ▪ ▪ Acne

42. A pregnant client has noticed an increase in her acne. Which of the following acne treatments would be contraindicated for the client?
    a. benzoyl peroxide preparations (Acne-Dome)
    b. isotretinoin (Accutane)
    c. topical erythromycin
    d. dermabrasion

43. Which statement by the client with acne indicates the need for further teaching?
    a. "My acne is caused by poor hygiene."
    b. "I should wash my face twice a day."
    c. "I should keep my hands away from my face."
    d. "I should eat a well-balanced diet."

▪ ▪ ▪ Pemphigus Vulgaris

44. Explain how plasmapheresis is beneficial to the client with pemphigus vulgaris.

45. Name six elements of discharge teaching the nurse should address for the client with pemphigus vulgaris.
    (a) _____
    (b) _____
    (c) _____
    (d) _____
    (e) _____
    (f) _____

▪ ▪ ▪ Toxic Epidermal Necrolysis

46. The cause of death in most clients with TENS is _____.

47. TENS is thought to be initiated by an immune or _____ response.

48. Identify four complications often developed by the client with TENS.
    (a) _____
    (b) _____
    (c) _____
    (d) _____

49. The client with TENS requires:
    a. contact isolation.
    b. reverse isolation.
    c. no special precautions.
    d. wound and skin precautions.

50. Which intervention is contraindicated when caring for a client with TENS?
    a. an alternating air flow mattress
    b. nutritional assessment and support
    c. teaching noninvasive pain measures
    d. offering warm fluids and foods

▪ ▪ ▪ Benign Skin Lesions

51. Which of the following statements by a client who has been diagnosed with a seborrheic keratosis would indicate that the client thoroughly understands the diagnosis?
    a. "These lesions occurred because I sit in the sun too much."
    b. "I have skin cancer."
    c. "It is unusual for these lesions to appear in adults."
    d. "I should monitor these lesions for an increase in size or a change in color."

52. A primary prevention strategy to prevent skin lesions is _____
    _____.

53. A secondary prevention strategy to detect skin lesions is _____
    _____.

54. An employee asks the employee health nurse to look at a skin lesion on his hand. He tells the nurse that the lesion bleeds easily and never seems to completely heal. It has been present for about 3 months, and he says it appears to be growing larger. The most appropriate recommendation by the nurse is that he:
    a. apply bacitracin twice a day.
    b. not worry; it is probably dermatitis.
    c. see a physician to have the lesion evaluated.
    d. continue to monitor the lesion for another month.

▪ ▪ ▪ Nonmelanoma Skin Cancer

55. The most common type of nonmelanoma skin cancer is:
    a. Kaposi's sarcoma.
    b. basal cell carcinoma.
    c. actinic keratosis.
    d. squamous cell carcinoma.

56. Which of the following environmental factors is most commonly implicated as the cause of nonmelanoma skin cancers?
    a. ultraviolet radiation
    b. viruses
    c. ionizing radiation
    d. physical trauma

57. A nurse researcher wants to examine tanning habits of cultural groups at high risk for skin cancer. Which group would the nurse most likely study?
    a. African Americans   b. Irish Americans   c. Asian Americans   d. Italian Americans

58. One characteristic of basal cell carcinomas is they:
    a. are always brown.
    b. are always flat.
    c. appear only on the face or neck.
    d. rarely metastasize.

59. A type of biopsy in which a section of the tumor and surrounding tissue is removed is called a(n) _____ biopsy.

60. When a portion of the tumor is removed by a surgical instrument such as a scalpel, the biopsy is called a(n) _____ biopsy.

61. When the entire tumor is removed for analysis, the biopsy is called a(n) _____ biopsy.

62. When the amount of tissue taken in a tumor sample does not extend below the dermis, this type of biopsy is called a(n) _____ biopsy.

63. A nurse is teaching the Sunshine School's PTA about skin health. Identify three strategies for skin care that he should include in his talk.

    (a) _____

    (b) _____

    (c) _____

▪ ▪ ▪ The Client with Malignant Melanoma

64. To assess the skin of the client with a nevus, the nurse uses the American Cancer Society's ABCD acronym. Identify what each letter of this acronym means.

    (a) _____   (c) _____

    (b) _____   (d) _____

65. If the Clark's level for staging malignant melanoma shows that a client's tumor is a level V, this indicates that the cancer has reached the:

    a. bone.   c. lungs.

    b. papillary dermis.   d. subcutaneous tissue.

66. Identify three topics the nurse should include when conducting a class in the prevention of malignant melanoma.

    (a) _____

    (b) _____

    (c) _____

▪ ▪ ▪ Pressure Ulcers

67. A client has developed a deep pressure ulcer on the trochanter. The ulcer involves full-thickness skin loss extending into, but not totally through, subcutaneous tissue or the underlying fascia. This wound would be described as:

    a. stage I.   c. stage III.

    b. stage II.   d. stage IV.

68. Which of the following should be included in the care of a client with a pressure ulcer?

    a. keep the head of bed at 90 degrees at all times

    b. massage reddened areas on the client's skin

    c. use a pull sheet when moving the client up in bed

    d. have the client sit on a donut-type of device

69. Which of the following dressings or products would be the best to use to debride a necrotic wound?

    a. hydrocolloid dressing

    b. dry, sterile dressing

    c. transparent dressing

    d. wet-to-damp dressing

Case Study

Hans Gunther, a 79-year-old male, has a 4 × 5 cm pressure ulcer that extends into the muscle and bone on his sacrum. He is being seen by the home health nurse for treatment of his pressure ulcer. He lives in a second floor walk-up apartment with his 75-year-old sister. Mr. Gunther had a fracture of his left hip, which was repaired with the insertion of a left hip prosthesis. He lives on Social Security.

70. When documenting an assessment of Mr. Gunther's pressure ulcer, the nurse should classify his ulcer as:

a. stage I.　　　　　b. stage II.　　　　　c. stage III.　　　　　d. stage IV.

71. Mr. Gunther has a pressure ulcer. What finding would indicate that it requires debridement?

_____

72. What assessments are important for the nurse to consider when developing a treatment plan for Mr. Gunther?

■ ■ ■ **Frostbite**

73. A nurse is skiing with a friend and notices that the tip of her friend's nose is white. The most appropriate intervention is to:

a. continue skiing.
b. apply firm pressure with a warm hand.
c. apply hot water compresses.
d. cover the nose with a scarf.

74. A client has experienced severe frostbite of his toes from winter hiking. When he is admitted to the hospital for rewarming, the nurse should anticipate:

a. immersing the affected extremities in cool water.
b. massaging the affected extremities.
c. rewarming the feet in circulating warm water.
d. wrapping the affected extremity tightly with compression bandages.

■ ■ ■ **Cutaneous and Plastic Surgery**

Identify the type of cutaneous surgical procedure described.

75. This type of cutaneous surgery results in the removal of the epidermis, dermis, and often some subcutaneous tissue. _____

76. This type of surgery is the removal of a lesion with a surgical instrument that cuts through soft or weak tissue but not through normal tissue. _____

77. This type of cutaneous surgery is done with an agent that causes inflammation with fibrosis of tissue. _____

78. This type of cutaneous surgery involves the destruction of tissue using high-frequency alternating currents. _____

79. This type of cutaneous surgery causes the destruction of tissue using cold or freezing agents.

_____

80. This type of cutaneous surgery involves the use of chemicals to cause peeling of the treated area.

_____

81. The major difference between a split-thickness skin graft and a full-thickness skin graft is that a full-thickness skin graft:
    a. can be placed on sites with poor blood supply.
    b. contains only epidermis.
    c. contains both epidermis and dermis.
    d. can be used on infected sites.

82. Postoperative nursing care of the client with a skin graft and/or flap includes which of the following interventions?
    a. palpating the graft site with a gloved hand to check the temperature of the graft
    b. positioning the client on a posterior graft site
    c. avoiding movement of the body part containing the donor site if possible
    d. changing the dressing on the donor site every 2 hours

■ ■ ■ Hair and Nail Disorders

Match the disorder (a–e) with the descriptions in questions 83–91. Disorders (a–e) may be used more than once.

_____ 83. This type of hair loss is genetically predetermined.

_____ 84. This is the total loss of hair on scalp. This condition is unresponsive to treatment and irreversible.

_____ 85. This type of hair loss often reverses without treatment.

_____ 86. This condition results in excessive hair growth.

_____ 87. The loss of hair over the central part of the scalp often due to elevated androgen levels.

_____ 88. This condition can result in defeminization (deepening of the voice, loss of breast tissue).

_____ 89. This type of hair loss begins at the temples and involves recession of the hairline and baldness of the crown.

_____ 90. This type of alopecia may be treated with oral contraceptives.

_____ 91. This type of alopecia responds to vasodilator drugs.

a. alopecia areata
b. hirsutism
c. alopecia totalis
d. male pattern baldness
e. female pattern alopecia

Case Study

Eliza Parker is a 32-year-old European American female who works for a networking company as an inside sales representative. She has just been promoted to an outside sales position, which will involve meeting customers and traveling to a number of cities in her sales region. Eliza looks forward to the increased responsibility and salary. Her greatest concern is related to her appearance. She has large areas of alopecia areata of the scalp and a birthmark covering her right cheek and part of her chin. She also suffers from exfoliating dermatitis of the hands, elbows, and feet. Both her exfoliative dematitis and alopecia have been recurrent problems since she was a teenager, and she has noticed that both are markedly worse in stressful situations.

92. Generate a list of "at risk for" and actual nursing diagnoses for Ms. Parker related to each of her conditions.

93. a. What is alopecia areata?

    b. Compare and contrast alopecia areata to alopecia totalis.

94. What nursing intervention would be appropriate to assist Ms. Parker with her problems?

95. Develop outcome statements that would help the nurse evaluate the effectiveness of the plan of care.

▪ ▪ ▪ Critical Thinking Exercises

96. Develop a teaching program for elders in the community on detecting skin cancer.

97. The nurse notices that a friend has a lesion on her leg that the nurse suspects might be a melanoma. What would be the most appropriate action?

98. Design a teaching program for high school students about sunscreen and how to make decisions about selecting from the various types and how to use them.

▪ ▪ ▪ Additional Learning Experiences

▪ Visit a community pharmacy. Explore the section of the store that displays topical ointments, creams, and lotions. Become more familiar with the various over-the-counter products.

▪ Ask your nursing instructor about attending a wound clinic or working with a wound and ostomy nurse.

Nursing Care of Clients with Burns

▪ ▪ ▪ Focused Study Tips

- Give examples of the four types of burn injury: thermal, chemical, electrical, and radiation, and describe prevention strategies for each type.

- Compare and contrast the physiologic changes, the goals of care, and the important nursing interventions for each phase of burn care.

- For a client with a burn, identify the major nursing interventions associated with respiratory care and the rationales for these interventions.

- Compare and contrast the different types of grafting and topical medications used to treat burns.

▪ ▪ ▪ The Client with a Major Burn

Match the type of burn injury (a–d) with the correct descriptions listed in questions 1–5. A type of burn injury (a–d) may be used more than once.

_____ 1. This type of burn occurs when acidic or basic agents come in direct contact with the skin.

_____ 2. This is the most common type of burn injury.

_____ 3. An example of this type of burn is a sunburn.

_____ 4. This type of burn results from exposure to moist heat.

_____ 5. The severity of this type of burn is difficult to assess because the destructive processes persist for weeks following the burn incident.

a. thermal
b. chemical
c. electrical
d. radiation

6. Which two groups face the highest risk of death from burns?
(a) _____   (b) _____

Read the statements below and determine if they are true or false. Correct any false statments.

_____ 7. A burn is an alteration in skin integrity resulting in tissue loss or damage.

_____ 8. A second-degree burn of less than 15% of the total body surface area in adults is known as a moderate burn injury.

_____ 9. All third-degree burns of 10% or greater of the total body surface area are known as major burns.

_____ 10. The American Burn Association (ABA) has classified burn injuries into three categories: minor, moderate, and major.

11. A nurse is planning a community education program to help decrease the incidence of burn injury. If the goal of the program is to target preventive strategies, which group of people should the program focus on?
    a. college students, 20–25 years old
    b. singles, 30–39 years old
    c. females, 40–49 years old
    d. seniors, 60–69 years old

12. The primary goal of an education program regarding burn injuries is _____.

Fill in the blanks in the following statements regarding pathophysiologic changes specific to major burn injuries.

13. Skin serves as a protective barrier for the body. Extensive loss of skin can result in: (a) _____ _____, (b) _____, and (c) _____.

14. _____ occurs when a massive amount of fluid shifts from the intracellular and intravascular compartments into the interstitium, thereby creating a state of hemodynamic instability.

15. (a) _____ and (b) _____ are the major goals of treatment during the early phases of the burn injury.

16. _____ is a frequent and often lethal complication of burns that results from exposure to asphyxiants, smoke, and heat, which initiate the pathophysiologic processes.

17. _____ is an acute ulceration of the stomach or duodenum that forms following a burn injury.

18. Two distinct phases characterize the body's metabolic response to the burn injury. The (a) _____ _____ lasts over the first 3 days of the injury and is manifested by decreased oxygen consumption, fluid imbalance, and shock. The (b) _____ occurs when adequate burn resuscitation has been accomplished.

19. A client is admitted with second- and third-degree burns. Which findings indicate that her resultant burn shock is reversing?
    a. blood pressure drops and urinary output deteriorates
    b. blood pressure drops and urinary output improves
    c. blood pressure increases and urinary output improves
    d. blood pressure drops and urinary output deteriorates

20. A client has a decrease in the T-cell counts following a major burn. This data supports which nursing diagnosis?
    a. *Knowledge Deficit*
    b. *Risk for Infection*
    c. *Ineffective Breathing Pattern*
    d. *Delayed Surgical Recovery*

Match the stages of burn injury (a–c) with the correct descriptions listed in questions 21–26. Stages (a–c) may be used more than once.

_____ 21. This stage begins with diuresis and ends with closure of the burn wound.

_____ 22. This stage lasts approximately 48–72 hours.

a. emergent/resuscitative stage
b. acute stage
c. rehabilitative stage

_____ 23. This stage begins with wound closure and ends when the client returns to the highest level of restoration.

_____ 24. During this phase, biopsychosocial adjustment is the primary focus of care.

_____ 25. Institution of fluid resuscitation therapy occurs in this stage.

_____ 26. Wound, nutrition, and pain management are major components of client care in this stage.

27. For which type of burn would a person "stop, drop, and roll"?
    a. chemical burn   b. electrical burn   c. thermal burn   d. radiation burn

28. Which of the following interventions would best maintain body temperature after a major burn injury?
    a. assess the client for respiratory status
    b. rinse the skin with warm saline
    c. replace the client's fluid volume by giving IV fluids
    d. cover the client with a blanket

▪ ▪ ▪ **Emergency Department Care**

29. Burns are classified by (a) _____
    and (b) _____.

30. Burns that involve only the epidermal layer of the skin are:
    a. superficial.   c. full thickness
    b. superficial partial thickness.   d. deep partial thickness.

31. Burns that involve all layers of the skin and may involve the underlying tissues such as muscle and bone are:
    a. superficial.   c. full thickness
    b. superficial partial thickness.   d. deep partial thickness.

32. Burns that involve the entire dermis and papillae of the dermis are classified as:
    a. superficial.   c. full thickness
    b. superficial partial thickness.   d. deep partial thickness.

33. A client is admitted with burns following a house fire. He has a burn area where there is no pain or sensation with light touch. What type of burn area is this?
    a. superficial.   c. full thickness
    b. superficial partial thickness.   d. deep partial thickness.

34. Name two formulas that can be used to classify the extent or percentage of burn injury.
    (a) _____
    (b) _____

35. The IV fluid of choice for resuscitating burn clients is:
    a. D5W.
    c. lactated Ringer's.
    b. normal saline.
    d. total parenteral nutrition.

Match the rationales (a–f) with the correct nursing interventions for ventilatory management of a burn client listed in questions 36–41.

_____ 36. maintain the head of the bed at 30 degrees

_____ 37. suction the client frequently

_____ 38. administer humidified oxygen

_____ 39. monitor the client's pulse oximetry

_____ 40. turn the client every 2 hours

_____ 41. administer mucolytic drugs as ordered

a. to maximize the client's ventilatory efforts
b. to help prevent drying of tracheal secretions
c. to keep the airway passages clear
d. to monitor the client's arterial oxygen saturation levels
e. to liquefy sputum and aid in expectoration
f. to prevent hypostatic pneumonia

▪ ▪ ▪ **Inpatient Collaborative Care**

42. List five responsibilities of the burn nurse.
    (a) _____
    (b) _____
    (c) _____
    (d) _____
    (e) _____

43. Name three members of the burn team other than the nurse.
    (a) _____   (c) _____
    (b) _____

44. For the client with a burn, indicate the significance of each of the following tests.
    (a) culture and sensitivity _____
    (b) urinalysis _____
    (c) hemoglobin _____
    (d) WBC _____
    (e) blood glucose _____

45. What is the rationale for ordering serial arterial blood gases (ABGs) for the client with a major burn?

46. Which of the following routes of pain management is contraindicated for a client hemodynamically unstable following a major burn?
    a. oral   b. intravenous   c. intramuscular   d. rectal

47. What are the three most commonly used topical antimicrobial agents for the treatment of burns?
    (a) _____   (c) _____
    (b) _____

48. Which of the following measures would be most appropriate to prevent Curling's ulcer in a burned client?
    a. turn and position the client every 2 hours
    b. use a pressure-reducing support mattress
    c. maintain the gastric pH below 5
    d. administer H₂ histamine blockers as scheduled

49. Although enteral feeding is the preferred nutritional therapy, this type of feeding is contraindicated when the client with burns develops which type(s) of complications?

50. For each of the following statements, identify the type of burn wound debridement described.
    (a) This type of debridement involves the use of a topical enzyme to dissolve the necrotic burned tissue. _____
    (b) Electrocautery is a common example of this type of debridement.

    _____

    (c) This type of debridement is performed during hydrotherapy.

    _____

51. A graft where skin is taken from a client's healthy skin and grafted to the burn site is called a(n):
    a. autograft.   b. allograft.   c. homograft.   d. heterograft.

52. A graft where skin from a cadaver is grafted to the burn site is called a(n):
    a. autograft.   b. allograft.   c. heterograft.   d. xenograft.

53. A graft where skin from an animal, usually a pig, is grafted to the burn site is called a(n):
    a. autograft.   b. allograft.   c. homograft.   d. heterograft.

Match the definitions (a–c) with the correct terms listed in questions 54–56.

_____ 54. hypertrophic scar

_____ 55. keloid

_____ 56. contracture

a. a permanent shortening of connective tissue
b. an overgrowth of dermal tissue that remains within the boundaries of the wound
c. a scar that extends beyond the boundaries of the original wound

Read the statements below and determine if they are true or false. Correct any false statements.

_____ 57. A goal of nursing care for the burn client is to maintain fluid balance.

_____ 58. Controlling infection is an important nursing goal in the care of the burn client.

_____ 59. A goal of the nurse caring for the burn client is to diminish mobility.

_____ 60. One goal of the nurse caring for the burn client is to reduce pain.

61. A nursing intervention on a burn client's care plan is to encourage the client to choose the time of dressing change. What is the related nursing diagnosis?
    a. *Pain*
    b. *Powerlessness*
    c. *Risk for Infection*
    d. *Impaired Physical Mobility*

Match descriptions (a–c) with the correct stage listed in questions 62–64.

_____ 62. early stage of recovery

_____ 63. intermittent stage of recovery

_____ 64. long-term stage of recovery

a. client undergoes intensive critical care
b. client returns to a state of physical stability
c. client leaves the hospital and returns to the community setting

▪ ▪ ▪ The Client with a Minor Burn Wound

65. What are two examples of a minor burn?
    (a) _____
    (b) _____

66. A client arrives at the clinic complaining of a red and painful back. She noticed her condition after awakening from a 3-hour nap in the sun. The nurse knows it is important to teach the client and her family:
    a. active range-of-motion (ROM) exercises.
    b. to identify and report signs and symptoms of impaired wound healing.
    c. pain management with use of narcotic analgesics.
    d. the importance of limiting fluid intake.

67. A client is being discharged from the hospital with healing second-degree burns affecting both of his arms. The discharge nurse should teach him to report:
    a. reddened healed skin.
    b. swelling and erythema.
    c. lessening pain and discomfort.
    d. increased range-of-motion.

68. A local volunteer fireman is admitted to the emergency room for smoke inhalation after rescuing a child. The priority nursing assessment in this situation is:
    a. extent and depth of burns.
    b. B/P, pulse, and distal circulation.
    c. respiratory rate and depth.
    d. patency of airway.

69. A client with extensive burns of his extremities is complaining of pain on movement. The most appropriate nursing intervention is to:
    a. encourage him to minimize activity to prevent pain and discomfort.
    b. apply deformity splints and reposition every 2–4 hours.
    c. perform active and passive ROM exercises to unaffected joints.
    d. perform active and passive ROM exercises to all joints.

70. After a 6-week hospitalization for major burns, the client complains of depression and intrusive thoughts about the burn injury. The most appropriate intervention by the nurse is to:
    a. encourage psychological counseling.
    b. tell the client that "better days are coming."
    c. encourage the client not to talk or think about the injury.
    d. ask the doctor to consider prescribing antidepressants.

Case Study

Jose Sanchez is a 57-year-old rancher who is recuperating from major burns on his legs, back, and right shoulder. He received these burns while fighting a brush fire. He has been transferred from the intensive care unit and is currently receiving daily hydrotherapy and applications of silver sulfadiazine in anticipation of skin grafting. He tells his family, "I just can't go to the tub any more. The pain is killing me."

71. What are the purposes of the client's current treatments?

    hydrotherapy

    silver sulfadiazine

72. Develop a teaching plan for the client and family regarding his treatments.

73. The client refuses to go to the whirlpool tub. What is the most appropriate action by the nurse?

74. Develop a plan of care to address the client's pain-related concerns.

75. What infection control principles should be observed now that the client leaves his room daily for hydrotherapy?

▪ ▪ ▪ Critical Thinking Exercises

76. Develop a plan of care for an adolescent who is recovering from extensive disfiguring burns, who is anticipating discharge to home within the next 10 days.

77. Imagine that you are a nurse in an acute care burn facility. Each day you are involved in providing care to clients in all phases of the recovery process. From a nursing perspective, identify the major challenges and issues involved in caring for this population.

▪ ▪ ▪ Additional Learning Experiences

- Visit your local fire station and find out about their fire prevention programs.
- Monitor your local newspaper and TV news reports. Note reports of burn injuries, and consider community programs that might prevent future injuries.

CHAPTER 19

Assessing Clients with Endocrine Disorders

■ ■ ■ **Focused Study Tips**

- Describe the normal anatomy, physiology, and assessment of each component of the endocrine system and the abnormal findings.

- Practice gathering endocrine system assessment data with family members and friends.

- Create a diagram illustrating each of the endocrine glands and their corresponding hormones.

■ ■ ■ **Anatomy and Physiology**

1. State the primary purpose of the endocrine system.

2. The endocrine system regulates which five major functions?

Match the endocrine glands (a–e) with their proper locations listed in questions 3–7.

_____ 3. behind the stomach, between the spleen and the duodenum

_____ 4. on top of the kidneys

_____ 5. beneath the hypothalamus

_____ 6. anterior to the upper part of the trachea

_____ 7. on the posterior surface of the lobes of the thyroid

a. pituitary gland
b. thyroid gland
c. adrenal glands
d. parathyroid glands
e. pancreas

8. The anterior pituitary gland secretes at least six major hormones. Which of the following is not in this group?
a. follicle-stimulating hormone
b. thyroid-stimulating hormone
c. growth hormone
d. aldosterone

Match the endocrine glands (a–h) with their corresponding hormones listed in questions 9–19. Endocrine glands (a–h) may be may used more than once.

_____ 9. antidiuretic hormone

_____ 10. somatotropin

_____ 11. androgens

_____ 12. aldosterone

_____ 13. prolactin

_____ 14. norepinephrine

_____ 15. parathormone

_____ 16. adrenocorticotropic hormone

_____ 17. insulin

_____ 18. progesterone

_____ 19. glucagon

a. thyroid gland
b. adrenal gland
c. parathyroid gland
d. gonads
e. pancreas
f. anterior pituitary gland
g. posterior pituitary gland
h. adrenal cortex

20. The release of mineralocorticoids is controlled by an enzyme called (a) _____. This substance acts on angiotensinogen and stimulates release of (b) _____ from the adrenal cortex.

21. Glucocorticoids are released during time of (a) _____. Excessive amounts of glucocorticoids (b) _____ the immune system.

22. The pancreas is both an (a) _____ gland and an (b) _____ gland. This means that the pancreas produces both (c) _____ and (d) _____.

23. (a) _____ are chemical messengers secreted by the (b) _____ glands and transported to (c) _____ cells in the body.

24. The hormonal mechanism in which increased levels of one hormone cause another gland to release a hormone is known as:
    a. hormonal release.   b. positive feedback.   c. homeostasis.   d. negative feedback.

25. The hormonal mechanism in which decreased levels of one hormone cause another gland to release a hormone is known as:
    a. hormonal release.   b. positive feedback.   c. homeostasis.   d. negative feedback.

Match the types of hormone release (a–c) with the corresponding stimulus listed in questions 26–28.

_____ 26. nerve fibers

_____ 27. hypothalamic hormones stimulating the anterior pituitary

_____ 28. fluctuations in serum levels, ions, and nutrients

a. hormonal release
b. humoral release
c. neural release

▪ ▪ ▪ Assessment of the Endocrine Function

29. Assessment of endocrine function is often more difficult than assessment of other body systems because _____
_____.

30. During the endocrine assessment interview, the nurse asks the client about conditions such as autoimmune disorders, hypertension, obesity, and tumors because:
    a. endocrine disorders may have a familial tendency.
    b. endocrine disorders may be directly caused by these conditions.
    c. these conditions are precursors of endocrine dysfunction.
    d. these conditions produce the type of long-term stress associated with endocrine dysfunction.

31. When assessing changes in behavior of a client, the nurse interviews the client and the _____
    _____.

Define the following terms.

32. stereognosis:

33. exophthalmos:

34. hirsutism:

Describe the technique used to assess each of the following:

35. Trousseau's sign:

36. Chvostek's sign:

37. If Trousseau's and Chvostek's signs are positive, what condition should the nurse suspect?
    a. hypercalcemia   b. hyperkalemia   c. hyponatremia   d. hypocalcemia

Match the hormonal disorders (a–i) with the corresponding abnormal findings listed in questions 38–47.
Hormonal disorders (a–i) may be used more than once.

_____ 38. smooth, flushed skin	a. Cushing's syndrome
_____ 39. variations in facial form	b. Addison's disease
_____ 40. exophthalmos	c. diabetes
_____ 41. goiter	d. dwarfism
_____ 42. carpal spasm	e. hyperthyroidism
_____ 43. diminished tendon reflexes	f. Grave's disease
_____ 44. peripheral neuropathies	g. acromegaly
_____ 45. short stature	h. hypothyroidism
_____ 46. hirsutism	i. hypoparathyroidism
_____ 47. hyperpigmentation	

48. The only endocrine organ that can be palpated is the:

    a. pancreas.   b. pituitary gland.   c. thyroid gland.   d. parathyroid gland.

49. List the order of the physical assessment of the endocrine system.

50. Which finding is not considered a normal variation of the older adult?

    a. decreased thyroid levels

    b. fibrotic anterior pituitary gland

    c. enlarged adrenal glands and increased weight

    d. thick, brittle, yellow nails

51. Which finding is not considered a normal variation of the older adult?

    a. increased female hormone production

    b. decreased anterior pituitary hormone output

    c. altered immune responses

    d. increased risk and infection

Case Study

Quinn Thomas is a 38-year-old client admitted for complaints of chronic fatigue, changes in appetite, and repeated bouts of insomnia. He has a family history of obesity, a recent health history of difficulty sleeping, and feelings of chronic fatigue. Mr. Thomas tells the nurse that no matter how much sleep he gets, he seems to feel tired and "dragged out." Mr. Thomas works as a computer programmer for a major software company and has been working very hard to meet the stringent deadlines for an important new software package. He confides in the nurse that he has felt "very stressed out" for the past 5 months while working on the project. He is currently taking no medications and denies allergies to food, medications, or environmental stimuli.

    The nurse's physical assessment reveals a well-nourished, 6'1" male weighing 245 lbs, whose rough, dry skin has a yellowish cast. Mr. Thomas' nails are brittle, dry, and thick, and he exhibits hyporeflexia on deep-tendon reflex assessment. Palpation of his thyroid reveals no apparent enlargement, and inspection of his musculoskeletal status finds him to be within the normal range. Both Trousseau's and Chvostek's signs are negative, indicating no abnormal findings in these areas.

52. List the subjective data, objective data, and possible etiologies of Mr. Thomas' condition.

    subjective findings:

    objective findings:

    possible etiologies:

53. List other assessment questions the nurse should ask Mr. Thomas.

54. Mr. Thomas is diagnosed with hypothyroidism and is started on Synthroid daily. Develop a teaching plan regarding his condition and medical therapy.

55. Develop a plan to assist Mr. Thomas to more effectively manage his stress.

▪ ▪ ▪ **Critical Thinking Exercises**

56. Prepare for a discussion group for senior citizens who have heard that they are more likely to experience thyroid disease and are interested in learning more about endocrine function.

57. Compare and contrast negative and positive feedback mechanisms related to hormone levels.

▪ ▪ ▪ **Additional Learning Experiences**

- Make flash cards of the various endocrine glands and the hormones they secrete.
- Draw a diagram that represents the feedback mechanisms of the various endocrine glands.

Nursing Care of Clients with Thyroid, Parathyroid, Adrenal, and Pituitary Disorders

CHAPTER 20

■ ■ ■ **Focused Study Tips**

- Compare and contrast the clinical manifestations of hyperthyroidism and hypothyroidism.

- Explain how the treatment of hyperthyroidism may result in hypothyroidism, and that medications given for hypothyroidism may result in signs and symptoms of hyperthyroidism.

- Describe the processes that occur in hyperparathyroidism.

- Review the pharmacologic interventions for hyperparathyroidism.

- Explain the physical characteristics of Cushing's syndrome and the electrolyte imbalances that occur with this syndrome.

■ ■ ■ **Hyperthyroidism**

1. Excessive amounts of thyroid hormone will result in which five physiologic responses?
   (a) _____   (d) _____
   (b) _____   (e) _____
   (c) _____

2. Another term for hyperthyroidism is _____.

3. The most common forms of hyperthyroidism are (a) _____ and
   (b) _____.

4. Graves' disease is classified as what type of disorder? _____
   _____

5. Toxic multinodular goiter is characterized by _____
   _____.

6. Name and describe the rare form of hyperthyroidism that can be life-threatening if left untreated.

7. Which condition can be the result of circulating immunoglobins or excess TSH stimulation and may cause body image disturbance? _____

8. Name the acute condition which, if it becomes chronic, can destroy the thyroid gland and lead to a hypothyroid state. _____

9. Which clinical manifestation occurs in hyperthyroidism and is characterized by a forward protrusion of the eyelids? _____

10. List the most common subjective and objective findings of hyperthyroidism.

    subjective:

    objective:

11. Which client statement may indicate a hyperthyroid state?
    a. "I have taken my pulse and it seems to be very slow."
    b. "I am always constipated."
    c. "My heart always feels as if it's racing."
    d. "I just can't seem to get warm no matter how much I cover up."

12. Which finding would be inconsistent with a diagnosis of hyperthyroidism?
    a. weight loss   b. elevated heart rate   c. a poor appetite   d. diarrhea

Match the medications (a–b) with their proper descriptions listed in questions 13–19. Medications (a–b) may be used more than once, and more than one medication may be appropriate for each description.

_____ 13. This medication may be prescribed for the   a. potassium iodide/sodium iodine
client prior to surgery to make the thyroid   b. propylthiouracil (PTU)/methimazole
gland less vascular.   (Tapazole)

_____ 14. The nurse administering this medication orally
should use a straw to prevent staining of the client's teeth.

_____ 15. When a client is taking Coumadin and this medication, an appropriate nursing intervention would be to place the client on bleeding precautions.

_____ 16. It is important to administer this medication at the same time every day.

_____ 17. A client discharged on this medication should be taught to monitor her menstrual cycle
for changes.

_____ 18. This medication must be diluted in orange juice prior to administering.

_____ 19. When this medication is prescribed, the nurse should teach the client that it may take a
few months to take effect and that the client must take the medication exactly as prescribed.

20. Following a total thyroidectomy, which statement by the client would indicate the need for fur-
    ther client teaching?
    a. " I need to take thyroid medication for the rest of my life."
    b. " I will require routine follow-up care."
    c. " I should report weight loss, palpitations, or nervousness to my physician."
    d. " I will need to take propylthiouracil and iodine for the rest of my life."

21. A client treated with radioactive iodine (^{131}I) may become (a) _____
    and require lifetime treatment with (b) _____.

22. While performing preoperative assessment on a client who is scheduled for a thyroidectomy, the nurse would be most concerned about which finding? The fact that the client:

    a. weighs 175 lbs.

    b. began smoking 2 months ago.

    c. had not received iodine preparations.

    d. has no palpitations.

23. The preoperative care for a client undergoing a subtotal thyroidectomy includes:

    (a) _____

    (b) _____

    (c) _____

24. A priority nursing intervention following a thyroidectomy is to determine:

    a. breathing pattern and respiratory rate.

    b. patency of airway.

    c. blood pressure and pulse.

    d. signs of hypokalemia.

25. To check for laryngeal nerve damage, the nurse should _____

    _____.

26 Following removal of the thyroid, the client may experience:

    a. hyperkalemia.   b. hypernatremia.   c. hypocalcemia.   d. thyroid storm.

27. Signs and symptoms of calcium deficiency include _____

    _____

28. What three tools should the nurse have available when assessing for respiratory distress immediately following a thyroidectomy?

    (a) _____

    (b) _____

    (c) _____

29. Nursing interventions for the person with Graves' disease and exophthalmos include:

    a. administering corticosteroid drops as prescribed.

    b. instilling artificial tears as prescribed.

    c. instilling otic antibiotic drops.

    d. administering saturated solution potassium iodide as prescribed to reduce exophthalmos.

30. An appropriate environment for a client with hyperthyroidism includes:

    a. maintaining adequate warmth.

    b. diversional activities.

    c. frequent rest periods.

    d. frequent physical activity.

31. Interventions to address a nursing diagnosis of *Altered Nutrition: Less than Body Requirements* for a client with hyperthyroidism include:

    (a) _____

    (b) _____

    (c) _____

Case Study

Michael August is visiting Susan Wong, a nurse practitioner, after experiencing palpitations, dyspnea, nausea, vomiting, and nervousness. Ms. Wong examines Mr. August and feels several nodules immediately adjacent to the sternocleidomastoid muscles. She decides to include a thyroid workup, among other tests.

32. If Mr. August has a thyroid disorder caused by an autoimmune process, he would have abnormalities in which laboratory test(s)? _____

_____

33. If Ms. Wong suspects that the thyroid abnormality is related to pituitary dysfunction, which laboratory data would she use to confirm this diagnosis? _____

▪ ▪ ▪ Hypothyroidism

34. In which client group is hypothyroidism often mistaken for a natural part of the developmental process?
    a. the young adult   b. the newborn   c. the older adult   d. the middle adult

35. In secondary hypothyroidism, the cause of the hypothyroid state:
    a. is the destruction of the gland by radiation.
    b. results from congenital defects.
    c. may be age-related changes.
    d. may be pituitary gland dysfunction.

36. Hypothyroidism can result from:
    a. age-related changes.   c. cardiac disease.
    b. treatment for hyperthyroidism.   d. treatment for diabetes mellitus.

37. The clinical manifestations of myxedema include _____

_____.

38. List the most common subjective and objective findings of hypothyroidism.
    subjective:

    objective:

39. List five factors that contribute to hypothyroidism.
    (a) _____
    (b) _____
    (c) _____
    (d) _____
    (e) _____

40. Identify and describe the extreme form of hypothyroidism that can be life-threatening if left untreated.

41. (a) _____ is the most common form of primary hypothyroidism. The gender it is most prevalent in is (b) _____.

42. Which client statement would indicate a hypothyroid state?
    a. "I'm eating less but still gaining weight."
    b. "My bowel pattern is unchanged."
    c. "My heart always feels as if it's racing."
    d. "I feel nervous and agitated."

43. Which assessment finding would be inconsistent with a diagnosis of hypothyroidism?
    a. heart rate of 54 BPM
    b. weight gain of 15 lb
    c. dry skin
    d. dehydration

44. In primary hypothyroidism, the TSH level is _____.

45. Which statement made by a client who is taking thyroid replacement hormones indicates learning has occurred?
    a. "I will minimize my intake of spinach, cabbage, carrots, and peaches."
    b. "I should stop the medication if I am going to have a dental procedure."
    c. "It is only necessary to take my thyroid medications for 6 to 8 weeks."
    d. "I am happy that I will no longer have to take insulin."

46. A client underwent a thyroidectomy in 1987. He was divorced last year, became severely depressed, and stopped taking his thyroid replacement medications. Which electrolyte imbalance should the nurse anticipate finding in the client?
    a. hyponatremia
    b. hypernatremia
    c. hypoglycemia
    d. metabolic alkalosis

47. When examining laboratory data for the client with myxedema coma, the nurse should find which three abnormalities?
    (a) _____
    (b) _____
    (c) _____

48. Strategies to maintain skin integrity for the client with hyperthyroidism include:
    a. frequent changing of position.
    b. bathing daily in a tub.
    c. applying alcohol-based lotions to the skin.
    d. avoiding use of sheepskins or foam cushions.

▪ ▪ ▪ Hyperparathyroidism

49. Clients with chronic hyperparathyroidism are at particular risk for:
    a. exophthalmos.   b. fractures.   c. hyperglycemia.   d. pancreatitis.

50. When caring for a client with hyperparathyroidism, the nurse should monitor which laboratory values closely?
    a. serum calcium and serum albumin
    b. serum calcium and serum magnesium
    c. serum calcium and serum phosphate
    d. serum calcium and serum sodium

51. To reduce the amount of serum calcium in a client with hyperparathyroidism, the nurse would expect to administer which of the following prescribed medications?
    a. calcium carbonate   b.digoxin   c. calcium chloride   d. Lasix (furosemide)

52. A high priority nursing diagnosis for a client with hyperparathyroidism is:
    a. *Fluid Volume Deficit.*
    b. *Risk for Injury.*
    c. *Altered Nutrition: More than Body Requirements.*
    d. *Anxiety.*

▪ ▪ ▪ Hypoparathyroidism

53. When caring for a client with hypoparathyroidism, the nurse should assess:
    a. skin turgor.   b. Chvostek's sign.   c. heart tones.   d. Homan's sign.

54. What is the most common cause of hypoparathyroidism?
    a. cancer of the parathyroids
    b. radiation therapy
    c. congenital defect
    d. removal during thyroid surgery

55. Numbness and tingling, muscle spasms, convulsions, and laryngeal spasm may be associated with (a) _____, which may result in (b) _____. Nursing assessment of hypocalcemia includes (c) _____ sign and (d) _____ sign.

56. Clinical manifestations of hypoparathyroidism include:
    a. numbness and tingling.
    b. constipation.
    c. oily skin.
    d. hypoactive reflexes.

57. The two therapies most commonly prescribed for a client with hypoparathyroidism are (a) _____ _____ and (b) _____.

▪ ▪ ▪ Adrenal Cortex Hyperfunction

Cushing's syndrome results in a disruption in glucose, protein, and fat metabolism. Describe how the nurse would observe how each of these alterations is manifested.

58. Altered glucose metabolism:

59. Altered protein metabolism:

60. Altered fat metabolism:

61. An iatrogenic form of Cushing's syndrome results from:

62. A common physical finding in the client with adrenal hyperfunction is:
    a. purple striae of the skin during inspection.
    b. a murmur heard on auscultation.
    c. edema of the lower extremities found on palpation.
    d. crackles heard on auscultation.

63. Which client is most at risk for Cushing's syndrome?
    a. a 25-year-old HIV-positive male who is taking AZT
    b. a 45-year-old female with diabetes mellitus who is taking insulin
    c. a 75-year-old female with rheumatoid arthritis who is taking hydrocortisone
    d. a 35-year-old male with a duodenal ulcer who is taking Tagamet (cimetidine)

64. The nurse assessing a client with Cushing's syndrome would expect to find which body type characteristics?
    a. round face, obese abdomen, and skinny legs
    b. edematous eyelids, large facial muscles, and extremely thin body
    c. elongated head, massive face, prominent nose, and cachectic appearance
    d. edematous extremities, thin face, and flattened abdomen

65. Which finding indicates complications related to Cushing's syndrome?
    a. weak, thready pulse
    b. sunken eyeballs
    c. hypotension
    d. weight gain

66. A client has normal adrenal function. Her serum cortisol level is drawn in the morning and in the evening. Which sample should be higher? _____

67. In Cushing's syndrome, serum levels of potassium, calcium, and glucose are _____ .

68. Which statement by a client who just underwent a bilateral adrenalectomy indicates the need for further client teaching?
    a. "I can eventually stop taking my dose of steroids."
    b. "My vital signs will be monitored very frequently during the first 48 hours after surgery."
    c. "I will eat a diet high in vitamins and proteins."
    d. "I will avoid individuals with infections."

69. The client with Cushing's syndrome is at risk for infection, injury, and _____
    _____ .

70. The most appropriate room placement for the client with Cushing's syndrome is _____
    _____ .

▪ ▪ ▪ Adrenal Cortex Hypofunction

Match the clinical manifestations (a–g) with the conditions associated with Addison's disease listed in questions 71–75. The clinical manifestations (a–g) may be used more than once or not at all.

_____ 71. hyperkalemia

_____ 72. excessive ACTH

_____ 73. hyponatremia

_____ 74. fluid volume deficit

_____ 75. hypoglycemia

a. confusion
b. syncope
c. hyperpigmentation of skin
d. cardiac arrhythmias
e. muscle weakness
f. postural hypotension
g. tremors

76. A common cause of Addison's disease is the sudden withdrawal of _____
    _____.

77. Which laboratory results are typical for the client who has experienced an Addison's crisis?
    a. sodium of 128 mEq/L
    b. serum glucose of 130 mg/dL
    c. serum potassium level 5.0 mEq/L
    d. serum cortisol level of 5 mcg/dL

78. A woman arrives comatose at the emergency department. Her laboratory data reveals that she is in Addison's crisis. An immediate nursing intervention is to: _____
    _____.

79. The client in question 78 has a serum sodium level of 120 mEq/L. Which nursing intervention is appropriate at this time?
    a. administer sodium chloride orally
    b. initiate fluid restriction
    c. initiate seizure precautions
    d. nothing; this is a normal sodium level

80. A client is diagnosed with adrenal insufficiency. During client teaching, the nurse should teach the client to:
    a. continue his usual diet.
    b. take his medications on an empty stomach.
    c. discontinue his medication and call the physician if he feels excessively fatigued.
    d. report any weight gain to his physician.

81. The client with Addison's disease is at risk for which complication?
    a. hypokalemia
    b. hypernatremia
    c. fluid volume deficit
    d. hypercalcemia

82. The nurse should teach the client with Addison's disease to:
    a. limit fluid and sodium intake.
    b. sit and stand slowly.
    c. take monthly weight measurements.
    d. eat a diet high in potassium.

▪ ▪ ▪ Adrenal Medulla Hyperfunction

83. Which symptoms are associated with pheochromocytoma?
    - a. weakness and fatigue
    - b. dizziness and orthostatic hypotension
    - c. always feeling cold
    - d. sweating and feeling of the heart racing

84. A client has been diagnosed as having a pheochromocytoma. She states that her physician told her that her symptoms are caused by tumors. She asks the nurse, "Do I have cancer?" The nurse's most appropriate response is:
    - a. "The tumors your doctor describes are often malignant."
    - b. "Talk with your physician about your concerns."
    - c. "The tumors your doctor describes are often benign."
    - d. "Yes, all tumors are cancerous."

▪ ▪ ▪ Pituitary Dysfunction

85. The most common cause of hyperpituitarism is _____.

86. Four possible causes of hypopituitarism are:
    - (a) _____
    - (b) _____
    - (c) _____
    - (d) _____

Match the pituitary hormones (a–b) with the proper clinical situations listed in questions 87–94. Pituitary hormones may be used more than once.

_____ 87. activity intolerance	a. growth hormone
_____ 88. acromegaly	b. prolactin
_____ 89. failure to lactate	
_____ 90. growth of bones	
_____ 91. amenorrhea	
_____ 92. decreased libido	
_____ 93. closure of epiphyseal plates	
_____ 94. body image disturbance	

95. Place a ✔ by the nursing interventions that would be appropriate for the client with syndrome of inappropriate antidiuretic hormone secretion (SIADH). More than one intervention is correct.

    _____ a. place client on fluid restriction

    _____ b. assess client for edema

    _____ c. withhold all diuretics

    _____ d. weigh client daily

    _____ e. allow liberal fluid intake

    _____ f. administer hypotonic sodium chloride

    _____ g. initiate seizure precautions

96. Which clinical manifestation indicates improvement in diabetes insipidus?
    a. increased urine output
    b. higher urine specific gravity
    c. worsening thirst
    d. hypernatremia

97. Treatment for diabetes insipidus may include administering IV hypotonic fluids, replacing ADH, and administering _____.

98. The treatment of SIADH includes:
    a. administering hypotonic saline.
    b. increasing oral fluids.
    c. administering hydrochlorothiazide.
    d. administering IV hypertonic saline.

99. Which of the following is contraindicated for a client with diabetes insipidus?
    a. restricting oral fluids
    b. monitoring specific gravity
    c. administering vasopressin
    d. administering hypotonic IV fluids

100. Which of the following is contraindicated for a client with SIADH?
    a. administering IV hypertonic saline
    b. monitoring specific gravity
    c. forcing oral fluids to 3000 cc/day
    d. monitoring for water intoxication

▪ ▪ ▪ Critical Thinking Exercises

101. The nurse is caring for a client whose treatment for hyperthyroidism has resulted in hypothyroidism. Develop a teaching program that explains this outcome to the client.

102. Develop a teaching plan for a client on long-term cortisol replacement.

103. Design a nursing care plan for a client with acromegaly.

▪ ▪ ▪ Additional Learning Experiences

▪ Develop a set of flash cards that organize the major signs and symptoms of the various endocrine disorders.

▪ Ask your clinical instructor about shadowing an endocrinologist for a day.

▪ If you care for a client on thyroid medication(s), ask them about their thyroid-related illness. Focus on its onset, evaluation, and treatment program.

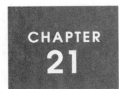

CHAPTER 21

Nursing Care of Clients with Diabetes Mellitus

■ ■ ■ ■ **Focused Study Tips**

- Describe the major metabolic problems in diabetic ketoacidosis (DKA): hyperglycemia, dehydration, accumulation of ketoacids, and osmotic diuresis.

- Discuss the usual clinical findings in hyperosmolar nonketotic coma (HNKC).

- Compare and contrast HNKC and DKA.

- State the onset of action, peak action, and duration of action for each type of insulin.

- Describe the key components of a teaching plan for a newly diagnosed client with Type 2 diabetes mellitus (DM).

■ ■ ■ ■ **Diabetes Mellitus**

1. Diabetes mellitus (DM) is not a single disorder, but a group of (a) _____ of the endocrine (b) _____.

2. Which of the following is the most common endocrine disorder?
   a. thyroid disorders
   b. Addison's disease
   c. hyperparathyroidism
   d. diabetes mellitus

3. When caring for clients with DM, a major role for the nurse is that of a(n) _____.

4. DM affects about (a) _____ million Americans. It is estimated that between (b) _____ and (c) _____ million Americans with DM are undiagnosed.

5. Worldwide, (a) _____ million individuals are affected by diabetes. It is one of the most serious chronic diseases, affecting (b) _____ to (c) _____ percent of the population.

6. DM occurs most commonly in:
   a. European Americans.
   b. African Americans.
   c. Native Americans.
   d. Hispanic Americans.

7. The fourth leading cause of death in the United States is (a) _____. Three common complications of this disorder are (b) _____, (c) _____, and (d) _____.

8. The islets of Langerhans produce hormones that are necessary for the metabolism and cellular utilization of (a) _____, (b) _____, and (c) _____.

9. The alpha cells of the pancreas produce (a) _____. The primary function of this hormone is to (b) _____.

10. The beta cells of the pancreas produce (a) _____. This hormone is responsible for (b) _____ and for decreasing blood glucose levels. This hormone also prevents (c) _____ _____.

11. Delta cells of the pancreas produce (a) _____. This substance inhibits the (b) _____.

Match the terms (a–e) with the proper descriptions listed in questions 12–16 below.

_____ 12. 70–110 mg/dL

_____ 13. stimulates the breakdown of glycogen

_____ 14. the breakdown of liver glycogen

_____ 15. facilitates the movement of glucose across the cell membrane

_____ 16. the formation of blood glucose from fats and proteins

a. glucagon
b. glycogenolysis
c. glyconeogenesis
d. insulin
e. normal blood sugar

17. The release of insulin is controlled by the (a) _____ level. After eating, the blood sugar level (b) _____, and so does the release of i - sulin. After eating, insulin levels peak in (c) _____ to (d) _____ minutes, and returns .o baseline within (e) _____ to (f) _____ hours.

Read the statements below and determine if they are true or false. Correct any false statements.

_____ 18. All body tissues and organs require a constant supply of glucose.

_____ 19. Brain, liver, intestinal, and renal tubule cells require insulin.

_____ 20. Skeletal and cardiac muscle, as well as adipose tissue, do not require insulin.

21. Other hormones that increase glucose in times of hypoglycemia, stress, growth, or increased metabolic demand include:
    (a) _____   (c) _____
    (b) _____   (d) _____

Match the types of DM (a–c) with the proper descriptions listed in questions 22–29. Types of DM (a–c) can be used more than once or not at all.

_____ 22. The onset of this DM is during pregnancy.

_____ 23. This type of DM usually has an onset in clients before the age of 30.

a. Type 1 DM
b. Type 2 DM
c. gestational diabetes

_____ 24. The client with this type of DM must have insulin to sustain life.

_____ 25. The onset of symptoms in this type of DM is slow.

_____ 26. The client with this type of DM is often obese, but may be of normal weight.

_____ 27. The onset of symptoms of this type of DM is rapid.

_____ 28. The onset of this type of DM is usually after age 35.

_____ 29. The client with this type of DM is usually thin.

Read the statements below and determine if they are true or false. Correct any false statment.

_____ 30. The client with Type 2 DM does not require insulin.

_____ 31. Women with gestational diabetes do not require treatment after pregnancy.

_____ 32. Diabetic complications may occur when the client requires insulin.

33. The factors that are believed to contribute to the destruction of the beta cells in Type 1 DM are:

    (a) _____   (c) _____

    (b) _____

34. The three classic signs of hyperglycemia in Type 1 DM are: (a) _____,

    (b) _____, and (c) _____.

35. Identify three other manifestations of Type 1 DM.

    (a) _____   (c) _____

    (b) _____

36. Explain why each of the following symptoms occurs:

    (a) polyuria:

    (b) glucosuria:

    (c) polydipsia:

    (d) polyphagia:

Read the statements below and determine if they are true or false. Correct any false statements.

_____ 37. The client with Type 1 DM requires insulin when oral agents are ineffective.

_____ 38. Complications of DM occur regardless of blood glucose control.

_____ 39. The causes of DM are well understood.

40. List three potential causes of diabetic ketoacidosis (DKA).

    (a) _____

    (b) _____

    (c) _____

41. The manifestations of DKA are the result of (a) _____ and

    (b) _____.

42. Treatment of DKA focuses on:

    (a) _____

    (b) _____

    (c) _____

43. Which laboratory finding is inconsistent with a diagnosis of DKA?

    a. blood glucose 350 mg/dL   c. presence of serum ketones

    b. plasma pH less than 7.3   d. plasma bicarbonate greater than 10 mEq/L

44. When caring for a client with diabetic ketoacidosis (DKA), the nurse will observe thirst, dry mucous membranes, and _____.

45. The risk factors for Type 2 DM include:
    (a) _____   (c) _____
    (b) _____

46. What two effects would weight loss have for the obese person with Type 2 DM?
    (a) _____
    (b) _____

47. The client with Type 2 DM does not experience ketosis because:
    a. the client's blood sugar never exceeds 300 mg/dL.
    b. the client does not require insulin.
    c. there is enough insulin present in the client's body to prevent the breakdown of fats.
    d. dehydration will occur before ketosis can occur.

48. Which of the following clinical manifestations is not commonly found in a client with Type 2 DM?
    a. polyuria   b. polydipsia   c. polyphagia   d. hyperglycemia

Read the statements below and determine if they are true or false. Correct any false statements.

_____ 49. Dehydration occurs in hyperosmolar nonketotic coma (HNKC).

_____ 50. HNKC is not as serious as DKA.

_____ 51. The onset of HNKC is slow and insidious.

_____ 52. Treatment is very similar for DKA and HNKC.

Match the clinical manifestations (a–e) with the proper descriptions listed in questions 53–57. Clinical manifestations (a–e) may be used more than once.

_____ 53. a morning rise in blood glucose to hyperglycemic
           levels following an episode of nocturnal hypoglycemia

_____ 54. a rise in blood glucose between 4 AM and 8 AM not in
           response to hypoglycemia

_____ 55. failure to secrete glucagon in response to a decrease in
           blood glucose

_____ 56. elevated blood sugar

_____ 57. low blood sugar

a. hyperglycemia
b Somogyi phenomenon
c. dawn phenomenon
d. insulin reaction
e. hypoglycemia
   unawareness

58. Which clinical manifestations will the nurse observe in the client with hypoglycemia?
    a. hunger and nausea   c. sweating and slowing pulse
    b. hypertension   d. dry skin

Read the statements below and determine if they are true or false. Correct any false statements.

_____ 59. Arteriosclerosis has an increased incidence and earlier onset in clients with DM when compared to those without DM.

_____ 60. DM protects the client from experiencing heart disease and strokes.

_____ 61. Gangrene from DM is the most common cause for nontraumatic amputations.

_____ 62. The incidence of blindness is not related to DM.

_____ 63. Diabetic retinopathy is the leading cause of blindness in individuals ages 25–74.

_____ 64. Diabetic nephropathy occurs in 75% of all diabetics.

_____ 65. Diabetic nephropathy is the most common cause for renal failure.

_____ 66. Diabetic neuropathy can affect sensory or motor function.

Define the following terms.

67. paresthesias:

68. mononeuropathies:

69. autonomic neuropathies:

70. Which clinical manifestation(s) would the nurse observe in a client with DM?
    a. excessive hair on the lower leg
    b. warm, moist skin
    c. dependent blanching and rubor on elevation
    d. intermittent claudication

Indicate whether clients with diabetes are at an increased (I) or decreased (D) risk for the following:

_____ 71. infection

_____ 72. periodontitis

_____ 73. arteriosclerosis

_____ 74. cardiovascular dysfunction

_____ 75. gastrointestinal dysfunction

_____ 76. sweating on hands and feet

_____ 77. sweating on face or trunk

_____ 78. ability to empty bladder

_____ 79. sexual dysfunction

80. When teaching the client with DM about foot care, the nurse should emphasize:
    a. the importance of inspecting the feet after walking barefoot.
    b. the fact that painless ulceration can occur and should be reported to the client's physician.
    c. accepting pain at rest because it is related to neuropathies.
    d. that thickened skin from cracks, fissures, and calluses helps prevent infection.

81. For each topic listed below, identify one important point the nurse should emphasize when performing client teaching for the young and middle adult with DM.
    (a) diet:
    (b) cigarette smoking:
    (c) exercise:

82. List five things the nurse should consider when planning care for the older client with DM.
    (a) _____
    (b) _____
    (c) _____
    (d) _____
    (e) _____

Indicate, using true or false, whether the following are diagnostic criteria for DM. Correct any false statements.

_____ 83. one measurement of a fasting plasma glucose level above 140 mg/dL

_____ 84. random plasma glucose level greater than 200 mg/dL with classic manifestations of DM

_____ 85. fasting plasma glucose level below 140 mg/dL but an abnormal response to two oral glucose tolerance tests

86. A client with Type 1 DM has an elevated glycosylated hemoglobin. This means that the client:
    a. requires less insulin.
    b. no longer requires iron supplements.
    c. needs better control of blood glucose.
    d. ingested too much sugar the day before the test.

87. In which of the following situations is urine or blood testing for the client with Type 1 DM not indicated?
    a. pregnancy
    b. while taking aspirin
    c. during illness
    d. while experiencing unexplained hyperglycemia

88. Which client statement about self-monitoring of blood glucose (SMBG) indicates the need for further teaching?
    a. "I will perform SMBG when my blood sugar is elevated."
    b. "I will perform SMBG if I suspect hypoglycemia."
    c. "I will perform SMBG more frequently during illness."
    d. "I will always perform SMBG at mealtimes."

89. If the client is not using a blood glucose monitor, which nursing assessment would be important to perform prior to teaching a client SMBG?
    a. visual acuity   b. color blindness   c. reading level   d. hearing ability

90. Which client statement indicates the need for further teaching about insulin?
    a. "I keep my insulin in the refrigerator."
    b. "I pinch up a fold of skin when giving myself insulin."
    c. "I keep a source of sugar available at all times."
    d. "I won't take my insulin on days when I feel ill."

91. For each of the following insulin types, give an example of an insulin preparation and its onset of action, peak of action (in hours), and duration of action (in hours).

Insulin Type	Insulin Preparation	Onset of Action	Peak of Action	Duration of Action
rapid-acting				
intermediate-acting				
long-acting				

92. Which is the only type of insulin that can be given intravenously? _____ _____

Read the statements below and determine if they are true or false. Correct any false statements.

_____ 93. U-100 is the most common concentration of insulin.

_____ 94. Regular insulin that is cloudy can be injected subcutaneously.

_____ 95. In U-100 insulin, there is 1 unit of insulin in 1 mL.

_____ 96. Insulin should be administered at room temperature.

_____ 97. The most rapid site of insulin absorption is the abdomen.

98. When performing an insulin injection, at what angle should the needle be inserted in a client of average or above average weight? _____

99. The nurse is teaching a client how to mix insulins in one syringe. Which of the following statements by the client indicates that the teaching has been successful?
    a. "I will withdraw the regular insulin and then the intermediate-acting insulin into the syringe."
    b. "I will withdraw the human insulin and then the animal insulin into the syringe."
    c. "I can mix U-100 NPH insulin and U-500 regular insulin in the same syringe."
    d. "NPH insulin should never be mixed with regular insulin."

100. When a client on insulin shows signs and symptoms of hypoglycemia such as shakiness, hunger, and nervousness, priority interventions by the nurse are to (a) _____ _____, and (b) _____.

101. A client is experiencing blurry vision immediately after being diagnosed with DM and starting insulin. The nurse advises the client to:
    a. immediately see an ophthalmologist as the client may be experiencing retinopathy.
    b. accept that blindness may occur from the microvascular changes that occur in diabetes.
    c. recognize that the blurry vision is related to fluid changes in the eye and will clear up in about 8 weeks.
    d. stop taking the insulin, as blurry vision may indicate an allergic reaction and may lead to blindness.

102. A client with Type 1 DM calls the Urgent Care Clinic complaining of symptoms of the flu. He cannot eat due to vomiting and is unsure about whether he should take his regular dose of insulin. What is the most appropriate response by the clinic nurse? _____

_____

_____

103. Lipodystrophy is defined as (a) _____,
whereas lipoatrophy is defined as (b) _____.
Two reasons these conditions may occur are (c) _____
and (d) _____. These conditions can lead to
(e) _____.

Case Study

Nelson Kujawa is taking oral hypoglycemic agents for Type 2 DM. For each of the following medications, indicate whether Mr. Kujawa's blood glucose level would increase (I) or decrease (D) if the medication was administered to him.

_____ 104. nonsteroidal anti-inflammatory agent (NSAID)

_____ 105. cimetidine

_____ 106. oral contraceptive

_____ 107. calcium channel blocker

_____ 108. glucocorticoid

_____ 109. sulfonamide antibiotic

_____ 110. beta-blocker

_____ 111. thiazide diuretic

112. For each of the following dietary considerations, provide the current recommendations that the client with DM should be taught.

(a) weight:

(b) calories:

(c) carbohydrates:

(d) protein:

(e) saturated fat and cholesterol:

(f) fiber:

(g) sodium:

(h) alcohol:

(i) sweeteners:

113. The nurse is teaching a client about food planning using an exchange list. If the client wants to exchange one tortilla for cooked rice, how much rice can he have?
    a. 1 cup
    c. ¼ cup
    b. ½ cup
    d. none; tortilla and rice cannot be exchanged

114. Which client statement indicates that the teaching about sick-day management has been successful?
    a. "I know that my blood glucose level will decrease when I am ill."
    b. "It is not necessary for me to perform SMBG when I am ill."
    c. "I should not take my regular dose of insulin when I am ill."
    d. "I should drink 8 to 12 ounces of fluid every hour when I am ill."

115. What is the net result of exercise on a person with DM?
    a. Exercise lowers blood glucose levels.
    b. Exercise raises blood glucose levels.
    c. Exercise has no effect on blood glucose levels.
    d. Exercise is contraindicated in clients with DM.

116. Which client statement indicates the need for further teaching regarding exercise and diabetes?
    a. "I should monitor my blood sugar before and after exercise."
    b. "High-impact aerobic exercise is the best exercise for my condition."
    c. "I will perform moderate exercises on a regular basis."
    d. "Fluid intake is important when I am exercising."

117. The client with Type 1 DM is at risk for which complications when undergoing surgery? Circle all that are appropriate.
    a. infection and delayed wound healing
    b. fluid and electrolyte imbalances
    c. hypoglycemia
    d. hyperglycemia
    e. DKA

118. Explain the 15/15 rule for treatment of hypoglycemia.

119. Which nursing intervention would be most appropriate for a client with DM who suddenly becomes unconscious and is suspected of being severely hypoglycemic?
    a. give the client a glass of orange juice
    b. have the client eat a slice of bread
    c. administer an intravenous bolus of 50% glucose
    d. give the client 1 mg of glucagon subcutaneous

120. Which client statement indicates the need for further teaching regarding foot care?
    a. "I cannot walk barefoot."
    b. "I should soak my feet in hot soapy water on a daily basis."
    c. "I must inspect my feet daily."
    d. "I will cut my toenails straight across after washing my feet."

121. The nurse should anticipate that on admission to the emergency department, the client with DKA would have a:
    a. normal K⁺ that rises quickly.
    b. low Na⁺ that decreases later.
    c. normal K⁺ that decreases later.
    d. normal Na⁺ that remains unchanged.

122. Because of changes in electrolyte values associated with the treatment of DKA, the nurse should assess for:
    a. knowledge deficits.
    b. cardiac dysrhythmias.
    c. anxiety.
    d. noncompliance.

123. In the client experiencing either DKA or HNKC, the nurse would observe hyperglycemia, dehydration, and _____.

124. An older client with DM calls his doctor's office complaining of an ingrown toenail. The nurse should advise the client to:
    a. soak the affected foot twice per day.
    b. trim the toenail straight across.
    c. wear soft shoes until the toenail improves.
    d. see a podiatrist as soon as possible.

125. List four components of dental care for the client with DM.
    (a) _____
    (b) _____
    (c) _____
    (d) _____

126. A common infection for women with diabetes is _____.

127. Diabetic clients must be taught how to recognize the signs and symptoms of key complications. List at least eight key signs and symptoms of hypoglycemia and hyperglycemia.

    hypoglycemia:

    hyperglycemia:

128. A 48-year-old male client with DM tells the nurse, "I am having trouble with my sex life." An appropriate response by the nurse is:
    a. "This happens with all adults as they age."
    b. "Most men with DM become impotent."
    c. "Tell me more about what you are experiencing."
    d. "You are probably a candidate for an implant."

129. List four priority client-teaching topics for the client with newly diagnosed Type 1 DM.
    (a) _____
    (b) _____
    (c) _____
    (d) _____

130. Describe five areas of consideration when teaching the older adult with diabetes.
    (a) _____
    (b) _____
    (c) _____
    (d) _____
    (e) _____

131. Identify three nursing interventions that may address issues and problems specific to the older adult with diabetes.
    (a) _____
    (b) _____
    (c) _____

■ ■ ■ Critical Thinking Exercises

132. The nurse is caring for a young college student with diabetes who is noncompliant with her prescribed diet. Develop a teaching plan to assist her in following her diet and meeting her nutritional needs.

133. The nurse is shopping at a mall when summoned to provide assistance to a person with diabetes who was found unresponsive in a large department store. The security officer tells the nurse that it will be at least 15 minutes before the EMTs will arrive. What should the nurse do while waiting for the ambulance?

134. Develop a teaching plan for people with diabetes who are experiencing somatic and visceral neuropathies.

■ ■ ■ Additional Learning Experiences

- Attend a support group for persons with diabetes.
- Surf the World Wide Web and identify resources for persons with diabetes.
- Visit your local pharmacy or a medical supplier. Determine the costs for various diabetic supplies and calculate those costs on an annual basis. Determine if any of these costs are reimbursable by insurance.

CHAPTER 22

Assessing Clients with Bowel Elimination Disorders

■ ■ ■ Focused Study Tips

- Describe the anatomy and physiology of each part of the lower gastrointestinal tract.

- Perform a thorough assessment of the gastrointestinal tract with your assigned clients whenever possible.

- Identify the function of each segment of the lower gastrointestinal tract.

- List and describe the components of a gastrointestinal assessment.

■ ■ ■ Anatomy and Physiology

1. List the three regions of the small intestine.
    (a) _____
    (b) _____
    (c) _____

2. Explain the purpose of the microvilli, villi, and circular folds in the small intestine. _____
   _____
   _____.

3. The three segments of the large colon are the:
    (a) _____
    (b) _____
    (c) _____

4. A common site of internal hemorrhoids in the large intestine is the _____
   _____.

5. The major function of the large intestine is to:
    a. eliminate undigestible food residue from the body.
    b. absorb nutrients through mucosal villi.
    c. produce enzymes used in the digestion of nutrients.
    d. secrete secretin and cholecystokinin.

6. The auscultation of _____ is a part of routine objective data collection on bowel function.

7. A 25-year-old woman has a current complaint of abdominal cramping and frequent loose stools. During her health assessment, she is questioned about her bowel movements. She appears flushed and hesitant to answer. Which of the following is the most appropriate response by the nurse performing the assessment?
   a. "Clients often feel embarrassed answering questions of this nature, but knowing your history and symptoms will help us choose the best treatment for you."
   b. "Believe me, I know how hard it is to be in your position, but if you answer these questions, we can get through this exam more quickly."
   c. "We see clients with these symptoms every day. There is no reason for you to be embarrassed."
   d. "Would you like me to find another nurse to do the assessment?"

Read the following statement and determine if it is true or false. Correct the statement if it is false.

_____ 8. Constipation is an expected finding in older adults.

9. The health assessment interview regarding bowel function should begin by inquiring about the client's:
   a. diet.
   b. elimination patterns.
   c. lifestyle patterns, including stress and/or history of depression.
   d. existing or previous medical conditions.

Match the causes (a–e) with the correct abdominal symptoms listed in questions 10–14.

_____ 10. lower abdominal pain

_____ 11. crampy, colicky pains

_____ 12. sudden abdominal cramping

_____ 13. left lower abdominal pain

_____ 14. rectal pain

a. distended colon filled with gas or fluid
b. stool retention and/or hemorrhoids
c. diverticulitis
d. diarrhea and/or constipation
e. obstruction of the colon

15. Constipation is often caused by medications. Which of the following categories of medication is least likely to cause constipation?
   a. anticholinergics   b. antibiotics   c. narcotics   d. tranquilizers

Case Study

During the physical examination of John Norton, the nurse collects the following objective data: generalized abdominal distention and faint, intermittent bowel sounds in all four quadrants.

16. What might be the cause of Mr. Norton's abdominal distention? _____
_____
_____

17. What condition does decreased or absent bowel sounds indicate? _____
_____

18. If Mr. Norton had normal bowel sounds, the nurse could expect to hear _____
_____ .

19. Movable, soft masses palpated in the anus and rectum may be:
    a. a prolapsed rectum.
    b. hemorrhoids.
    c. diverticulum.
    d. polyps.

20. Colonic atrophy occurs after the age of:
    a. 40 years.   b. 60 years.   c. 75 years   d. 90 years.

21. Name the three characteristics of feces for which the nurse assesses when inspecting feces.
    (a) _____   (c) _____
    (b) _____

22. Watery, diarrhea stools are present in which bowel disorders?
    a. malabsorption syndromes
    b. spastic colon
    c. bowel obstruction
    d. ingestion of oral iron

23. Black, tarry stools, which often occur with upper gastrointestinal bleeding, are referred to as ___
_____.

24. Greasy, yellow, frothy stools may appear in which of the following gastrointestinal problems?
    a. lactose intolerance
    b. fat malabsorption
    c. irritable bowel syndrome
    d. ulcer disease

25. *Circle the correct choice:* Blood from the colon due to ulcerative colitis, diverticulosis, or tumors
    presents (on/within) the stool.

26. Bowel function is assessed through a(n):
    (a) _____
    (b) _____
    (c) _____

27. A complete bowel assessment also includes:
    (a) _____
    (b)_____

28. A 50-year-old woman presents with a complaint of constipation. She is scheduled for a complete
    assessment of her abdomen. In preparing the client for a rectal exam, the nurse should instruct
    the client to turn to the (a) _____ position. This position is also
    known as the (b) _____.

29. During the rectal exam, the client states, "Stop! I'm going to have a bowel movement!" The best
    response by the nurse is:
    a. "We are almost done. Just take some deep breaths and try to think of something else."
    b. "What you are experiencing is a normal sensation that clients often experience during a
       rectal exam. Taking slow, deep breaths will help you to relax."
    c. "Don't worry. That almost never happens."
    d. "Although that feeling is normal, we will interrupt the exam and allow you to use the
       bathroom."

30. The student nurse assigned to a client hears high-pitched, rushing, and growling bowel sounds upon auscultation of the client's abdomen. Two possible explanations are (a) _____ _____ and (b) _____.

31. Identify three precipitating factors leading to decreased bowel elimination in the older client.
    (a) _____
    (b) _____
    (c) _____

32. Fecal incontinence is _____.

33. Name two ways the older client can decrease the risk of constipation.
    (a) _____
    (b) _____

34. Abnormal findings during the inspection of the perineal area include:
    (a) _____.
    (b) _____.
    (c) _____.

Read the statements below and determine if they are true or false. Correct any false statements.

_____ 35. Movable, soft masses felt when palpating the anus and rectum may be polyps.

_____ 36. Hard, firm, irregular embedded masses felt when palpating the anus and rectum may indicate carcinoma.

_____ 37. When examining the anus and the rectum, rotate the index finger to the right side to palpate any lesions or masses.

_____ 38. It is possible to examine the prostate or cervix at the same time the anus and rectum are examined.

_____ 39. Lubricant should not be used when examining the anus and rectum as it could affect the results of the test for occult blood.

Case Study

Tina Russell is a 49-year-old European American female admitted with a 3-day history of nausea and vomiting. Her admitting physician suspects she may have a bowel obstruction.

40. What subjective assessment data should the nurse collect?

41. What objective assessment data should the nurse collect?

42. Which assessment findings would indicate that the client's bowel obstruction is resolving?

▪ ▪ ▪ Critical Thinking Exercises

43. Develop a teaching plan for a group of older adults who are concerned about constipation.

44. The nurse is interviewing a client who tells the nurse that she has diarrhea 20 times a day. What other assessment questions should the nurse ask? What is the best way to validate the client's complaint?

▪ ▪ ▪ Additional Learning Experiences

- Practice listening to the normal bowel sounds of willing family members and friends.
- Consult with your nursing instructor about opportunities to observe activities in an endoscopy department.
- Monitor TV and print media commercials for laxatives and anti-diarrheal agents.

Nursing Care of Clients with Bowel Elimination Disorders

▪ ▪ ▪ Focused Study Tips

- Discuss the different causes of diarrhea in adult clients and the pharmacologic preparations used to treat diarrhea.

- Describe the nursing care required before and after each diagnostic test that might be ordered for a client with a bowel disorder.

- Discuss the common nursing diagnoses, interventions, and rationales for caring for a client with an infectious disease of the bowel.

- Compare and constrast ulcerative colitis and Crohn's disease.

- Compare and contrast the nursing care of a client with a colostomy or an ileostomy.

- Compare and contrast the care of clients with diverticulosis and the care of clients with diverticulitis.

▪ ▪ ▪ Disorders of Intestinal Motility

1. List direct and indirect effects on the gastrointestinal tract.
   direct:

   indirect:

▪ ▪ ▪ The Client with Diarrhea

2. Define diarrhea. _____

_____

3. Even though diarrhea is rarely a primary disorder, it can have devastating results. Identify three imbalances that can occur in a client with diarrhea.
   (a) _____
   (b) _____
   (c) _____

Case Study

Arthur Jones is a 60-year-old male who has experienced diarrhea for 1 week. He arrives at his primary care practitioner's office complaining of "weakness and fatigue." Rose, the family nurse practitioner, completes a history and physical exam on Mr. Jones and is unable to discover the cause of the diarrhea.

4. Identify three tests the nurse practitioner should order for Mr. Jones.
   (a) _____
   (b) _____
   (c) _____

5. a. A sigmoidoscopy has been scheduled for Mr. Jones. Describe the procedure for performing a sigmoidoscopy.

  b. After the sigmoidoscopy, Mr. Jones complains of abdominal pain and some bleeding. The most appropriate advice for the nurse to give is:

6. Initial dietary management of a client with acute diarrhea should include:
   a. soft, bland foods.
   b. small, frequent feedings.
   c. no solid food for the first 24 hours.
   d. drink milk to soothe the stomach.

7. Which of the following indicates the client has been successfully taught the information about taking antidiarrheal preparations?
   a. "I will swallow the bismuth subsalicylate tablets after each loose stool."
   b. "I will not take aspirin while I'm taking bismuth subsalicylate tablets."
   c. "I will call the physician immediately if my tongue becomes darkened while taking bismuth subsalicylate tablets."
   d. "I will take my bismuth subsalicylate tablets for 1 week."

For each of the following nursing diagnoses, give at least three nursing interventions and their rationales for care of a client with diarrhea.

8. *Risk for Fluid Volume Deficit*
   Nursing interventions and rationales
   (a) _____
   _____
   (b) _____
   _____
   (c) _____
   _____

9. *Risk for Impaired Skin Integrity*
   Nursing interventions and rationales
   (a) _____
   _____
   (b) _____
   _____
   (c) _____
   _____

▪ ▪ ▪ The Client with Constipation

10. (a) _____ is defined as the infrequent or difficult passage of stools. In older adults, this condition and its accompanying complications of gas and impaction are called (b) _____. Teaching older adults about the above focuses on (c) _____.

11. Identify three causes of constipation.

    (a) _____

    (b) _____

    (c) _____

12. A client undergoes a colonoscopy with polyp removal. He wants to return to work in his job in shipping and receiving at a local manufacturer. The most appropriate instructions for the nurse to give are:

    a. "You may return to your full activities after 48 hours if you experience no bleeding."

    b. "You may return to full activities when you have your first bowel movement."

    c. "You may not do any heavy lifting or straining for 7 days."

    d. "You may eat a high-fiber diet and should drink plenty of fluids."

13. Which of the following client statements indicates that the client correctly understands the teaching about the dietary management for preventing constipation?

    a. "I will eat more refined foods."

    b. "I will reduce the amount of fiber in my diet."

    c. "I will drink 6 to 8 glasses of fluid daily."

    d. "I will avoid eating raw fruits and vegetables."

14. Which type of enema is least irritating to the bowel?

    a. phosphate enema

    b. saline enema

    c. soap suds enema

    d. tap water enema

15. Which of the following statements indicates the need for further client teaching about how to take calcium polycarbophil (FiberCon), a bulk-forming agent?

    a. "I will drink 6 to 8 glasses of water every day."

    b. "I will mix this drug in a glass of fruit juice."

    c. "I will take this drug right before going to bed at night."

    d. "I will check with my health care provider before increasing the amount of bran in my diet."

▪ ▪ ▪ **The Client with Irritable Bowel Syndrome**

16. A 38-year-old client has irritable bowel syndrome. Which statement by the client indicates that he needs further client teaching?

    a. "I have reduced my intake of milk and milk products."

    b. "I stopped drinking apple juice."

    c. "I no longer drink caffeinated beverages."

    d. "I drink grape juice instead of grape soda."

Read the following statement and determine if it is true or false. Correct the statement if it is false.

_____ 17. When teaching the client with irritable bowel syndrome, the nurse should emphasize that although no organic disease is present, the client's symptoms are very real.

▪ ▪ ▪ The Client with Fecal Incontinence

18. Which of the following nursing interventions would be least effective in helping to manage the care of a client with fecal incontinence?
    a. teaching the client Kegel exercises
    b. encouraging the client to eat a high-residue diet
    c. taking loperamide (Imodium) as ordered
    d. using biofeedback therapy

Provide the rationales for the following nursing interventions, which are often used in the care of a client with bowel incontinence.

19. Insert a glycerine suppository 15 to 20 minutes before toileting the client.
    Rationale: _____
    _____

20. Place the client on the toilet at the same time each day.
    Rationale: _____
    _____

21. Clean the skin thoroughly with soap and water after each bowel movement.
    Rationale: _____
    _____

22. Apply a skin cream after each bowel movement.
    Rationale: _____
    _____

▪ ▪ ▪ The Client with Appendicitis

Read the following statement and determine if it is true or false. Correct the statement if it is false.

_____ 23. The appendix is usually located in the left iliac region at McBurney's point.

24. Preoperative care of a client scheduled for an appendectomy should include:
    a. a diet of clear fluids.
    b. an enema to prepare the bowel for surgery.
    c. administering IV antibiotics.
    d. applying a heating pad to the abdomen to decrease pain.

25. A primary goal in caring for a client with appendicitis is to _____
    _____ in both the preoperative and postoperative periods.

26. Which of the following findings in a client with appendicitis would indicate perforation or peritonitis?
    a. slowed pulse rate
    b. elevated blood pressure
    c. normal temperature
    d. rapid, shallow breathing

27. Which of the following white blood counts is indicative of appendicitis?
    a. 3000/mm^3 b. 5000/mm^3 c. 9000/mm^3 d. 13000/mm^3

28. A client is admitted to the emergency department complaining of nausea and right lower quadrant pain of 6-hour duration. The client's urinalysis report indicates large numbers of bacteria as well as many white and red blood cells. These findings are consistent with:
    a. the diagnosis of acute appendicitis.
    b. a urologic cause for her problem.
    c. normal findings in a menstruating adolescent.
    d. a contaminated urine specimen.

■ ■ ■ **The Client with Peritonitis**

29. Identify four clinical manifestations that would support a diagnosis of peritonitis.
    (a) _____
    (b) _____
    (c) _____
    (d) _____

30. Which of the following is not a sign of peritonitis in an older, chronically ill client?
    a. diffuse abdominal pain
    b. confusion and restlessness
    c. decreased urinary output
    d. vague abdominal complaints

Read the statements below and determine if they are true or false. Correct any false statements.

_____ 31. Peritonitis is easily treated and rarely serious.

_____ 32. A white blood count of 18,000/mm^3 is consistent with peritonitis.

_____ 33. Blood cultures are performed in peritonitis to assess for bacteremia.

_____ 34. Septicemia causes peritonitis.

_____ 35. Free air under the diaphragm is a normal finding.

_____ 36. The purpose of a Cantor tube is to relieve abdominal distention.

_____ 37. Taking fluids during an episode of paralytic ileus promotes peristaltic activity.

38. A client is undergoing treatment for peritonitis. He is experiencing a fluid volume deficit. Which of the following interventions is not appropriate for his condition?
    a. Assess his skin turgor every 1 to 2 hours.
    b. Monitor intake and output every 2 hours.
    c. Measure or estimate any fluid losses.
    d. Obtain a weight daily using the same scale.

■ ■ ■ **The Client with a Viral or Bacterial Infection**

39. List four causes of gastroenteritis.
    (a) _____
    (b) _____
    (c) _____
    (d) _____

40. The effects of a bacterial or viral infection of the gastointestinal tract are the result of:

    (a) _____

    (b) _____

Match the following statements (41–47) with the specific disorders (a–g).

_____ 41. onset is usually 2 to 8 hours after consuming contaminated food

_____ 42. diplopia and loss of accommodation are common initial symptoms

_____ 43. client may experience up to 10 loose stools each day

_____ 44. the incubation is 1 to 4 days

_____ 45. causes violent diarrhea, 8 to 48 hours after eating raw or improperly cooked meat, poultry, eggs, or dairy

_____ 46. has an incubation of 1 to 3 days and results in watery, grey, cloudy stools

_____ 47. results in severe abdominal cramping and watery, grossly bloody diarrhea

a. shigellosis
b. salmonellosis
c. *E coli* hemorrhagic colitis
d. traveler's diarrhea
e. staphylococcal food poisoning
f. botulism
g. cholera

48. The most common etiologic agent responsible for traveler's diarrhea is:

    a. *Entamoeba*   b. *Escherichia coli*   c. *Salmonella*   d. *Shigella*

49. _____ is a severe, life-threatening form of food poisoning.

50. Which of the following nursing diagnoses is the primary focus of the care of a client with an infectious bowel disorder causing diarrhea?

    a. *Activity Intolerance*
    b. *Risk for Aspiration*
    c. *Fluid Volume Deficit*
    d. *Altered Nutrition: Less than Body Requirements*

▪ ▪ ▪ The Client with a Protozoal Infection of the Bowel

Match the following statements (51–56) with the specific disorders (a–c).

_____ 51. most common protozoal pathogen in the United States

_____ 52. chiefly found in the tropics

_____ 53. contaminated water is a frequent source of infection

_____ 54. symptoms may include abdominal cramps, flatulence, and intermittent, bloody diarrhea

_____ 55. causes severe diarrhea in individuals with HIV and AIDS

_____ 56. incubation period may be 1 to 3 weeks

a. cryptosporidiosis
b. giardiasis
c. amebiasis

57. A nurse is providing teaching related to prevention to a client with a recent parasitic infection. Which of the following statements by the client indicates a need for further teaching?

    a. "I should avoid foods that cannot be cooked or peeled."
    b. "I should avoid rectal contact during sexual activity."
    c. "I should take these medications to prevent protozoal infections."
    d. "I should ensure that the water source is safe."

▪ ▪ ▪ The Client with a Helminthic Disorder

58. Which of the following infections is commonly known as pinworm?
    a. ascariasis   b. enterobiasis   c. trichinosis   d. strongyloidiasis

59. Which of the following lab values would be increased in a client with helminthic disease?
    a. eosinophils   b. hemoglobin   c. hematocrit   d. monocytes

60. Which statement by a client with a helminthic disorder indicates the need for further client teaching?
    a. "I should cook all meats and fish adequately and peel or cook vegetables."
    b. "When I travel, I should drink bottled water or use water purification tablets."
    c. "I should avoid handling the feces of domestic and wild animals."
    d. "Handwashing will not prevent the spread of a helminthic disorder."

61. Which disease has a portal of entry through the skin, usually of the feet?
    a. enterobiasis   c. trichinosis
    b. hookworm disease   d. ascariasis

62. Which round worm disease causes diarrhea, cramps, and malaise?
    a. enterobiasis   c. trichinosis
    b. hookworm disease   d. ascariasis

▪ ▪ ▪ The Client with a Ulcerative Colitis

63. Which of the following clinical findings is consistent with a diagnosis of ulcerative colitis?
    a. fever   c. frequent bloody stools
    b. fistulas   d. cobblestone appearance of the bowel

64. The nurse is teaching a client with ulcerative colitis about sulfasalazine (Azulfidine). Which of the following client statements indicate that further teaching is necessary?
    a. "I will drink at least 2 quarts of fluid per day."
    b. "I will take extra vitamin C while taking this drug."
    c. "I will not use my oral contraceptive; instead, I will use an alternate method of contraception."
    d. "I will use sunscreen to prevent any burn when I'm in the sun."

65. Initial dietary management of a client hospitalized with acute ulcerative colitis would be:
    a. a low-residue diet.
    b. a diet free of milk products and gas-producing foods.
    c. a regular diet with bulk-forming agents added.
    d. npo status with total parenteral nutrition (TPN).

Match the descriptions (a–c) with the correct types of ileostomies listed in questions 66–68.

_____ 66. total proctocolectomy with permanent ileostomy

_____ 67. Kock's ileostomy

_____ 68. loop ileostomy

a. often used to eliminate feces and allow tissue healing for 2 to 3 months
b. involves removal of the colon, rectum, and anus
c. involves construction of an intra-abdominal reservoir

69. Which of the following client behaviors indicates that teaching of self-care for a permanent ileostomy has been successful?
    a. The client shaves the skin around the stoma with a straight razor.
    b. The client follows a low-sodium diet.
    c. The client cuts the opening for the flange ¼ inch larger than the stoma.
    d. The client assumes a knee-chest position to relieve food blockage.

▪ ▪ ▪ The Client with Crohn's Disease

Reads the statements below and determine if they are true or false. Correct any false statements.

_____ 70. Crohn's disease only affects the terminal ileum and right colon.

_____ 71. Crohn's disease is a full-thickness inflammatory disease of the bowel.

_____ 72. Unlike ulcerative colitis, Crohn's disease is never associated with extraintestinal manifestations.

_____ 73. The peak ages of onset of Crohn's disease are 20 years and 40 years.

_____ 74. Uncommon complications of Crohn's disease are intestinal obstruction, abscess, and fistula formation.

75. A client is undergoing an outpatient evaluation for Crohn's disease. His physician told him to go to the pharmacy and purchase and take a routine bowel prep prior to a colonoscopy. The most appropriate intervention for the nurse is to tell the client to:
    a. take one-half of the usual amount of the bowel prep.
    b. not to take the bowel prep because of recent diarrhea.
    c. follow the physician's instructions and call with any problems
    d. contact the physician and clarify the instructions.

76. What type of diet is prescribed for the client with Crohn's disease?

77. Develop a teaching plan to help a client with Crohn's disease meet nutritional requirements.

▪ ▪ ▪ Malabsorption Syndromes

78. Which of the following is a systemic manifestation of malabsorption?
    a. diarrhea   c. steatorrhea
    b. abdominal distention   d. weight loss

79. Three common malabsorption disorders in adults are:
    (a) _____
    (b) _____
    (c) _____

■ ■ ■ The Client with Sprue

80. _____ is a chronic hereditary disorder characterized by sensitivity to the gliadin fraction of gluten.

81. _____ is an acquired chronic disease that is manifested by a sore tongue, diarrhea, and weight loss.

82. Gluten is found in which four cereals?
    (a) _____
    (b) _____
    (c) _____
    (d) _____

Match the following descriptions (83–88) with the specific laboratory/diagnostic tests (a–e).

_____ 83. This test is used to evaluate intestinal absorption.

_____ 84. This test is reduced in the client with celiac disease.

_____ 85. This test is used to rule out other causes for malabsorption and anemia.

_____ 86. This test requires the client to collect feces for a 72-hour period.

_____ 87. Blood and urine measurements are taken to evaluate the absorptive ability of the intestine.

_____ 88. This test allows direct visualization of the upper small intestine.

a. serum complement
b. enteroscopy
c. Schilling test
d. D-xylose absorption test
e. fecal fat

89. Develop a teaching plan for a client with steatorrhea and diarrhea.

■ ■ ■ The Client with Lactose Intolerance

90. The client from which of the following cultural groups is least likely to have a lactase deficiency?
    a. Asian American   b. African American   c. Native American   d. European American

91. Symptoms of lactose intolerance include _____
_____.

92. Nursing care for a client with lactose intolerance includes:
    (a) _____
    (b) _____

■ ■ ■ The Client with Short Bowel Syndrome

93. Short bowel syndrome is a condition that may result when _____
_____

94. Describe components of nursing care for a client with short bowel syndrome.

▪ ▪ ▪ The Client with Polyps

95. In which of the following types of polyps is the risk of malignancy almost 100%?
    a. pedunculated polyps
    b. familial polyposis
    c. villous polyps
    d. sessile polyposis

Match the following descriptions (96–99) with the correct type of polyp (a–c).

_____ 96. attached by a broad membranous base

_____ 97. a globelike structure

_____ 98. an uncommon autosomal dominant genetic disorder

_____ 99. may be called tubular adenomas

a. familial polyposis
b. villous polyp
c. pedunculated polyp

100. A client who has had a colorectal polyp removed states, "Well, I am glad I do not have to worry about that again." The most appropriate response by the nurse is:
    a. "Regular follow-up is crucial to detect any future problems."
    b. "Be sure to contact your doctor if you have similar problems in the future."
    c. "Yes, it is a relief that this problem is resolved and you don't have to worry."
    d. "You need to have a colonoscopy every 3 months for the next 5 years."

▪ ▪ ▪ The Client with Colorectal Cancer

101. In a client with bowel cancer, _____ is often the initial manifestation that prompts the client to seek medical care.

102. The most common permanent colostomy performed is a:
    a. double-barrel colostomy.
    b. sigmoid colostomy.
    c. transverse loop.
    d. Hartmann procedure.

103. An irrigation has been ordered for a client with a loop colostomy. Which stoma should be irrigated?
    a. distal
    b. proximal
    c. both distal and proximal
    d. neither distal nor proximal

104. The nurse is teaching a client with a permanent colostomy about diet management. Which of the following foods will increase stool odor?
    a. eggs   b. beer   c. bananas   d. pasta

105. Which member of the health care team is usually responsible for visiting the client preoperatively to determine stoma placement?
    a. oncologist
    b. gastroenterologist
    c. enterostomal therapist
    d. social worker

106. A client has a sigmoid colostomy. Which statement indicates that further client teaching is needed about colostomy irrigation?
    a. "I will use 1000 mL of water."
    b. "I allow the fluid to flow in quickly—in less than 5 minutes."
    c. "I always lubricate the cone before inserting its tip into my stoma."
    d. "I hold the irrigation bag at a height of 12 inches."

107. Which statement about emptying a colostomy bag is correct?
    a. The bag should be changed each time it is full.
    b. The bag should be emptied when it is three-quarters full.
    c. The bag should be emptied when it is no more than one-third full.
    d. The bag should be changed when it is one-half full.

108. A client has just had an abdominal perineal resection with colostomy. Which statement indicates a need for further teaching?
    a. "I should not use rectal suppositories."
    b. "I will have a colostomy the rest of my life."
    c. "My colostomy is only temporary."
    d. "I should not use a rectal thermometer."

109. A client has just returned from surgery that resulted in a colostomy. The nurse would expect to observe a:
    a. pink/red, moist stoma.
    b. stoma flush with the skin.
    c. brown stoma and copious amount of brown effluent.
    d. stoma that protrudes about 4 cm from the abdominal wall.

■ ■ ■ The Client with a Hernia

110. If the blood supply to hernia contents is compromised, the result is a _____ _____.

111. Which of the following nursing diagnoses has the highest priority for a client with an inguinal hernia?
    a. *Altered Tissue Perfusion: Gastrointestinal*   c. *Urinary Retention*
    b. *Impaired Skin Integrity*   d. *Altered Role Performance*

112. Differentiate indirect hernias from direct hernias.

113. Two conditions that contribute to umbilical hernias are:
    (a) _____
    (b) _____

114. What is the best way to observe an incisional or ventral hernia?

115. Describe the teaching plan for the postoperative client following an inguinal hernia repair.

▪ ▪ ▪ The Client with an Intestinal Obstruction

116. In a functional obstruction or (a) _____, peristalsis stops as a result of either neurogenic or muscular impairment. With a (b) _____, the bowel lumen is obstructed by a physical barrier, such as scar tissue or a tumor.

117. The most common cause of mechanical bowel obstruction is from (a) _____ They are usually acquired from (b) _____ or (c) _____.

118. Manifestation of a small bowel obstruction includes:

119. The most common manifestations of a large bowel obstruction are:

120. Identify at least four major complications associated with bowel obstruction.

▪ ▪ ▪ The Client with Diverticular Disease

121. A condition where a client has saclike projections of mucosa on the muscular layer of the colon is called (a):
    a. diverticula.   b. diverticulosis.   c. diverticulitis.   d. strangulated hernia.

122. The nurse is doing discharge teaching for a client with diverticulosis. Which of the following dietary options should be reinforced to the client?
    a. high fiber   b. low residue   c. low fiber   d. npo status

123. A client is being discharged on a high-fiber, high-residue diet. Which one of the following diet choices is the most appropriate?
    a. oatmeal, an apple, whole wheat bread, and orange juice
    b. cream of wheat, a banana, apple juice, and white toast
    c. shredded wheat, strawberries, whole grain toast, and an orange
    d. corn flakes, applesauce, a bagel, and a banana

124. Identify the manifestations of diverticulitis.

125. Compare and contrast the care for uncomplicated diverticulosis and acute diverticulitis.

▪ ▪ ▪ Anorectal Disorders

126. A client has just undergone perianal surgery. Which of the following actions in his plan of care should the nurse question?
    a. Keep fresh ice packs over the rectal dressing.
    b. Use a flotation pad when the client is sitting.
    c. Limit daily fluid intake to 1000 mL orally.
    d. Give stool softeners as prescribed.

127. When asymptomatic, _____ these varices of the anus and anal canal are considered to be a normal condition found in all adults.

Match the descriptions (a–c) with the correct terms listed in questions 128–130.

_____ 128. anal fissure

_____ 129. anorectal abscess

_____ 130. anorectal fistula

a. occurs when the epithelium of the anal canal over the internal sphincter becomes abraded
b. invasion of the pararectal spaces by pathogenic bacteria
c. a tunnel or tubelike tract with one opening in the anal canal and the other usually in the perianal skin

Read the following statement and determine if it is true or false. Correct the statement if it is false.

_____ 131. Clients with anorectal disorders should be taught to maintain a low-fiber diet and restrict fluid intake.

▪ ▪ ▪ Critical Thinking Exercises

132. The nurse is caring for a homebound client who frequently experiences fecal incontinence. Develop a nursing care plan to assist the client in managing this problem.

133. The nurse's friend calls and tells the nurse that she thinks she may have appendicitis. She does not have insurance and is worried about paying for an unnecessary doctor's visit. What questions should the nurse ask to help her determine the seriousness of her current complaint? If her symptoms are consistent with appendicitis, how might the nurse convince her to seek medical care?

134. Your community is experiencing an epidemic of giardiasis. Develop a community program to help address this epidemic and limit its spread.

135. Develop a dietary plan for a client with a recent colostomy.

▪ ▪ ▪ Additional Learning Experiences

- Practice teaching about self-care of an ileostomy or colostomy to a willing friend or family member.
- Confer with your nursing instructor about the possibility of observing clients undergoing diagnostic testing related to bowel disorders.
- Identify resources for clients who have a new ostomy.
- Attend an ostomy support group.

CHAPTER 24

Assessing Clients with Urinary Elimination Disorders

▪ ▪ ▪ Focused Study Tips

- Describe the mechanisms of fluid, electrolyte, and acid/base balance regulation by the kidney and within the body.

- Describe the components of a health assessment related to urinary function.

- Identify the characteristics of normal urine.

- Differentiate normal and abnormal laboratory findings for clients with urinary disorders.

▪ ▪ ▪ Anatomy and Physiology

1. List the four main functions of the urinary system.
   (a) _____
   (b) _____
   (c) _____
   (d) _____

2. The dense connective tissue that surrounds the kidney is known as the:
   a. renal capsule.
   b. hilum.
   c. renal fascia.
   d. middle adipose capsule.

3. List four functions of the kidney.
   (a) _____
   (b) _____
   (c) _____
   (d) _____

4. Briefly describe the functions of each of the three distinct regions of the kidneys:
   (a) cortex: _____
   (b) medulla: _____
   (c) renal pelvis: _____

5. The tuft of capillaries contained in each nephron is known as:
   a. a glomerulus.
   b. Bowman's space.
   c. the renal corpuscle.
   d. the major calyx.

Match the description (a–h) with the correct anatomic structures of the kidney listed in questions 6–13.

_____ 6. external urethral sphincter

_____ 7. detrusor muscle

_____ 8. ureters

_____ 9. urinary bladder

_____ 10. external urethral orifice

_____ 11. internal urethral sphincter

_____ 12. loop of Henle

_____ 13. urethra

a. a U-shaped structure actively involved in the reabsorption of some filtrate substances
b. muscular tube that channels urine outside the body
c. allows bladder size to adjust based on urine volume
d. storage site for urine
e. also called the urinary meatus
f. transports urine from kidney to bladder
g. skeletal bladder muscle under voluntary control
h. bladder muscle that relaxes in response to a full bladder and signals the need to urinate

14. Explain the process of glomerular filtration, including the three factors that influence filtration rate.

15. In healthy adults, the bladder can hold how many mL of urine before the urge to void occurs?
    a. 100–200   b. 200–300   c. 300–500   d. 500–800

16. In females, the length of the urethra is (a) _____ inches long, and in males the urethra is about (b) _____ inches long.

17. A client is admitted with an abdominal complaint. His urinalysis report includes a WBC of >5000/hpf. The nurse should suspect that the client:
    a. has a normal urinalysis.
    b. has mucus in his urine.
    c. has a urinary tract infection.
    d. did not collect a clean-void specimen.

18. A client is admitted with pneumonia. The nurse receives a report that her urinalysis indicates a specific gravity of 1.040. The most appropriate action by the nurse is to:
    a. restrict fluids.
    b. encourage fluids.
    c. increase the IV rate.
    d. do nothing; this value is normal.

19. Identify four normal characteristics of urine.
    (a) _____
    (b) _____
    (c) _____
    (d) _____

20. As an important part of urine formation in healthy kidneys, virtually all organic nutrients are returned to the body by the transepithelial process known as _____.

21. The dilution or concentration of the urine is largely determined by the:
    a. renal plasma clearance time.
    b. osmolality of the filtrate.
    c. countercurrent exchange system.
    d. action of antidiuretic hormone (ADH).

22. Hormones that are either activated or synthesized by the kidneys include (a) _____ _____ and (b) _____.

23. Briefly describe the action of erythropoietin and natriuretic hormone.

▪ ▪ ▪ Assessment of Urinary System Function

Match the terms (a–f) with the correct definitions listed in questions 24–29.

_____ 24. voiding excessive amounts of urine

_____ 25. blood in the urine

_____ 26. bacteriuria

_____ 27. excessive urination at night

_____ 28. voiding scant amounts of urine

_____ 29. painful urination

a. dysuria
b. hematuria
c. nocturia
d. oliguria
e. polyuria
f. pyuria

30. Health assessment information about cigarette smoking, usual fluid intake, and current medications belongs to which of the following categories?
    a. nutrition/metabolic
    b. health perception/health management
    c. activity/exercise
    d. physical assessment

31. A client comes into the emergency department (ED) complaining of back pain. He asks why the nurse wishes to collect a urine specimen. The most appropriate response by the nurse would be:
    a. "It is a routine test for all ED clients."
    b. "The doctor ordered it; we will have to ask him."
    c. "We want to make sure you do not have any urinary problems."
    d. "We are checking for abnormalities."

32. The correct order of physical assessment for clients with known or suspected urinary system problems is:
    a. auscultation, inspection, palpation, percussion.
    b. inspection, auscultation, percussion, palpation.
    c. inspection, palpation, percussion, auscultation.
    d. auscultation, palpation, inspection, percussion.

33. An accumulation of crystals is found on the skin of a client with untreated renal failure. This phenomenom is known as _____.

34. A 28-year-old mother of two has been admitted for complaints of excruciating pain in her right upper back, just below her rib cage. She has been unable to relieve her pain with the use of Advil (ibuprofen), heat, or rest. Auscultation of the left and right upper abdominal quadrants is quiet. The nurse notes increased pain and tenderness upon percussion and palpation of the client's kidneys. Auscultation of the kidneys is performed to:
    a. determine presence of systolic arterial bruits.
    b. rule out the possibility of cardiac or gastrointestinal causes of pain.
    c. detect enlargement.
    d. establish presence of normal renal veins.

35. Which of the following is not a normal age-related variation in urinary system assessment findings of the older adult?
    a. frequency and urgency
    b. urinary incontinence
    c. decrease in bladder capacity
    d. nocturia

36. A common urinary system problem in postmenopausal women is (a) _____ _____, while urinary retention in older men is most commonly caused by (b) _____.

37. By age 70, the rate of filtrate formation in the older adult is _____ that of the middle adult.
    a. one-half of
    b. equal to
    c. one-quarter of
    d. one-third of

38. List three common symptoms related to physiologic changes in urinary function in older adults.

    _____

Case Study

A client has come to the outpatient clinic complaining of urinary frequency and urgency. She describes dysuria when voiding. Her urinalysis report shows large numbers of white blood cells and bacteria. She tells the nurse she stopped drinking fluids 24 hours ago so she would not have to void. She has tenderness over the suprapubic area and her kidneys are nontender to palpation and percussion.

39. List the subjective findings.

40. List the objective findings.

41. What additional assessment questions should be asked?

▪ ▪ ▪ Critical Thinking Exercises

42. Develop a presentation for nursing assistants that will assist them in understanding the importance of intake and output and what they need to observe when they are measuring urine output.

43. The nurse is caring for a client with only one kidney. He asks the nurse if one kidney can do the work of two kidneys. Provide him with an explanation of the urinary tract and how this is possible.

▪ ▪ ▪ Additional Learning Experiences

- Identify resources for a client with urinary incontinence.
- Visit your local drugstore and explore the aisle with the products for urinary incontinence.
- Consult with your clinical instructor about an observational experience in a urology clinic.

CHAPTER 25

Nursing Care of Clients with Urinary Tract Disorders

■ ■ ■ **Focused Study Tips**

- Describe the different diagnostic tests that are used to rule out structural and excretory functions of the urinary tract, and discuss the nursing care required before and after each test.

- Compare and contrast the different categories of incontinence and the nursing care associated with each.

■ ■ ■ **The Client with Urinary Tract Infection**

1. Which of the following factors is least important for maintaining the sterility of the urinary tract?
   a. complete bladder emptying
   b. an adequate urine volume
   c. position of urethra when voiding
   d. free flow of urine from the kidneys through the urinary meatus

2. To prevent infection of the urinary tract, is it more favorable to have urine that is acidic or alkaline? _____.

3. The most common organism found in urinary tract infections is:
   a. *Enterobacter.*   b. *Klebsiella.*   c. *Staphylococcus.*   d. *Escherichia coli.*

4. The two ways urinary catheters promote urinary tract infections are:
   (a) _____
   (b) _____

5. Which of the following factors increases the risk of a urinary tract infection in the older male client?
   a. a short urethra
   b. a long urethra
   c. increase in prostatic secretions
   d. decrease in prostatic secretions

6. The nurse practitioner suspects that an 82-year-old client has cystitis. List five possible symptoms the client may have.
   (a) _____
   (b) _____
   (c) _____
   (d) _____
   (e) _____

7. A urinary sample that is indicative of infection must have a bacterial cell count of:
   a. 100 (10^2) /mL.
   b. 1000 (10^3) /mL.
   c. 10,000 (10^4) /mL.
   d. 100,000 (10^5) /mL.

8. A nurse has submitted a clean-catch urine sample for Gram's stain and culture and sensitivity. Explain the purpose of each of these tests.
   (a) Gram's stain _____

   _____

   (b) Urine culture and sensitivity _____

   _____

9. Prior to which of the following examinations would the nurse be sure to check the client's record for allergy to iodine?
   a. cystoscopy
   b. intravenous pyelogram (IVP)
   c. prostate examination
   d. ultrasound of the kidneys

Case Study

Gabrielle Larson is taking Bactrim (trimethoprim-sulfamethoxazole) and Pyridium (phenazopyridine hydrochloride) for a urinary tract infection. She has Type 2 diabetes mellitus and takes Coumadin (warfarin) for a mechanical heart valve.

10. The nurse should teach Ms. Larson to avoid which of the following beverages while she is taking Bactrim?
    a. milk
    b. carbonated beverages
    c. cranberry juice
    d. coffee

11. The nurse empties Ms. Larson's bedpan and notices that her urine is orange. The next action by the nurse should be to:
    a. hold the next dose of Bactrim (trimethoprim-sulfamethoxazole).
    b. inform the physician STAT.
    c. insert a Foley catheter.
    d. nothing; this is an expected finding.

12. All of the following nursing orders have been entered into Ms. Larson's nursing care plan. Identify the rationale of each.
    (a) Have client drink 1000–2000 mL of fluid/24 hours.
       Rationale: _____

       _____

    (b) Fingerstick client each shift for blood glucose level.
       Rationale: _____

       _____

    (c) Assess skin for bruising and hematomas every shift.
       Rationale: _____

       _____

13. Clients taking Macrodantin (nitrofurantoin), a urinary anti-infective, should be closely monitored for changes in which of the following body systems?
    a. respiratory
    b. cardiac
    c. gastrointestinal
    d. hematological

14. The nurse practitioner is treating a client with an uncomplicated UTI. Identify three reasons why the nurse practitioner would prescribe only a single-dose or three-day course of antibiotics.

    (a) _____

    (b) _____

    (c) _____

15. The pain of pyelonephritis is typically located:
    a. around the urinary meatus.
    b. in the suprapubic area.
    c. in the flank area.
    d. in the central abdominal region.

16. A 23-year-old client, who has been a new mother for 3 weeks, arrives at the emergency department with complaints of sudden onset of chills, vomiting, temperature of 102.8F, flank pain, and costovertebral tenderness. A diagnosis of acute pyelonephritis is made. What would be the results of the client's laboratory test?

17. A client has been diagnosed with acute pyelonephritis. He is receiving his second dose of antibiotics and tells the nurse, "The pain is so severe, I can't take it anymore." The most appropriate and therapeutic response by the nurse is:
    a. "There is nothing I can do. The pain will subside in 24 to 48 hours."
    b. "Perhaps the physician will order a heating pad which will make you feel better."
    c. "A sitz bath will make the pain go away."
    d. "I will call your physician to tell him the antibiotic is not working."

18. In a health promotion class for women, the nurse should teach participants which of the following methods for preventing urinary tract infection?
    a. wear nylon briefs
    b. void before and after sexual intercourse
    c. use feminine hygiene sprays
    d. clean the perineal area from back to front after voiding

19. Discharge instructions for the client who has completed anti-infective therapy should include:
    a. limiting the amount of vitamin C ingested daily.
    b. avoiding sexual intercourse for 10 days.
    c. drinking cranberry juice and/or orange juice daily.
    d. voiding only when bladder is full to increase the force of the stream.

■ ■ ■ The Client with Urinary Calculi

20. The most important factor in the prevention of urolithiasis is:
    a. a proper diet.
    b. adequate hydration.
    c. early ambulation.
    d. preventive drugs.

21. The rationale for administering anticholinergic drugs to the client with urolithiasis is to:
    a. increase peristalsis through the ureters.
    b. diminish the use of mucous production in the ureters.
    c. reduce vasospasm of the ureters.
    d. decrease urinary flow.

22. The rationale for straining all urine for stones that a client has passed is to:
    a. analyze the stones for information concerning possible preventive measures.
    b. determine if the client will require surgical interventions.
    c. analyze for indications of cancerous conditions.
    d. know if and when the stone has been "passed."

23. Dietary modification for the client with urinary calculi includes which of the following?
    a. increase acidic foods
    b. decrease alkaline-ash foods
    c. increase fluids
    d. eat a well-balanced diet

24. A procedure in which renal calculi are crushed either by percutaneous ultrasonic or laser technique or by extracorporeal shock wave technology is called (a) _____.
    In the initial postoperative period, the client must be monitored for (b) _____
    and _____. Urine is often bright (c) _____ for the first two days.
    (d) _____ urine may indicate the presence of an infection.

25. The primary outward manifestation of urolithiasis is:
    a. hematuria.
    b. pain.
    c. palpable mass in the lower left or right abdominal quadrants.
    d. oliguria.

26. Severe renal colic often causes a sympathetic response associated with what other three symptoms?
    (a) _____   (c) _____
    (b) _____

27. Beside each complication of urinary calculi, write the signs and symptoms that the client may exhibit.
    (a) UTI _____
    (b) Trauma to the urinary tract _____
    (c) Obstruction _____
    _____

28. A new nurse on the nephrology unit is assigned to care for a postoperative client who has had a nephrolithotomy with a ureteral stent placement. The nurse states that he has never cared for a ureteral stent. What information should the nurse preceptor provide the new nurse about each of the following?
    (a) why ureteral stents are placed _____
    _____
    (b) labeling all drainage tubes _____
    _____
    (c) maintaining the client's fluid intake, encouraging fluids that acidify urine _____
    _____

29. A 64-year-old client has been ordered a 24-hour urine collection starting today at 10:00 AM. Which nursing action would be following the correct procedure?
    a. discard the voided urine at 10:00 AM today, collect all urine in a container for a 24-hour period, and save the voided urine at 10:00 AM tomorrow
    b. save the urine voided at 10:00 AM today, collect all urine in a container for a 24-hour period, and discard the voided urine at 10:00 AM tomorrow
    c. send each voided specimen to the lab for analysis for 24 hours
    d. collect only the midstream portion of each voided specimen for 24 hours

▪ ▪ ▪ The Client with a Tumor of the Urinary Tract

30. What two major factors are implicated in the development of bladder cancer?

    (a) _____

    (b) _____

31. Exposure to which of the following substances is not associated with the development of bladder cancer?

    a. dyes

    b. cigarette smoke

    c. leather finishers

    d. coal dust

32. What is the presenting sign in 75% of urinary tract tumors?

    a. midabdominal pain

    b. sudden weight loss

    c. gross or microscopic hematuria

    d. urinary retention

33. The collaborative treatment plan for the client with a tumor of the urinary tract focuses on which three goals?

    (a) _____

    (b) _____

    (c) _____

34. A client is to have Thiotepa instilled into her bladder for the first time for superficial tumors of the bladder. Which statement by the client would indicate that further teaching is needed?

    a. "I must fast for 8–12 hours before the treatment."

    b. "The solution will be instilled by a catheter."

    c. "The solution will remain in the bladder for 2 hours."

    d. "I must stay very still during the time the solution is in the bladder."

Match the diagnostic studies for detecting urinary tract tumors (a–f) with the correct descriptions listed in questions 35–40.

_____ 35. allows visualization of the ureters with an endoscope inserted transurethrally

_____ 36. used to detect minor differences between tissues and tissue boundaries

_____ 37. allows direct visualization, assessment, and biopsy of identified lesions of the urethra and bladder

_____ 38. microscopic examination of cells within the urine for abnormalities

_____ 39. assesses for the presence of blood cells in the urine

_____ 40. noninvasive test that can reveal the presence of tumors or hydronephrosis

a. computed tomography

b. urine cytology

c. ureteroscopy

d. cystoscopy

e. renal ultrasound

f. urinalysis

41. Which of the following urinary diversions is considered a continent diversion?

    a. ileal conduit

    b. ureterosigmoidostomy

    c. Kock's pouch

    d. colon conduit

42. Two days following a client's surgery for bladder cancer, a nurse is providing care to the client's stoma. When the nurse cleanses the stoma with normal saline, it begins to bleed slightly. Her most appropriate action at this time is to:
    a. call the physician immediately.
    b. stop the procedure and position the client in the shock position.
    c. stop the procedure, apply a dressing, and monitor vital signs every 15 minutes.
    d. nothing; this is a normal finding two days postoperatively.

43. Four days postoperatively, the nurse prepares to clean the stoma. She finds the stoma to be dark purple. Her most appropriate action at this time is to:
    a. call the physician.
    b. stop the procedure and position the client in the shock position.
    c. stop the procedure, apply a dressing, and monitor vital signs every 15 minutes.
    d. nothing; this is a normal finding four days postoperatively.

44. A client has a urinary stoma device and is going to be discharged in 3 days. The nurses have been attempting to involve the client in his care, but he refuses to even look at the surgical site. A nursing diagnosis of *Body Image Disturbance* is entered into his record. Identify two nursing interventions with rationales that the nurses might utilize.
    (a) _____
    _____
    (b) _____
    _____

45. A client is being discharged after having a cystectomy with an ileal conduit. How will her discharge teaching differ from that of a client who has a Koch's pouch for bladder cancer?

▪ ▪ ▪ The Client with Urinary Retention

46. It is important to teach clients not to overfill their bladders because urinary retention can lead to loss of:
    a. the ability to urinate.
    b. detrusor muscle tone.
    c. the sensation of the need to urinate.
    d. the ability to fill it over time.

47. List four common causes of urinary retention.
    (a) _____
    (b) _____
    (c) _____
    (d) _____

48. How does each of the following interventions help to prevent urinary retention?
    (a) placement of an indwelling urinary catheter following surgery _____
    _____
    (b) administration of cholinergic medications _____
    _____
    (c) placement of the client in normal voiding position _____
    _____

▪ ▪ ▪ The Client with Neurogenic Bladder

49. The stimulus of more than (a) _____ mL of urine in the bladder normally signals empty-ing. Diseases or (b) _____ to the (c) _____ or (d) _____ nervous systems may interfere with normal mechanisms, resulting in (e) _____ bladder. Peripheral (f) _____ may cause some degree of hyporeflexia of the bladder. (g) _____ is the most common cause of peripheral bladder neuropathy.

50. A variety of drugs can be used to treat neurogenic bladder. For each class of drug listed below, explain the effects on the urinary bladder or other structures. Give an example of each.
    (a) alpha-adrenergic stimulants: _____
    _____

    Example: _____
    (b) cholinergic drugs: _____
    _____

    Example: _____
    (c) anticholinergic drugs: _____
    _____

    Example: _____
    (d) anticholinesterase drugs: _____
    _____

    Example: _____
    (e) alpha-receptor blocking drugs: _____
    _____

    Example: _____

51. Care must be exercised when executing or teaching the Credé method in clients with spinal cord injuries in order to prevent:
    a. a urinary tract infection. b. autonomic dysreflexia. c. renal calculi. d. urinary retention.

▪ ▪ ▪ The Client with Urinary Incontinence

52. Which structural and mechanical factors maintain continence?
    (a) _____
    (b) _____

Match the type of urinary incontinence (a–f) with the definition listed in questions 53–57.

_____ 53. an inability to empty the bladder, resulting in overdistention and frequent loss of small amount of urine

_____ 54. an involuntary loss of moderate volume of urine without stimulus or warning

_____ 55. an incontinence that results from physical, environmental, or psychosocial factors

_____ 56. urine is lost through increased intra-abdominal pressure as occurs when sneezing, coughing, or lifting

_____ 57. inability to inhibit urine flow long enough to reach toilet after urge sensation

a. reflex
b. functional
c. overflow
d. urge
e. stress
f. total

58. Identify the most common physical findings in male and female clients with incontinence.
    (a) male clients _____
    (b) female clients _____

59. A test to determine how completely the bladder is emptied with voiding is called:
    a. an intravenous pyelogram.
    b. a cystometrography.
    c. a post-void residual.
    d. a uroflowmetry.

60. A 67-year-old client is scheduled for a suspension of the bladder neck for stress incontinence. The nurse performing preoperative teaching should include which four important points?
    (a) _____
    (b) _____
    (c) _____
    (d) _____

61. During the postoperative assessment of the above client, the nurse should notify the physician for which of the following three indications of hemorrhage?
    (a) _____
    (b) _____
    (c) _____

62. What will the client in question 60 need to be taught about catheter care when she is discharged with a urethral catheter?

    _____

    _____

63. Describe how to perform Kegel exercises.

64. What diet and fluid intake modifications should be made to avoid stress and urge incontinence?

▪ ▪ ▪ **Critical Thinking Exercises**

65. Develop a presentation that addresses urinary health for junior high school students enrolled in a health class.

66. Develop a system for triaging outpatients with a suspected urinary tract infection. What indications would require an office visit? What should be included in client teaching?

67. Develop a nursing care plan for a 79-year-old woman who has become socially isolated related to her urinary incontinence.

▪ ▪ ▪ **Additional Learning Experiences**

▪   Ask your clinical instructor about opportunities to observe a lithotripsy or ileal conduit surgery.

▪   Visit the World Wide Web and identify resources for adults with urinary problems.

Nursing Care of Clients with Kidney Disorders

■ ■ ■ **Focused Study Tips**

- List the disorders that are the leading causes of renal failure in the United States.

- Discuss hypertension and renal artery occlusion and their effects on renal function.

- Identify the causes of prerenal, intrarenal, and postrenal failure.

- Compare and contrast the pharmacologic therapies associated with acute renal failure, including diuretics, renal perfusers, exchange resins, and phosphate binders.

- Describe the laboratory tests used to track disease processes in the kidney.

■ ■ ■ **Kidney Disorders**

1. In North America, (a) _____ people are affected by kidney and urinary tract disease. Each year (b) _____ in (c) _____ Americans develop(s) end-stage renal disease.

2. Urea and creatinine are considered ideal substances for evaluating renal function because:
   a. both are bound to glucose.
   b. neither is reabsorbed in the tubules.
   c. both are measured using random urine testing.
   d. neither is influenced by other disease states.

3. The normal ratio of BUN to creatinine is (a) _____ to (b) _____.

4. In renal disease, the BUN rises at a _____ rate than the serum creatinine.

5. Identify three factors that decrease the glomerular filtration rate (GFR) in the older client.
   (a) _____
   (b) _____
   (c) _____

6. By age 80, the GFR may be less than _____ of what it was at age 20.

7. The _____ is the most sensitive indicator of an older adult's GFR.

8. List four common classes of medications that are affected by a decreased GFR.
   (a) _____
   (b) _____
   (c) _____
   (d) _____

■ ■ ■ Congenital Kidney Malformation

Match the conditions (a–d) with the correct descriptions listed in questions 9–12.

_____ 9. underdevelopment of the kidney

_____ 10. places client at risk for stasis, infection, and lithiasis

_____ 11. causes distention of the renal pelvis and calyces with urine

_____ 12. absence of an organ

a. agenesis
b. hypoplasia
c. horseshoe kidney
d. abnormal kidney position

■ ■ ■ The Client with Polycystic Kidney Disease

13. In the adult with polycystic kidney disease, the nurse would be sure to include assessments of which body system?
    a. gastrointestinal   b. visual   c. cardiac   d. musculoskeletal

14. The client with polycystic kidney disease typically shows symptoms between the ages of _____ _____.

15. Common symptoms of polycystic kidney disease are (a) _____,
    (b) _____, (c) _____,
    (d) _____, and (e) _____.

16. Clients with polycystic kidney disease are usually good candidates for renal transplant because they _____.

17. Following a CT scan of the kidneys with contrast, which nursing intervention should be implemented?
    a. maintaining npo status for 4 hours
    b. medicating the client for pain
    c. removing conductive gel from flanks
    d. encouraging oral intake of fluids

18. Which statement by the client with polycystic kidney disease indicates the need for further teaching?
    a. "I should restrict my fluid intake."
    b. "I should report burning, frequency, or urgency."
    c. "I should check with my doctor before taking any new medicine."
    d. "My family may require screening for this problem."

■ ■ ■ The Client with Hydronephrosis

19. Define vesicoureteral reflux.

20. Hydronephrosis must be treated promptly to _____.

21. A client is diagnosed with hydronephrosis, and the physician has inserted a percutaneous nephrostomy tube to relieve the urinary obstruction. The client has denied pain or discomfort for 24 hours after the procedure. While the nurse is teaching him about home care of the drainage system in preparation of discharge, the client starts complaining of acute colicky pain radiating to the groin, nausea, and abdominal pain. An appropriate intervention by the nurse is to:
   a. administer prn medications.
   b. irrigate the nephrostomy tube.
   c. assess the tube for patency.
   d. recognize his anxiety regarding self-care.

▪ ▪ ▪ The Client with a Disorder of the Glomerulus

22. Which of the following is not a normal constituent of urine?
   a. cast   b. protein   c. hydrogen ions   d. creatinine

23. The most common precipitating factor that places a client at risk for acute glomerulonephritis is
   _____.

24. The urinalysis of a client with acute glomerulonephritis would have which of the following findings?
   a. cast cells   c. proteinuria
   b. pH of 3.0   d. a specific gravity of 1.020

25. The nephrotic syndrome is characterized by which four clinical findings?
   (a) _____
   (b) _____
   (c) _____
   (d) _____

26. A client is about to undergo a renal biopsy. Which of the following nursing interventions is not appropriate for this client?
   a. Tell the client that the procedure takes about an hour and is painful.
   b. Maintain the client's npo status from midnight before the procedure.
   c. Tell the client not to breathe when the needle is inserted.
   d. Tell the client that a local anesthetic is used at the injection site, but no sedation is given.

27. Azotemia is:
   a. hematuria and proteinuria.
   b. increased blood levels of nitrogenous waste products.
   c. oliguria and hypoalbuminemia.
   d. oncotic pressure and increasing GFR.

28. A 14-year-old client is recovering from strep throat. Her mother calls and asks the office nurse if it is normal for her daughter to be experiencing hematuria and fluid retention. The nurse's most appropriate response is:
   a. "Make sure she drinks plenty of fluids."
   b. "The antibiotic she is taking causes these effects."
   c. "Don't worry, these symptoms can occur with strep."
   d. "Please bring her in to see the doctor."

29. List at least five symptoms of acute glomerulonephritis.

(a) _____

(b) _____

(c) _____

(d) _____

(e) _____

30. A 28-year-old client is admitted with Goodpasture's syndrome. He tells the nurse he has been coughing up small amounts of blood. In setting priorities, the nurse should:

a. recognize these symptoms as part of the syndrome.

b. monitor respiratory status and assess for bleeding.

c. tell him to swallow the sputum to prevent excess blood loss.

d. recognize that bleeding is a sign that death is imminent.

31. An erythrocyte sedimentation rate is performed on clients with renal disease because it is a(n):

a. specific test for kidney disease.

b. indicator of inflammatory response.

c. indicator of damage to the erythrocytes.

d. measure of protein in the blood.

32. A KUB evaluates the (a) _____, (b) _____, and (c) _____.

33. A client is going to collect a 24-hour urine for creatinine clearance. She will start collecting the urine at 10:00 AM. So that the specimen is timed and collected accurately, the nurse should tell her to: _____

_____

_____

_____

34. A normal BUN is (a) _____ mg/dL. A normal serum creatinine is (b) _____ mg/dL for a female and (c) _____ mg/dL for a male.

35. A client is taking Imuran (azathioprine) for her renal disease. Which statement by the client indicates a need for further client teaching?

a. "I should avoid crowds while taking this medication."

b. "This medication will prevent pregnancy."

c. "I should avoid aspirin or ibuprofen while taking this medication."

d. "I should report coughing or breathing problems."

36. A client has a glomerular disease, severe edema, and hypertension. Which nursing intervention is appropriate regarding the client's fluid intake?

a. encourage fluids to increase urine output

b. increase IV rate in relationship to urine output

c. maintain ordered fluid restriction

d. offer foods high in sodium to minimize edema

37. The above client is suffering from severe fatigue. The nurse should advise him:
    a. that fatigue is something he has to accept.
    b. to balance activity and rest to minimize fatigue.
    c. that the fatigue will lessen in time.
    d. that eating high-calorie foods will give him more energy.

38. Compared to individuals without renal disease, the client with renal disease is at:
    a. no additional risk for infection.
    b. a much lower risk for infection.
    c. a higher risk for infection.
    d. a lower risk for HIV.

39. A client has severe glomerular disease. She tells the nurse, "My family expects me to do more around the home." The most appropriate response by the nurse is:
    a. "I will tell your family that they cannot expect you do household chores."
    b. "You should tell your family that you are sick and cannot possibly do household work."
    c. "Tell me more about how you are feeling and the expectations of your family."
    d. "Perhaps the doctor should talk to your family and set some limits."

■ ■ ■ **The Client with a Vascular Disorder of the Kidneys**

40. The single most important contributor to healthy kidney function is:
    a. acid-base balance.
    b. vasomotor tone.
    c. sufficient electrolytes.
    d. adequate blood supply.

41. Which of the following kidney disorders is implicated in secondary hypertension?
    a. glomerulonephritis
    b. renal vein occlusion
    c. renal artery stenosis
    d. lupus nephritis

42. In malignant hypertension, the diastolic pressure is in excess of (a) _____ mm Hg and can be as high as (b) _____ mm Hg.

43. A 28-year-old client has a blood pressure reading of 190/96, and the nurse hears a bruit over his epigastric area. The most appropriate action by the nurse is to:
    a. refer him for evaluation as soon as possible.
    b. monitor his blood pressure for the next 3 weeks.
    c. assess his stress level at work and home.
    d. teach him relaxation exercises.

■ ■ ■ **The Client with a Neoplastic Disorder of the Kidneys**

44. The most common clinical symptom that is seen in the client with renal cell cancer is:
    a. proteinuria.   b. hematuria.   c. cloudy urine.   d. painful urination.

45. Three systemic symptoms of renal carcinomas include:
    (a) _____   (c) _____
    (b) _____

46. Following a radical nephrectomy for renal cell carcinoma, the priority concern for the nurse is:
    a. pain management.
    b. discharge teaching.
    c. managing anxiety.
    d. turning and positioning.

47. The nurse is caring for a client who just had a nephrectomy. The nurse observes bright red blood in the urinary catheter drainage system. An appropriate action by the nurse is to:
    a. start a continuous bladder irrigation.
    b. assess vital signs and report bleeding.
    c. note bleeding and continue to monitor.
    d. recognize that hematuria is expected following nephrectomy.

48. Following a nephrectomy, fluid intake should be:
    a. 2000–2500 mL each day.
    b. less than 2000 mL each day.
    c. over 3000 mL each day.
    d. equal to urinary output.

49. The nurse is teaching a client about home care following a nephrectomy. Which statement by the client indicates a need for further teaching?
    a. "I should urinate before and after intercourse."
    b. "I should drink 2000 to 2500 mL each day."
    c. "I can return to gymnastics 6 weeks after surgery."
    d. "I should report burning, frequency, or urgency."

▪ ▪ ▪ The Client with Renal Failure

For each statement, identify whether the cause of renal failure is prerenal, intrarenal, or postrenal.

50. A client is in a motor vehicle accident and ruptures the bladder. _____

51. A client overdoses on a nephrotoxic drug. _____

52. A client has pregnancy-induced hypertension. _____

53. A client is found to have urinary obstruction secondary to uric acid crystals. _____

54. A client has systolic heart failure. _____

55. A client has anasarca secondary to hypoalbuminemia. _____

56. The nurse is examining the specific gravity in the urinalysis of a client in acute renal failure (ARF). Typically, the specific gravity result would show that the:
    a. urine is concentrated, having a specific gravity of 1.045.
    b. urine is dilute, having a specific gravity of 1.000.
    c. specific gravity is equal to that of plasma, 1.010.
    d. urine contains brownish pigmented casts.

57. When teaching a client who is prescribed an aminoglycoside, the nurse should be certain to instruct the client:
    a. to drink at least 2–3 L of water per day.
    b. to discontinue taking the medication when symptoms subside.
    c. to expect changes in the frequency and amount of urination.
    d. to hold the medication for one day if the urine becomes concentrated.

58. When a client is receiving an aminoglycoside antibiotic, the nurse should monitor which three laboratory values?

    (a) _____

    (b) _____

    (c) _____

59. Which client is at the highest risk for the development of postrenal failure?

    a. a 29-year-old pregnant female

    b. a 75-year-old male

    c. a 15-year-old male with diabetes

    d. a 16-month-old hospitalized infant

60. Which of the following urine patterns is seen in the maintenance phase of acute renal failure?

    a. anuria

    b. polyuria

    c. oliguria

    d. hypovolemia

61. Which of the following electrolyte imbalances is characteristic of the maintenance phase of acute renal failure?

    a. hyperkalemia

    b. hypokalemia

    c. hypophosphatemia

    d. hypercalcemia

62. Explain why the client in the diuretic phase of acute renal failure continues to have impaired renal function.

63. Dopamine (Itropin) is prescribed to the client in acute renal failure to:

    a. increase the intravascular volume.

    b. dilate the urinary bladder.

    c. dilate the blood vessels of the kidney.

    d. raise the client's blood pressure.

64. The desired outcome in the client receiving sodium polystyrene sulfonate (Kayexalate) is:

    a. several loose stools.

    b. an increase in the potassium level.

    c. an increase in the sodium level.

    d. an increase in the volume of urine produced.

65. The primary purpose of administering aluminum hydroxide to a client in acute renal failure is:

    a. to prevent the client from developing ulcers.

    b. to reduce the amount of potassium in the serum.

    c. to wash out the kidney of nephrotoxic metabolites.

    d. to reduce the amount of phosphate in the serum.

66. A nurse is caring for a client in acute renal failure. He receives an order to restrict his client's fluid. To calculate the client's daily intake, the nurse adds the previous urine output to the client's insensible losses. Insensible losses (respiration, perspiration, and bowel) are allotted:

    a. 250 mL.   b. 500 mL.   c. 750 mL.   d. 1000 mL.

67. The primary difference between hemodialysis (HD) and peritoneal dialysis (PD) is that:
    a. fluid is removed with HD and not with PD.
    b. PD uses the client's peritoneum as the dialyzing membrane.
    c. HD is the only procedure that removes nephrotoxins.
    d. PD cannot be used in the client with acute renal failure.

68. A client in acute renal failure has life-threatening hyperphosphatemia. Which of the following findings is least likely for this client?
    a. hyporeflexia
    b. hyperreflexia
    c. paresthesia
    d. tetany

69. A client is in acute renal failure. She asks her mother to bring her coffee from her favorite coffee shop. The best response by the nurse at this time is:
    a. "That's fine. Having something she enjoys would make her feel better."
    b. "I'm sorry, but your daughter is not able to have any fluids at this time."
    c. "That would be fine; however, I must know how much she is drinking."
    d. "Coffee is a diuretic, and your daughter may not have any diuretics at this time."

70. A client is being discharged during the maintenance phase of acute renal failure. It is important for the nurse to teach the client that she:
    a. can resume the diet that she consumed prior to going into acute renal failure.
    b. should now consume a large amount of protein to help regain her strength.
    c. should record all of her urine output, and ingest twice as much fluid as she is voiding.
    d. should continue to follow all of the fluid and dietary recommendations she has learned thus far.

71. Which of the following cultural groups has the highest incidence of end-stage renal disease?
    a. European Americans
    b. Asian Americans
    c. Native Americans
    d. Hispanic Americans

72. In the client with chronic renal failure, the most common cardiovascular clinical manifestation is:
    a. edema.
    b. hypertension.
    c. cardiac arrhythmias.
    d. cardiomyopathy.

73. The nurse completes a motor assessment of a client with progressive uremia. The nurse would enter which of the following nursing orders into the client's plan of care?
    a. ambulate client 4 times every shift
    b. when in bed, maintain side rails up at all times
    c. do not provide range-of-motion exercises
    d. maintain client on bed rest at all times

74. The advantage of using peritoneal dialysis (PD) when compared with hemodialysis (HD) is that:
    a. HD is more effective for removing fluid than PD.
    b. HD is less expensive than PD.
    c. PD offers the client control over his or her problem.
    d. PD requires less client involvement than HD.

75. A client is receiving a left arm arteriovenous fistula for long-term hemodialysis. Which of the following preoperative nursing interventions would not be appropriate?
    a. aggressively hydrate client prior to surgery
    b. assess the client's respiratory function
    c. check that informed consent has been obtained
    d. restrict venipuncture and blood pressure to the left arm

76. Three common problems seen with AV fistulas are:
    (a) _____   (c) _____
    (b) _____

77. A client has acute renal failure. Her hematocrit is 24.5%. In this situation, the nurse knows that:
    a. unexplained bleeding can occur in ARF.
    b. erythropoietin levels are reduced.
    c. edema has resulted in hemodilution.
    d. a transfusion is indicated.

78. A client just underwent an aortic aneurysm repair. She has had only 15 mL of urine output since surgery. The nurse knows that the client:
    a. will increase her urine output when intraoperative fluid losses have been replaced.
    b. may be suffering from early symptoms of acute renal failure.
    c. needs to have her catheter removed and discontinued.
    d. requires more vigorous fluid replacement and the nurse should call for orders.

79. A client is taking Lasix (furosemide). Which statement by the client indicates a need for further teaching?
    a. "I should rise slowly from a sitting or lying position."
    b. "I should take this with food or milk."
    c. "I should take this at bedtime."
    d. "I should avoid nonsteroidal anti-inflammatory drugs."

80. While caring for a client with ARF, the nurse should monitor the client for signs and symptoms of:
    a. hyperkalemia, hyponatremia, and hyperphosphatemia.
    b. hypokalemia, hypernatremia, and hypophosphatemia.
    c. hyperkalemia, hypernatremia, and hypophosphatemia.
    d. hypokalemia, hyponatremia, and hyperphosphatemia.

81. The nurse is caring for a client on hemodialysis. The client has not voided in 24 hours. The most appropriate action by the nurse is to:
    a. obtain an order to catheterize the client.
    b. encourage more fluids.
    c. use suggestive voiding techniques.
    d. continue to monitor voiding.

▪ ▪ ▪ Renal Transplantation

82. A client experiencing an acute rejection of a transplanted kidney would have which of the following physical findings?
    a. diarrhea
    b. tenderness at the graft site
    c. periumbilical discoloration
    d. increase in urine output

83. Identify two nursing interventions that are appropriate following renal transplantation.

    (a) _____

    (b) _____

84. Discuss two priorities when the nurse is providing care to a client who is in the preoperative phase prior to renal transplantation.

    (a) _____

    (b) _____

85. List complications associated with long-term immunosuppression.

    (a) _____

    (b) _____

    (c) _____

■ ■ ■ **Critical Thinking Exercises**

86. The nurse is caring for a client who is on a 1000-cc oral fluid restriction. Develop a plan to assist the client in complying with this restriction.

87. Develop a presentation related to fatigue to assist clients with renal failure in coping with this side effect.

88. The nurse is caring for a client who just underwent a nephrectomy. He asks the nurse how he should manage his care after discharge. Develop a discharge instruction sheet for him to take home.

■ ■ ■ **Additional Learning Experiences**

■ Consult with your clinical instructor about observing clients undergoing outpatient hemodialysis.

■ Attend a support group for clients with renal failure.

■ Interview clients who have undergone radiologic procedures to diagnose a kidney problem.

Assessing Clients
with Cardiac Disorders

■ ■ ■ **Focused Study Tips**

- Discuss the anatomy and physiology of the heart, including the normal blood flow through the chambers and valves, as well as coronary circulation and conduction.

- Listen to heart sounds and differentiate between normal and abnormal sounds.

■ ■ ■ **Anatomy and Physiology**

1. The apex of the heart is located:
   a. midline with the sternum.
   b. beneath the second rib.
   c. near the left lower lobe of the lung.
   d. approximate with the left fifth intercostal space, midpoint to the clavicle.

2. Which of the following structures is not adjacent to the heart?
   a. lungs   b. sternum   c. liver   d. diaphragm

Match the descriptions (a–j) with the correct anatomical structures of the heart listed in questions 3–12.

_____ 3. pulmonary valve

_____ 4. tricuspid valve

_____ 5. chordae tendineae

_____ 6. ventricles

_____ 7. mitral valve

_____ 8. pericardial sac

_____ 9. semilunar valves

_____ 10. myocardium

_____ 11. coronary arteries

_____ 12. atria

a. a covering over the heart
b. the middle layer of the heart wall
c. vessels that encircle the myocardium
d. connect the ventricles to the great vessels
e. the atrioventricular valve on the right side of the heart
f. joins the right ventricle with the pulmonary artery
g. pumping chambers of the heart
h. structures that control the movement of the AV valves
i. hollow upper chambers of the heart
j. another name for the bicuspid valve

13. The amount of blood pumped by the ventricles into the pulmonary and systemic circulation in 1 minute is known as:
   a. cardiac output.   b. stroke volume.   c. ejection fraction.   d. systolic heart rate.

14. The (a) _____ nervous system increases heart rate, while the (b) _____ nervous system slows heart rate.

15. The percentage of the blood emptied from the ventricle during contraction (systole) is known as the _____.

16. The amount of blood ejected by the left ventricle at each heartbeat is known as the _____ _____.

17. Which of the following statements is true? Correct any false statements.
    a. Preload is the amount of cardiac muscle fiber tension that exists at the end of systole.
    b. Preload is measured as systemic vascular resistance.
    c. Afterload is the force the ventricles must overcome to eject their blood volume.
    d. Afterload is influenced by venous return and the compliance of the ventricles.

18. The inherent capability of the cardiac muscle fibers to shorten is known as:
    a. elasticity.   b. contractility.   c. excitability.   d. ischemia.

19. Describe the conduction of electricity through the heart, beginning with the sinoatrial node.

20. _____ is the process by which sodium, potassium, and calcium ions are exchanged across the cardiac muscle cell membrane, causing the intracellular electrical charge to change to a positive state.

21. The cellular action potential of the heart serves as a basis for what diagnostic test?
    a. phonocardiography   c. electrocardiography
    b. stress testing   d. angiographic studies

22. The best indicator of how effective the heart is as a pump is _____.

▪ ▪ ▪ Assessment of Cardiac Function

23. The assessment of the cardiac system begins with an exploration of the client's _____ _____.

24. Which of the following is the least significant assessment area for the interview of a client with a disorder of cardiac function?
    a. history of recurrent infections
    b. history of previous surgeries
    c. family history of neoplastic disorders
    d. family history of coronary artery disease

25. During the physical assessment, the nurse does *not* inspect the precordial area of the client's chest for the following movements:
    (a) _____
    (b) _____
    (c) _____
    (d) _____

Match the cardiac disorders (a–k) with the correct heart sounds listed in questions 26–36.

_____ 26. fixed splitting

_____ 27. diminished S2

_____ 28. atrial gallop

_____ 29. accentuated S2

_____ 30. abnormal splitting of S1

_____ 31. friction rub

_____ 32. ventricular gallop

_____ 33. diminished S1

_____ 34. paradoxical splitting

_____ 35. wide splitting of S2

_____ 36. opening snap

a. myocardial failure and ventricular overload

b. atrial septal defect

c. mitral stenosis or cor pulmonale

d. stenotic mitral valve

e. left bundle branch block

f. mitral regurgitation

g. hypertension, cardiomyopathy

h. right bundle branch block, premature ventricular contraction

i. aortic and pulmonic stenosis

j. first-degree heart block

k. pericarditis

Case Study

Julius Janovich is a 72-year-old client who is admitted for recurring episodes of tachycardia accompanied by lightheadedness, vertigo, and transient numbness in his left arm. Upon interviewing the client, the nurse obtains the following information: Mr. Janovich has smoked a pack of cigarettes daily for 35 years, has noticed increasing fatigue in his activities of daily living, and is short of breath at night. He has found that using an extra pillow when he goes to bed helps with his difficulty breathing. His father and brother both died of heart disease in their early 60s. He attributes his "good health" to the fact that he doesn't eat red meat and drinks a "shot of vodka every day."

On examination, the nurse determines that Mr. Janovich is 6'4" tall and weighs 228 lbs. His vital signs are: pulse 106 at rest, B/P 150/98, respirations 20, and temperature 98.4F. On inspection, the nurse notes slight retraction of the precordium. On auscultation, the nurse notes bigeminy and atrial and ventricular gallops.

37. Identify the significant cardiac assessment findings and describe the implications of each finding.

38. The increased anteroposterior diameter of the chest in older adults may make the _____ _____ difficult to locate.

39. The sounds made by turbulent blood flow through the heart are known as:

a. ejection sounds.

b. sinus dysrhythmia.

c. bruits.

d. murmurs.

40. Describe three steps to utilize as guidelines for cardiac auscultation.

(a) _____

(b) _____

(c) _____

Match the following descriptions (41–47) with the grade or characteristic of murmurs (a–i).

_____ 41. loudest

_____ 42. loud

_____ 43. barely heard

_____ 44. clearly heard

_____ 45. low, medium, high

_____ 46. crescendo/decrescendo

_____ 47. harsh, blowing, or musical

a. Grade I
b. Grade II
c. Grade III
d. Grade IV
e. Grade V
f. Grade VI
g. pitch
h. quality
i. pattern

48. List three common age-related changes of the cardiovascular system experienced by older adults.

(a) _____

(b) _____

(c) _____

Read the statements below and determine if they are true or false. Correct any false statements.

_____ 49. The heart rate of an older adult may be over 100, especially if the client is sedentary.

_____ 50. The risk of arteriosclerosis of the coronary arteries decreases as one ages.

_____ 51. As one ages, the heart valves thin and there is an increase in cardiac reserve.

_____ 52. The apical impulse is easier to locate as the chest wall thins.

▪ ▪ ▪ Critical Thinking Exercises

53. The nurse is caring for a 48-year-old client who is worried about heart disease. Identify assessment questions that will help the nurse determine her current heart health and risk state.

54. A client is told by the cardiologist that his ejection fraction is low. Explain what this means to the client.

55. The client is starting on medications that will affect his preload and afterload. His wife asks, "What does that mean?" How would the nurse explain these concepts to her and the client?

▪ ▪ ▪ Additional Learning Experiences

- Practice cardiac assessments on every client you encounter and on willing family members.
- Consult with your instructor about attending a cardiac rehabilitation program.
- Visit the World Wide Web and identify resources for clients trying to minimize risk factors for cardiac disease.

CHAPTER 28

Nursing Care of Clients with Cardiac Disorders

■ ■ ■ **Focused Study Tips**

- Identify normal sinus rhythm, sinus tachycardia, sinus bradycardia, ventricular tachycardia, and premature ventricular contractions.

- Describe the principles and procedures for cardiopulmonary resuscitation.

- Compare and contrast the various classifications of medications used for dysrhythmias, angina, myocardial infarction, and congestive heart failure. Describe the modes of action of

each classification, their side effects, adverse effects, and toxic effects.

- Identify the risk factors for various cardiac disorders, especially disorders of myocardial perfusion and cardiac failure.

- Discuss the relationships of activity, rest, and oxygen requirements during acute episodes of cardiac illness, recovery, and rehabilitation.

■ ■ ■ **The Client with a Cardiac Dysrhythmia**

1. The primary pacemaker of the heart is the (a) _____, which usually fires at a rate of (b) _____ times per minute. The impulse is slowed when it reaches the (c) _____. This delay allows the atria to contract, delivering a bolus of blood to the (d) _____ before they contract; this extra amount of blood accounts for the (e) _____. The electrical conduction pathways through the ventricle include (in order) the (f) _____, (g) _____, and finally the (h) _____. In the event that there is failure of the primary pacemaker, secondary pacemakers located in the (i) _____ or (j) _____ will take over. In this instance, the heart rate will be (k) _____ than that resulting from the usual pacemaker.

Match the definitions (a–j) with the correct terms listed in questions 2–11.

_____ 2. automaticity

_____ 3. conductivity

_____ 4. contractility

_____ 5. depolarization

_____ 6. excitability

_____ 7. myocardial working cells

_____ 8. pacemaker cells

_____ 9. polarized

_____ 10. refractory period

_____ 11. sarcomere

a. the ability of a cell to transmit an impulse from cell to cell

b. portion of myocardial cell where calcium ions act on actin and myosin, causing myocardial contraction

c. the ability of a cardiac working cell to respond to an electrical impulse

d. cells that spontaneously generate an electrical impulse

e. myocardial cells that contract in response to an impulse

f. the natural ability of myocardial fibers to shorten in response to an electrical stimulus

g. the condition of a cell in the resting state with positive and negative ions aligned on either side of the cell membrane

h. the stage in which a cell is resistant to stimulation

i. ability of the pacemaker cell to spontaneously initiate an electrical impulse

j. the change in a membrane potential from a negative to a positive state

Match the descriptions (a–f) with ECG terms listed in questions 12–16.

_____ 12. P wave

_____ 13. P-R interval

_____ 14. QRS complex

_____ 15. QT interval

_____ 16. ST segment

a. represents ventricular repolarization

b. represents atrial depolarization and contraction

c. total time for ventricular depolarization and repolarization

d. represents ventricular depolarization and contraction

e. represents time needed for sinus impulse to reach the AV node and enter the bundle branches

f. represents the beginning of ventricular depolarization

17. An alteration in conductivity that results in a delay in or failure of impulse transmission is a ____
_____.

18. Sinus tachycardia has all of the characteristics of a normal sinus rhythm (NSR) except that the rate is _____.

19. Sinus bradycardia may be the result of:
    a. stimulation of the sympathetic nervous system.
    b. a fever.
    c. vagal stimulation.
    d. acute blood loss.

20. Paroxysmal supraventricular tachycardia (PSVT) results in manifestation of decreased cardiac output because PSVT causes (a) _____ and (b) _____.

21. The sawtooth or picket fence appearance of the P wave on an ECG is indicative of _____
_____.

22. Which of the following clients does not require continuous cardiac monitoring?
    a. a 24-year-old male who is 6 hours posttonsillectomy
    b. a 43-year-old female with chest pain of unknown etiology
    c. a 78-year-old male with a dissecting thoracic aortic aneurysm
    d. a 25-year-old female with multiple trauma of the legs, pelvis, and possibly the head

23. A 55-year-old male is diagnosed with myocardial infarction (MI). After having occasional premature ventricular contractions (PVCs), the cardiac monitor shows a 35-second run of ventricular tachycardia (VT). The drug most likely to be given for this is:
    a. digoxin (Lanoxin).
    b. diltiazem (Cardizem).
    c. atropine.
    d. lidocaine (Xylocaine).

24. A coronary care unit (CCU) nurse is caring for a client known to have cardiac dysrhythmias. The monitor alarm sounds and the monitor is displaying a flat line. The nurse's first action should be to:
    a. call a code.
    b. assess the client.
    c. prepare epinephrine.
    d. page the physician STAT.

25. During emergency external defibrillation, it is of vital importance that:
    a. there is continuous heart and lung auscultation during the procedure.
    b. the paddles be positioned precisely at the heart's apex and over the xiphoid process.
    c. no one is touching the client when the "all clear" signal is called.
    d. a second shock is not administered for at least 90 seconds.

26. Which intervention is contraindicated when caring for the client following pacemaker insertion?
    a. monitoring pacemaker function, heart rate, and rhythm
    b. maintaining sterile dressing and keeping the incision clean and dry
    c. encouraging active and full range of motion of the affected shoulder
    d. providing analgesics and positioning for comfort

27. A 49-year-old client tells the nurse that she has had "electrical problems" with her heart. She states that the doctor is going to implant a device that will recognize life-threatening changes in her cardiac rhythm and automatically deliver an electric shock. Based on these statements, the nurse recognizes that the physician is planning on inserting:
    a. a pacemaker.   b. an AICD.   c. a defibrillator.   d. a cryoprobe.

28. Identify three safety precautions required when caring for the client with an external pacemaker.
    (a) _____
    (b) _____
    (c) _____

■ ■ ■   **The Client with Sudden Cardiac Death**

29. A home care nurse proficient in basic cardiac life support finds a client who is unresponsive and without a palpable peripheral pulse or respiratory movement. The nurse's first action in this situation is to:
    a. dial 911.
    b. give two breaths to the clients.
    c. perform five chest compressions.
    d. give adrenalin intravenously.

30. Because most instances of sudden cardiac death result from ventricular fibrillation, immediate _____ is appropriate.

31. The monitor technician tells the nurse that a client's monitor pattern is ventricular tachycardia with a heart rate of 250 bpm. The client is alert, oriented, and sitting up in the chair talking. An appropriate response by the nurse is to:
    a. prepare the client for an emergency cardioversion.
    b. immediately defibrillate the client at 200 joules.
    c. administer to the client a bolus of lidocaine and start a lidocaine drip.
    d. return the client to bed and assess her vital signs.

■ ■ ■   **The Client with Coronary Artery Disease (CAD)**

32. Define CAD. _____
    _____

33. The highest incidence of CAD in the United States is found in:
    a. African American males under 25 years of age.
    b. females of all races under 65 years of age.
    c. European American females after menopause.
    d. European American males over 45 years of age.

34. A modifiable risk factor for CAD is:
    a. gender.　　　　b. age.　　　　c. smoking.　　　　d. race.

35. Obesity is a risk factor for CAD if the client is (a) _____ % above ideal body weight and the fat stores are primarily in the (b)_____ area.

36. (a) _____ is considered "bad" cholesterol because it deposits cholesterol on the artery walls. In contrast, (b) _____ is considered "good" cholesterol because it helps clear cholesterol from the arteries, transporting it to the liver for excretion.

37. A client tells the nurse that he does not have to worry about heart disease. He states, "My cholesterol is only 198." He also reports a two-pack-per-day smoking history. The most appropriate response by the nurse is:
    a. "You are right, a desirable cholesterol is under 200."
    b. "You should have your low density lipoprotein and high density lipoprotein checked."
    c. "Your number one risk factor for heart disease is smoking."
    d. "Keep up the good work; but try to cut down on smoking."

38. List five modifiable lifestyle risk factors for coronary artery disease and at least one nursing intervention to help a client modify the risk factor.
    (a) _____
    (b) _____
    (c) _____
    (d) _____
    (e) _____

39. A client tells the nurse that his cholesterol is 220 mg/dL. He asks if this is normal. The most appropriate response by the nurse is:
    a. "It is borderline high, and you should have it retested in 3 years."
    b. "It is within acceptable normal limits, and you should have it retested next year."
    c. "It is borderline high, and a low-fat, low cholesterol diet may help to decrease it."
    d. "Don't worry about your cholesterol level, the only test we worry about is your triglyceride level."

40. A client is on a low-fat, low cholesterol diet. Which diet selection is most appropriate for breakfast?
    a. scrambled eggs, home fries, dry toast, marmalade, and orange juice
    b. oatmeal, a banana, a bran muffin, and apple juice
    c. cold cereal, low-fat milk, whole wheat toast and jelly, and grapefruit juice
    d. a bagel with low-fat cream cheese, orange juice, and dried fruit

41. A client is taking lovastatin to lower his cholesterol. He tells the nurse he is experiencing muscle aches and pains. He believes it is related to his age and a recent increase in activity. The most appropriate response by the nurse is:
    a. "You are probably right, take it easy with your exercise, and see how you feel."
    b. "Try taking some ibuprofen on a regular basis when you exercise."
    c. "Contact your physician, and let him know that you are experiencing aches and pains."
    d. "Let your physician know about these symptoms if they are not relieved by ibuprofen."

▪ ▪ ▪ The Client with Angina Pectoris

42. Angina pectoris is the result of a temporary imbalance between myocardial oxygen (a) _____ _____ and (b) _____.

43. Which of the following statements is true about angina pectoris?
    a. It consistently follows physical activity.
    b. It may be described as a tight, heavy, or squeezing sensation.
    c. It begins over the the heart and radiates to the epigastric region.
    d. It usually lasts about 30 minutes per episode.

44. During periods of myocardial ischemia, the ECG will show an ST segment which is (a) _____ _____ and a T wave which is (b) _____ or (c) _____.

45. An exercise electrocardiogram is considered positive if the client:
    a. has any premature atrial or ventricular contractions.
    b. has a 20% increase in the heart rate.
    c. has muscle pain in the calves.
    d. has ST depressions on the tracing.

46. The drug of choice for treatment of an acute anginal attack is (a) _____, taken by the (b) _____ route.

47. Which of the following is appropriate teaching for a client who is prescribed sublingual nitroglycerin for acute angina?
    a. Take one dose. If that does not relieve the pain, repeat it after 5 minutes. If after another 5 minutes the pain is still present, take a third dose and call 911.
    b. Notify your physician or go to the emergency room immediately after you have found it necessary to take a dose of nitroglycerin.
    c. If the first dose does not relieve the pain, call your physician and go to the emergency room or the physician's office or clinic.
    d. Take one dose. If that does not relieve the pain, repeat it after 5 minutes. After taking the second dose, seek out medical help.

48. For the client who is prescribed transdermal nitroglycerin, the incidence of tolerance can be reduced by instructing the client to _____.

49. Identify the four common side effects of nitrate therapy.
    (a) _____
    (b) _____
    (c) _____
    (d) _____

50. A client experiences bradycardia with a heart rate of 40 bpm during sheath removal. The most important intervention by the nurse is to:
    a. know that this is an expected, transitory experience.
    b. administer atropine IV according to protocol.
    c. apply oxygen and maintain bedrest.
    d. use an ammonia inhaler as a noxious stimuli.

51. A client complains of chest pain following a percutaneous transluminal coronary angioplasty (PTCA). The most appropriate action by the nurse is to:
    a. recognize this is a common experience following this procedure.
    b. administer analgesics as ordered for procedure-related pain.
    c. teach the client to expect this type of discomfort for a few days.
    d. apply oxygen, administer nitroglycerin as ordered, and contact the physician.

52. A client is recovering from a coronary artery bypass graft. She complains of chest pain. The most appropriate action by the nurse is to:
    a. administer oral narcotics for incisional pain.
    b. apply oxygen and administer nitroglycerin.
    c. differentiate this pain as incisional or anginal.
    d. assess her vital signs and contact the physician.

53. A client has just been extubated following open heart surgery. Her oxygen saturation is 87%. The most appropriate action by the nurse is to:
    a. re-intubate her and administer oxygen.
    b. assist her to sit up and deep breathe.
    c. take off the nasal oxygen and put on a face mask.
    d. suction her vigorously and assess her skin color.

■ ■ ■ The Client with Acute Myocardial Infarction

54. A client is scheduled for a cardiac catheterization with a PTCA of the right coronary artery (RCA). When performing preprocedure teaching, the nurse will inform the client that:
    a. he will be npo after 6 AM on the morning of the procedure.
    b. chest pain or shortness of breath experienced during the procedure is normal and he should not be concerned.
    c. he may have a sensation of flushing and a metallic taste in his mouth when the dye is administered during the procedure.
    d. he will be asleep during the procedure.

55. Identify at least three immediate assessment priorities for the above client following the PTCA.
    (a) _____
    (b) _____
    (c) _____

56. Knowing that the angioplastied lesion was the RCA, an occlusion of that vessel would manifest itself in the _____ leads.

57. Lab values that are important to check postangioplasty or postcardiac catheterization include (a) _____, (b) _____, (c) _____, (d) _____, and (e) _____.

Read the following statement and determine if is true or false. Correct the statement if it is false.

_____ 58. For the client who has undergone a coronary artery bypass graft (CABG), speaking will not be possible while the endotracheal tube is in place.

59. The underlying pathology of most myocardial infarctions is:
    a. the presence of atherosclerotic plaques in a coronary artery.
    b. noncompliance with a treatment regimen.
    c. genetic predisposition to hyperlipidemia.
    d. a type A personality resulting in coronary artery spasm.

60. Coronary artery occlusion and myocardial ischemia is usually caused by a _____ _____ developing at a site of arterial narrowing.

61. Myocardial infarctions occur most often in the (a) _____ as a result of an occlusion of the (b) _____.

62. Describe how manifestations of a myocardial infarction differ from the manifestations of an acute anginal attack.

63. The most common complication of a myocardial infarction is _____.

64. The risk of developing pump failure and cardiogenic shock following a myocardial infarction is greatest when the infarct involves the:
    a. left atrium.   b. left ventricle.   c. right ventricle.   d. posterior septum.

65. The specific cardiac isoenzyme that peaks most rapidly after acute myocardial damage is:
    a. CK-BB.   b. LDH.   c. CK-MB.   d. LD1.

66. A 75-year-old client is admitted to the emergency department (ED) with chest pain and ECG changes indicative of an acute anterior MI. Which of the following findings from the client's history is not a contraindication for thrombolytic therapy?
    a. The client's chest pain began 2 hours prior to admission to the ED.
    b. The client had surgery for colon cancer 3 weeks ago.
    c. Hypertension was diagnosed 3 years ago and has not been adequately controlled.
    d. The client has diabetes and a history of hemorrhagic retinopathy.

67. The drug of choice for relief of the above client's acute chest pain is morphine sulfate. It does not:
    a. stimulate the sympathetic nervous system to counter hypotension.
    b. decrease the client's anxiety as well as the perception of pain.
    c. decrease the preload and afterload of the heart.
    d. decrease the rate and depth of respirations.

■ ■ ■ **The Client with Congestive Heart Failure**

68. The definition of heart failure is _____ _____.

69. Research indicates that chronic heart failure among African Americans is related to:
    a. hypertension.
    b. obesity.
    c. diabetes mellitus.
    d. congenital heart defects.

70. Identify the three compensatory mechanisms activated in heart failure.
    (a) _____
    (b) _____
    (c) _____

71. The earliest manifestation of left-sided heart failure usually is:
    a. rhonchi throughout the lung fields.
    b. fatigue with activity intolerance.
    c. marked dyspnea.
    d. dependent edema.

72. The most common cause of right-sided heart failure is _____.

73. Which of the following is not a manifestation of right-sided heart failure?
    a. abdominal distention
    b. rapid, thready pulse
    c. jugular venous distention
    d. peripheral edema

74. Foods prohibited for a client who is on a low-salt diet include:
    a. salad greens.
    b. rye breads.
    c. jelly and jams.
    d. canned soups and meats.

75. The pulmonary artery catheter is used to assess _____
    _____.

76. A client is recovering from an acute MI. He calls for the nurse and reports that he is experiencing air hunger and a sense of impending doom. The nurse should recognize that he is most likely experiencing:
    a. an extension of his MI.
    b. a dysrhythmia.
    c. acute anxiety.
    d. pulmonary edema.

77. A client suffers from congestive heart failure. He has gained 3 pounds in the last 2 days. The nurse should instruct him to:
    a. increase his diuretic dose.
    b. decrease his oral intake.
    c. go to the emergency room.
    d. contact his physician.

78. A client is taking digoxin for his congestive heart failure. He starts experiencing nausea and blurred vision. The most appropriate action by the nurse is to:
    a. advise him to stop his digoxin immediately.
    b. tell him to take his pulse and report it if it is under 60 bpm.
    c. advise him to contact his health care provider.
    d. instruct him to reduce his dose by one-half.

79. What components should be included in a teaching plan for a client with CHF?

80. Compare and contrast the clinical manifestations and causes of right- and left-sided heart failure.

▪ ▪ ▪ **The Client with Pulmonary Edema**

81. The primary goals for treatment of acute pulmonary edema are:
    a. decreasing the sodium level and maintaining the potassium level.
    b. reducing excess pulmonary system fluid and improving gas exchange.
    c. controlling the tachypnea and tachycardia and keeping the client in an upright position.
    d. reducing the client's anxiety and administering oxygen.

82. The drug of choice for treating anxiety, hypertension, and tachypnea of pulmonary edema is (a) _____, given initially by the (b)_____ route.

83. It is 3 AM and a client is complaining of symptoms consistent with pulmonary edema. The most appropriate action by the nurse is to:
    a. call the physician immediately.
    b. wait until the morning to call the physician.
    c. give the client prn medications.
    d. monitor the client and assess for further problems.

Read the following statements and indicate if they are true or false. Correct any false statements.

_____ 84. Morphine is contraindicated in acute pulmonary edema.

_____ 85. Loop diuretics should be administered intravenously in acute pulmonary edema.

_____ 86. Vasodilators will only increase the severity of pulmonary edema.

_____ 87. In acute pulmonary edema, place the client in a high-Fowler's position with legs dangling.

_____ 88. Emergent care in acute pulmonary edema focuses on relieving anxiety and removing excess fluids.

▪ ▪ ▪ **The Client with Valvular Disorders**

89. Most often, the earliest manifestation of stenosis of the mitral valve is:
    a. pedal edema.
    c. jugular venous distention.
    b. dyspnea on exertion.
    d. paroxysmal nocturnal dyspnea.

90. Mitral stenosis often leads to atrial fibrillation as a result of chronic atrial distention. The nurse must be aware that this places the client at particular risk for:
    a. ascites.
    c. palpitations.
    b. pulmonary edema.
    d. cerebral vascular accident (CVA).

91. Which of the following statements is not true about aortic stenosis?
    a. Aortic stenosis is often asymptomatic in the early stages, but usually progresses.
    b. Left ventricular hypertension is a compensatory mechanism of aortic stenosis.
    c. Pulse pressure widens to greater than 50 mm Hg in the later stages of aortic stenosis.
    d. Aortic stenosis produces a harsh systolic murmur, heard best at the second intercostal space to the right of the sternum.

92. All persons who have valvular disease must be instructed to inform other health care providers, especially their dentist, of their valvular disorder. Why is this necessary? _____
    _____
    _____ .

93. In caring for a client having a balloon valvuloplasty, the nurse knows that the postprocedure care is similar to that given to a client with CAD who has undergone _____ .

94. In caring for a client after valve replacement surgery, the nurse observes carefully for indications of decreasing cardiac output. Manifestations of this complication include:
    a. a rising systolic pressure with a stable diastolic pressure.
    b. increasing respiratory crackles and dyspnea.
    c. acute weight loss.
    d. decreasing pulmonary artery and wedge pressures.

Match the etiologies (a–c) with the classifications of cardiomyopathy listed in questions 95–97.

_____ 95. dilated

_____ 96. hypertrophic

_____ 97. restrictive

a. amyloidosis; radiation
b. heredity; chronic hypertension
c. idiopathic; possibly alcoholism or myocarditis

98. Identify two nursing goals for care of a client with dilated or restrictive cardiomyopathy.
    (a) _____
    (b) _____

■ ■ ■ The Client with Cardiomyopathy

99. Differentiate between primary and secondary cardiomyopathies.

100. What is the prognosis for an individual diagnosed with dilated cardiomyopathy?

101. What three findings on a chest x-ray are consistent with cardiomyopathy?
    (a) _____
    (b) _____
    (c) _____

102. Develop a teaching plan for a client with cardiomyopathy.

▪ ▪ ▪ The Client with Inflammatory and Infective Cardiac Disorders

103. The disorder or condition which is most likely to result in diseases of the cardiac valves is:
    a. rheumatic fever.
    b. myocardial infarction.
    c. ventricular dysrhythmias.
    d. cardiomyopathy.

104. Rheumatic fever is the result of an altered immune response following an infection caused by:
    a. *Staphylococcus aeries.*
    b. *Treponema pallidum.*
    c. *Hemophilus influenza.*
    d. Group A *Streptococcus.*

105. Persons who are at greatest risk for the development of infective endocarditis are those with a history of:
    a. coronary artery disease.
    b. congestive heart failure.
    c. valve disorders.
    d. cardiac dysrhythmias.

106. Manifestations of infective endocarditis include flulike symptoms. Peripheral signs include:
    a. petechiae on the lower parts of the legs and the feet.
    b. splinter hemorrhages under fingernails and toenails.
    c. enlarged, nontender lymph nodes of the axilla.
    d. angina pectoris.

107. The most frequent presenting manifestation of acute pericarditis is _____.

108. A client with pericarditis is usually most comfortable in which position? _____.

109. Which of the following is not a potentially fatal complication of pericarditis?
    a. pericardial effusion
    b. cardiac tamponade
    c. cor pulmonale
    d. constrictive pericarditis

110. Pain management for clients with acute pericarditis is usually accomplished by:
    a. administering NSAIDs on a regular, round-the-clock schedule.
    b. administering meperidine or morphine by the intramuscular route as needed.
    c. positioning in high-Fowler's position in bed, or in a recliner.
    d. controlling the inflammatory process with corticosteroids and antibiotics.

111. Discharge teaching for a client who is recovering from pericarditis should include:
    a. avoiding the use of aspirin and other nonsteroidal anti-inflammatory agents.
    b. daily fluid intake must be restricted to the amount of urinary output plus 500 mL.
    c. recurrence of pericarditis is a very remote possibility.
    d. activity will be gradually increased as the inflammatory process decreases.

▪ ▪ ▪ Drug Therapies

Match the cardiac drugs (a–h) with the effects listed in questions 112–119.

_____ 112. decreases the rate and depth of respirations

_____ 113. affects the PTT (partial thromboplastin time)

_____ 114. is a positive inotrope

_____ 115. used to decrease heart rate and blood pressure

_____ 116. used to decrease blood pressure and to treat some dysrhythmias

_____ 117. decreases reload and afterload

_____ 118. vasodilates coronary arteries

_____ 119. modifies platelets

a. digoxin
b. calcium channel blockers
c. ACE inhibitors
d. beta-blockers
e. heparin
f. morphine
g. nitroglycerin
h. aspirin

▪ ▪ ▪ Critical Thinking Exercises

120. Develop a teaching plan for a client who is taking acebutolol, verapamil, and digoxin. What side effects might be observed? What symptoms should the client report to the physician?

121. A client died as a result of a sudden cardiac death. His wife asks, "How could that happen? He was fine when he saw the cardiologist last week." Develop an explanation that would assist her in understanding this cause of death.

122. Develop a presentation for fifth-grade students who want to learn how to prevent heart disease.

123. Explain how the experience of an MI may differ for an older adult compared to a younger adult.

▪ ▪ ▪ Additional Learning Experiences

▪ Consult with your instructor about observing a cardiac catheterization or electrophysiology studies.

▪ Interview clients who are attending cardiac rehabilitation about their experiences with heart disease.

▪ Visit your local chapter of the American Heart Association and explore the resources they provide.

CHAPTER 29

Assessing Clients with Peripheral Vascular and Lymphatic Disorders

▪ ▪ ▪ Focused Study Tips

- Discuss the anatomy and physiology of each part of the peripheral vascular and lymphatic systems.

- Compare and contrast the etiology and related nursing care for the various peripheral vascular and lymphatic disorders.

▪ ▪ ▪ Anatomy and Physiology

1. The two main components of the peripheral vascular system are the arterial and venous networks. Blood flows through these networks from the aorta to the (a) _____ to the (b) _____ to the (c) _____ to the (d) _____ to the (e) _____ to the (f) _____.

2. Which of the following describes what the nurse feels when assessing a client's pulse?
   a. changes in abdominal and thoracic pressure that occur with breathing
   b. the highest pressure exerted against arterial walls at the peak of ventricular contraction
   c. a pressure wave caused by the alternate expansion and contraction of an artery as the heart beats
   d. the resistance to blood flow as the channels become more distant from the heart

3. Identify three factors affecting peripheral vascular resistance.
   (a) _____
   (b) _____
   (c) _____

4. The highest pressure exerted against the arterial walls at the peak of ventricular contraction is called the:
   a. diastolic blood pressure.
   b. mean arterial blood pressure.
   c. pulse pressure.
   d. systolic blood pressure.

5. Identify the pattern of blood pressure findings (hypertensive, hypotensive, or normotensive) that the nurse would expect when assessing clients with the following conditions.
   (a) High cardiac output and high peripheral vascular resistance. _____
   (b) High cardiac output and low peripheral vascular resistance. _____
   (c) Low cardiac output and high peripheral vascular resistance. _____
   (d) Low cardiac output and low peripheral vascular resistance. _____

Match the physiologic effects on the vascular system (a–c) with the factors that influence arterial blood pressure listed in questions 6–11. Physiologic effects may be used more than once.

_____ 6. the sympathetic nervous system

_____ 7. warm temperatures

_____ 8. epinephrine

_____ 9. the parasympathetic nervous system

_____ 10. alcohol and histamine

_____ 11. the renin-angiotensin mechanism

a. vasoconstriction

b. vasodilation

c. no effect

12. Which of the following statements best describes the purpose of the lymphatic vessels?
    a. to protect the upper respiratory and digestive tracts from foreign pathogens
    b. to collect and drain excess tissue fluid that accumulates at the venous end of the capillary bed
    c. to cleanse the lymph of foreign materials, tumor cells, and infectious organisms
    d. to filter blood by breaking down old red blood cells and storing or releasing their by-products to the liver

13. Identify the five major lymphoid organs in the body.
    (a) _____
    (b) _____
    (c) _____
    (d) _____
    (e) _____

■ ■ ■ Assessment of Peripheral Vascular and Lymphatic Function

14. Identify three areas the nurse should assess when performing a health history on a client with a peripheral vascular system disorder.
    (a) _____
    (b) _____
    (c) _____

15. A 75-year-old male client has been admitted for complaints of numbness, tingling, and pain in his lower left leg. Upon inspection, his lower left leg appears pale with smooth, shiny skin. His toenails appear thickened and when placed in a dependent position his left foot becomes dusky red in color. Upon palpation his skin is cool to the touch, pulses are diminished, and capillary refill time is 3 seconds. The nurse should suspect that the client is suffering from:
    a. arterial insufficiency.
    b. aortic aneurysm.
    c. thrombophlebitis.
    d. venous insufficiency.

16. Which of the following is the least important interview question to ask a client who presents with enlarged lymph nodes and fatigue?
    a. "Do you use intravenous drugs?"
    b. "Have you ever been exposed to radiation or toxic chemicals?"
    c. "Do you notice that the glands in your neck became swollen after an infection of any kind?"
    d. "Are you currently experiencing a chronic illness such as cardiovascular disease or renal disease?"

17. The techniques used to assess the peripheral vascular system include auscultation of the (a) _____ _____, palpation of the major (b) _____ of the body, and inspection of the (c) _____ for changes such as (d) _____, and (e) _____ or alterations in (f) _____ and (g) _____.

18. A client's blood pressure is charted as 120/72/64. Explain the significance of each number.
   120:
   72:
   64:

19. Identify four sources of error when auscultating a client's blood pressure.
   (a) _____
   (b) _____
   (c) _____
   (d) _____

20. Identify three steps the nurse performs when assessing a client's lower extremities.
   (a) _____
   (b) _____
   (c) _____

21. A pulsatile mass in the upper abdomen is suggestive of:
   a. decreased cardiac output.   c. venous insufficiency.
   b. partially occluded iliac arteries. d. an aortic aneurysm.

Match the following peripheral vascular conditions (a–l) with the correct descriptions listed in questions 22–29.

_____ 22. a silent interval between systolic and diastolic BP

_____ 23. a decrease in systolic BP over 15 mm Hg and a drop in diastolic pressure on standing

_____ 24. a dusky red coloring suggesting arterial insufficiency and delayed venous return

_____ 25. a murmuring or blowing sound heard over stenosed peripheral vessels

_____ 26. blood pressure readings over 140/90 in adults

_____ 27. the difference between systolic and diastolic blood pressures

_____ 28. a pulse over 100 beats per minute at rest

_____ 29. palpable fine vibrations

a. hypertension
b. thrills
c. sinus arrhythmia
d. auscultatory gap
e. pulse pressure
f. tachycardia
g. hypotension
h. rubor
i. orthostatic hypotension
j. capillary refill
k. bruit
l. bigeminal pulse

30. Normal variations in the peripheral vascular assessment findings of the older person may include (a) _____, (b) _____, and (c) _____.

31. Lesions of the lower extremities with wide, diffuse margins, brown pigmentation of the skin, and edema are known as _____.

Match the terms (a–e) with the correct descriptions listed in questions 32–36.

_____ 32. a taut swelling of the face associated with hypothyroidism

_____ 33. swelling due to lymphatic obstruction

_____ 34. a bacterial infection of the lymph nodes

_____ 35. an enlargement of lymph nodes without tenderness

_____ 36. an inflammation of a lymphatic vessel

a. lymphangitis
b. lymphedema
c. lymphadenopathy
d. myxedema
e. lymphadenitis

37. Name at least six characteristics that should be considered during the examination of regional lymph nodes.

(a) _____ (d) _____

(b) _____ (e) _____

(c) _____ (f) _____

38. Enlargement of the left supraclavicular nodes is suggestive of _____

_____.

39. Axillary lymphadenopathy is associated with _____.

Match the terms (a–g) with the correct descriptions listed in questions 40–46.

_____ 40. loss of hair, thickened toenails, ulcerations

_____ 41. bluish discoloration of the skin and mucous membranes

_____ 42. abnormal accumulation of fluid in interstitial fluids

_____ 43. absence of color of the skin

_____ 44. the result of ischemia and hypoxia of tissue

_____ 45. tortuous and dilated veins with incompetent valves

_____ 46. necrosis that occurs as the loss of blood supply and infection

a. pallor
b. cyanosis
c. edema
d. varicose veins
e. atrophic changes
f. gangrene
g. pressure ulcers

47. A positive Homan's sign indicates that the client has:
   a. a thrombophlebitis.
   b. calf pain on dorsiflexion.
   c. no calf pain on dorsiflexion.
   d. an arterial occlusion.

48. When assessing capillary refill, the nurse notes that the capillary time is 5 seconds. The most appropriate action by the nurse is to:
   a. recognize this finding as normal.
   b. assess circulation, sensation, and motion of the extremities.
   c. continue to monitor capillary refill every 15 minutes.
   d. assess for pulsus paradoxus.

49. A pulse deficit means that:
   a. there is no ulnar pulse.
   b. the radial pulse is faster than the apical pulse.
   c. the radial pulse is slower than the apical rate.
   d. the client has thromboangitis obliterans.

50. Pulsus paradoxus occurs with which three conditions?

(a) _____

(b) _____

(c) _____

Determine whether the following statements are true or false. Correct any false statements.

_____ 51. An older adult's skin may become thinner and drier with age.

_____ 52. Decreased arterial flow in older adults results in increased hair growth in affected areas.

_____ 53. There is a decrease in the number and size of lymph nodes in older adults.

_____ 54. Systolic hypertension and orthostatic hypotension are rare occurrences in older adults.

_____ 55. The older adult is more likely to experience chronic venous insufficiency.

Case Study

Mr. Issacs is admitted with a cyanotic right foot and an ulcerated area on his right great toe. He denies pain or discomfort and tells the nurse the foot has been "funny colored for a few days." He tells the nurse that he thought he had bruised it, but when he went to the doctor, he was admitted to the hospital. He has a weak pedal pulse in the left foot and there is no palpable pulse in the right foot. He tells the nurse he has diabetes and forgets to test his blood sugar regularly. His blood sugar is 298 mg on admission. His blood pressure is 138/98.

56. List the subjective findings for Mr. Issacs.

57. List the objective findings for Mr. Issacs.

58. What other assessments should be made on admission for Mr. Issacs?

▪ ▪ ▪ Critical Thinking Exercises

59. The nurse is caring for a 59-year-old woman who is admitted with a black toe. What assessment questions should the nurse ask her on admission?

60. Compare and contrast the vascular system to the lymphatic system.

▪ ▪ ▪ Additional Learning Experiences

▪ Practice interviewing friends and family members about their peripheral vascular and lymphatic systems.

▪ Consult with your instructor about observing radiologic procedures for clients with peripheral vascular disease.

Nursing Care of Clients with Peripheral Vascular and Lymphatic Disorders

■ ■ ■ **Focused Study Tips**

- Compare and contrast the various classifications of medications used to treat hypertension. Discuss the modes of action of each classification, their side effects, adverse effects, and how each is used to reduce blood pressure.

- Compare and contrast the disorders of the peripheral arteries.

- Describe the mechanism(s) involved for each disorder of the peripheral vascular system, and identify the clinical manifestations that differentiate one disorder from the other.

- Describe the common disorders of venous circulation and their related nursing care.

■ ■ ■ **Blood Pressure Regulation**

1. Identify four major processes that interfere with the normal flow of peripheral blood and lymphatic fluids.

  (a) _____   (c) _____

  (b) _____   (d) _____

■ ■ ■ **The Client with Hypertension**

2. Essential hypertension is often called the "silent killer" because:
  a. the pathophysiology of essential hypertension remains unknown.
  b. individuals usually display no signs and symptoms of the disease.
  c. there is little or no correlation between the disease and known risk factors.
  d. the diagnosis of the disease must be validated by laboratory testing.

3. A 77-year-old client has a blood pressure reading of 168/94. Which of the following statements by the nurse is the most appropriate in this case?
  a. "Your BP is normal for your age. Have it checked again in 1 year."
  b. "Your BP is elevated. I'll check it again right now."
  c. "Your BP is slightly elevated. Make an appointment to see your doctor and have it checked again."
  d. "Your BP is very elevated. See your doctor immediately."

4. According to the National Institutes of Health, a client is considered hypertensive when the systolic blood pressure reading is above:
  a. 140.   b. 150.   c. 160.   d. 170.

5. Which ethnic group has the highest prevalence of hypertension?
  a. European Americans   c. Asian Americans
  b. African Americans   d. Native Americans

6. A client confides in the nurse that he knows he should refrain from drinking alcohol given his history of hypertension. However, he states that he enjoys having a glass of wine with dinner. The most appropriate response by the nurse is:
   a. "You must refrain from all alcohol to manage your disease."
   b. "It is okay for you to continue to have one glass of wine with dinner."
   c. "It is okay for you to have one glass with each meal."
   d. "You can drink as much alcohol as you want, so long as it doesn't include beer or hard liquor."

7. Conservative management of hypertension would include which of the following strategies?
   a. dietary modifications
   b. compliance with diuretic therapy
   c. switching to low-tar cigarettes
   d. compliance with antihypertensive drug therapy

8. List three dietary modifications recommended for hypertensive clients.
   (a) _____
   (b) _____
   (c) _____

9. The treatment of choice for decreasing stress in the client with essential hypertension is:
   a. biofeedback techniques.   c. therapeutic touch.
   b. anti-anxiety medications.   d. regular aerobic exercise.

Match the categories of anti-hypertensives (a–f) with the correct nursing interventions listed in questions 10–15.

_____ 10. monitor BUN and creatinine levels

_____ 11. administer first dose at bedtime to avoid "first dose syncope"

_____ 12. instruct the client to avoid activities that require full alertness

_____ 13. instruct client to change position slowly to avoid dizziness and prevent falls

_____ 14. assess lungs for crackles and wheezes

_____ 15. monitor blood glucose levels, since these drugs can mask hypoglycemic episodes

a. beta-blockers
b. central-acting sympatholytics
c. vasodilators
d. alpha-adrenergic blockers
e. calcium channel blockers
f. angiotensin-converting enzyme inhibitors

16. Identify three nursing interventions that are appropriate when planning care for a hypertensive client with a nursing diagnosis of *Decreased Cardiac Output*.
   (a) _____
   (b) _____
   (c) _____

17. When planning and implementing nursing care for clients with hypertension, it is essential that the nurse begins with:
   a. dietary modification.   c. mutually established goals.
   b. activity restrictions.   d. stress reduction strategies.

18. Which of the following clients is at highest risk for the development of secondary hypertension?
    a. a 75-year-old African American male
    b. a 58-year-old male with a high stress job
    c. a 36-year-old female taking oral contraceptives
    d. a 45-year-old female who is 30 lbs overweight

19. Name five causes of secondary hypertension.
    (a) _____   (d) _____
    (b) _____   (e) _____
    (c) _____

20. A rare tumor of the adrenal medulla that causes persistent or intermittent hypertension is called
    _____.

21. A client is admitted to the hospital with a blood pressure of 245/135. An appropriate action by
    the nurse is to:
    a. recognize that admission anxiety can elevate the blood pressure.
    b. recheck the client's blood pressure in 1 hour.
    c. call the physician immediately and report the blood pressure.
    d. recognize that this may be the client's normal blood pressure.

22. The (a) _____ is used to obtain an accurate B/P in older adults be-
    cause it helps differentiate between (b) _____ hypertension and actual hypertension.

▪ ▪ ▪   **The Client with Peripheral Arteriosclerosis**

23. Arterial occlusion that causes pain in the calves of the legs, thighs, and buttocks and is relieved
    by rest is called:
    a. an aneurysm.   c. deep vein thrombosis.
    b. intermittent claudication.   d. varicose veins.

24. A diagnosis of peripheral arterial occlusion can be best supported by which of the following ob-
    jective data?
    a. hypotension   c. dependent rubor
    b. poor skin turgor   d. peripheral edema

25. A nurse is unable to palpate dorsalis pedal pulses in her 85-year-old client. There is no cyanosis
    present. To assist with her assessment, the nurse uses an electronic stethoscope to amplify the
    sound of blood flowing through her client's arteries. This technique is called a(n):
    a. Doppler ultrasound.   c. digital subtraction angiography.
    b. oscillometry.   d. plethysmography.

26. The primary reason for prescribing low-dose aspirin to the client with peripheral vascular dis-
    ease is to:
    a. reduce the amount of pain.
    b. reduce the risk of blood clot formation.
    c. prevent the formation of ulcers.
    d. reduce the client's temperature.

27. Health teaching for the client experiencing intermittent claudication includes:
    a. limiting activities and teaching the significant other to perform passive range-of-motion exercises.
    b. ingesting three baby aspirin prior to engaging in any activity.
    c. demonstrating to the client how to alter gait so that no weight is placed on the affected extremity.
    d. walking each day to the point of pain, resting until the pain ceases, then walking again.

Case Study

Michael Washington, a 69-year-old client, has peripheral vascular disease complicated by several ischemic lesions on the medial and dorsal surfaces of the feet.

28. Mr. Washington's physician has scheduled him for a lumbar sympathectomy. Mr. Washington asks the nurse what this means. What is the nurse's most appropriate response?
    a. "The nerve ganglia will be removed in order to increase blood flow."
    b. "A graft will be inserted to divert blood flow past an occluded artery."
    c. "An incision will be made to remove a thrombus that has occluded an artery."
    d. "A balloon will be used to widen the lumen of an occluded arterial lesion."

29. Following his lumbar sympathectomy, Mr. Washington's legs should be kept:
    a. elevated at 25 degrees.
    b. in a dependent position.
    c. gatched at the knee.
    d. in the position of comfort.

30. Following his surgery, Mr. Washington begins to complain of severe pain in his right foot. The priority intervention by his nurse is to:
    a. medicate him for pain.
    b. elevate his foot.
    c. assess the distal circulation, sensation, and motion.
    d. apply ice to the affected area.

▪ ▪ ▪ The Client with Arterial Thrombus or Embolism

31. To diminish the amount of pain that a client with arterial occlusive disease is experiencing, the most appropriate intervention by the nurse is to:
    a. elevate the client's legs.
    b. place the client in a high-Fowler's position.
    c. place the client's legs in a dependent position.
    d. apply cool compresses to the client's legs.

32. When caring for the client with peripheral arterial occlusive disease, which of the following nursing interventions is not appropriate?
    a. place socks on lower extremities; check skin integrity every shift
    b. maintain client's feet in the dependent position
    c. apply heating pads to the affected extremity as tolerated
    d. wash affected extremity once daily, apply moisturizing lotions liberally

33. During a home visit, an 86-year-old client with a history of atrial fibrillation tells the nurse that she feels "pins and needles" down her left leg, with pain in the foot. The nurse notes that the client's left foot and leg are cold, pale to mottled in color, and have diminished peripheral pulses. The nurse should immediately suspect:
    a. arterial embolism.
    b. thrombophlebitis.
    c. aneurysm.
    d. varicose veins.

34. When assessing a client's left lower extremity after arterial reconstruction surgery, the nurse notices that every 20 minutes there is a brief (less than 10 seconds) period of cyanosis, followed by hyperemia. The nurse notifies the surgeon, who orders a calcium channel blocker. The rationale for this is the client may:
    a. be hypertensive; this drug lowers blood pressure.
    b. have vasospasm; this drug relaxes vascular smooth muscle.
    c. have arterial vasoconstriction; this drug blocks the uptake of sympathomimetics.
    d. be hypotensive; this drug raises blood pressure.

35. Postoperative nursing care of the client with arterial reconstruction should include which of the following?
    a. flexing the client's leg postoperatively
    b. ensuring the bedcover fits snugly over the affected extremity
    c. restraining the affected extremity
    d. elevating the foot of the bed no more than 30 degrees

36. Identify four conditions that promote the development of arterial thrombosis.
    (a) _____
    (b) _____
    (c) _____
    (d) _____

37. Which statement by the client with peripheral arteriosclerosis indicates a need for further teaching?
    a. "I should not cross my legs."
    b. "I should examine my feet daily."
    c. "I should wear nylon socks."
    d. "I should avoid sunburning my legs or feet."

38. List six manifestations of unusual bleeding related to anticoagulants.
    (a) _____
    (b) _____
    (c) _____
    (d) _____
    (e) _____
    (f) _____

■ ■ ■ The Client with Buerger's Disease

39. The most important factor the nurse should include when teaching a client with Buerger's disease is the importance of:
    a. weight control.
    b. meticulous foot care.
    c. smoking cessation.
    d. stress reduction.

40. Buerger exercises involve (a) _____ and (b) _____ the extremities. Each of (c) _____ repetitions take about (d) _____ minutes. The client should be instructed to (e) _____
_____.

■ ■ ■ **The Client with Raynaud's Disease**

41. Which of the following individuals is most likely to be affected by Raynaud's phenomenon and/or disease?
    a. 64-year-old hypertensive male with a stressful job
    b. 22-year-old female who works outdoors in cold weather
    c. 48-year-old obese female who lives a sedentary lifestyle
    d. 78-year-old male who smokes and enjoys three beers a day

42. Raynaud's disease is referred to as the blue-white-red disease. Identify the physiological process that is occurring in the affected extremity with each color.
    a. Blue: _____
    b. White: _____
    c. Red: _____

43. When experiencing an attack as a result of Raynaud's disease, a client should _____
_____
_____.

■ ■ ■ **The Client with an Aneurysm**

44. The major risk factor for the development of an aneurysm is:
    a. age.   b. weight.   c. female gender.   d. history of hypertension.

45. The primary difference between a true aneurysm and a false aneurysm is that:
    a. a false aneurysm involves only the intima layer of the vessel wall.
    b. a true aneurysm involves the three layers of the vessel wall.
    c. a false aneurysm is a pathologic weakening of the arterial wall.
    d. a true aneurysm is most often caused by trauma to the vessel wall.

46. A client with a history of Marfan's disease who is complaining of severe anterior chest pain is most likely suffering from:
    a. myocardial infarction.   c. pulmonary embolus.
    b. dissecting thoracic aneurysm.   d. dissecting abdominal aneurysm.

47. The severity of an abdominal aortic aneurysm is best determined by:
    a. the intensity of the pain a client has.
    b. the client's age and the location of the aortic aneurysm.
    c. the amount of peripheral edema a client has.
    d. whether the intima, media, or adventitia is involved.

48. When antihypertensive medications are prescribed for a client with a dissecting aneurysm, the desired outcome is to achieve a systolic blood pressure of no more than:
    a. 75.   b. 100.   c. 120.   d. 135.

49. A client is being discharged after having an abdominal aortic aneurysm repaired. Discharge teaching should include:

(a) _____

(b) _____

(c) _____

(d) _____

50. Preoperatively, which of the following medications would not be indicated for a client with a dissecting aortic aneurysm?

a. Colace (docusate sodium)

b. Inderal (propranolol)

c. Nipride (nitroprusside)

d. morphine

■ ■ ■ The Client with Thrombophlebitis

51. Identify the three pathologic factors, known as Virchow's triad, that are associated with thrombophlebitis.

(a) _____

(b) _____

(c) _____

52. Which of the following clinical manifestations would the nurse not expect to observe in a client diagnosed with deep vein thrombosis?

a. cyanosis of the affected extremity

b. absent peripheral pulses

c. pain with walking

d. tenderness in the affected extremity

53. Which of the following examinations is the most valuable in the detection of thrombosis of large and superficial veins?

a. ascending phlebography

b. Doppler ultrasound

c. plethysmography

d. visualization by x-ray

54. Conservative therapy for a client with a superficial venous thrombosis includes:

(a) _____

(b) _____

55. Which of the following nursing interventions is appropriate when caring for the client with a venous occlusion of the calf?

a. massaging the affected extremity

b. maintaining bed rest and providing range-of-motion exercises

c. ambulating and maintaining mobility

d. maintaining the client's legs in a dependent position

56. Preventive measures aimed at decreasing the risk of deep vein thrombosis (DVT) in postoperative clients would not include:

a. regular leg exercises.

b. anticoagulation therapy.

c. use of elastic or pneumatic stockings.

d. early ambulation.

57. Which of the following activated partial thromboplastin time (APTT) levels indicates effective anticoagulation therapy for deep vein thrombosis?

a. control 20, client 48

b. control 22, client 28

c. control 24, client 60

d. control 18, client 36

58. A 47-year-old client with thrombophlebitis is being discharged on warfarin. Teaching by the discharge nurse regarding the use of warfarin should include:
    (a) _____
    (b) _____
    (c) _____

59. A client is told that she has a venous thrombus and must be on bed rest. She tells the nurse that she is much too busy and can't stay on bed rest. The best response by the nurse is:
    a. "The rest will be beneficial to you."
    b. "Activity and exercise may cause life-threatening complications."
    c. "There is no other treatment for the problem that you have."
    d. "Bed rest is necessary to reduce venous inflammation and edema."

60. Which nursing intervention is inappropriate for the client with deep vein thrombosis?
    a. elevating extremities at all times
    b. maintaining compression stockings continuously
    c. encouraging position changes every 2 hours
    d. increasing fluid and fiber intake

61. Identify four nursing interventions that are appropriate nursing actions when caring for the client with DVT.
    (a) _____
    (b) _____
    (c) _____
    (d) _____

▪ ▪ ▪   The Client with Chronic Venous Insufficiency

62. The presence of stasis ulcers in the client with chronic venous insufficiency can best be explained by:
    a. the lack of exercise in the affected extremity.
    b. congestion of blood in the affected extremity.
    c. pressure applied to the affected extremity.
    d. increased temperature in the affected extremity.

63. List four clinical manifestations of chronic venous insufficiency.
    (a) _____
    (b) _____
    (c) _____
    (d) _____

64. Which statement by the client with chronic venous insufficiency indicates the need for further teaching?
    a. "I should elevate my legs while resting or sleeping."
    b. "I should walk as little as possible."
    c. "I should not wear anything that pinches my legs."
    d. "I should keep the skin on my legs clean, soft, and dry."

▪ ▪ ▪ The Client with Varicose Veins

65. A nurse is teaching a health education class. A participant asks how she can prevent varicose veins. The nurse should tell her that the best prevention is to:
    a. walk regularly and daily.
    b. perform isometric exercises.
    c. take one aspirin daily.
    d. visit the podiatrist regularly.

66. List at least five clinical manifestations of varicose veins.
    (a) _____
    (b) _____
    (c) _____
    (d) _____
    (e) _____

67. List two important conservative interventions for clients with varicose veins.
    (a) _____
    (b) _____

▪ ▪ ▪ The Client with Lymphedema

68. Which of the following clinical findings most clearly distinguishes lymphedema from edema of cardiac causes?
    a. The client has no pain.
    b. There is massive swelling of the involved extremity.
    c. The edema is soft and pitting.
    d. The edema causes progressive client disability.

69. For the client undergoing a lymphangiography, the nurse should assess the client's:
    a. respiratory status.
    b. record for an allergy to penicillin.
    c. prothrombin time.
    d. BUN and creatinine.

70. List five conservative measures to maintain normal lymphatic circulation.
    (a) _____
    (b) _____
    (c) _____
    (d) _____
    (e) _____

71. Appropriate nursing actions when caring for the client with lymphedema include:
    (a) _____
    (b) _____
    (c) _____

72. A client is suffering from severe lymphedema following breast surgery. She tells the nurse, "My arm is so ugly, I just can't go out in public." The most appropriate response by the nurse is:
    a. "Wear long sleeves and no one will notice."
    b. "If you follow the treatment plan the edema will resolve."
    c. "You will learn to accept this change in time."
    d. "Tell me more about how you are feeling."

73. A client has elephantiasis. He ask the nurse what this means. The nurse responds that elephantiasis is (a) _____. He also asks what causes this condition. The nurse responds that it is caused by (b) _____ _____.

▪ ▪ ▪ **Critical Thinking Exercises**

74. The nurse is caring for an elderly homebound client with Raynaud's disease. Develop a plan of care to assist him in managing his condition.

75. Develop a plan of care for a client who is experiencing a hypertensive crisis.

76. The nurse is caring for a client with hypertension who is experiencing high levels of stress. Develop a stress-reduction program for the client.

▪ ▪ ▪ **Additional Learning Experiences**

▪ Consult with your clinical instructor about visiting a wound clinic that manages wounds associated with peripheral vascular disease.

▪ Visit the World Wide Web and identify resources for clients with hypertension.

▪ Consult with your instructor about conducting a hypertension screening.

Nursing Care of Clients with Hematologic Disorders

■ ■ ■ Focused Study Tips

- Identify the normal laboratory results for complete blood count and state the terminology associated with size, color, and number of the various types of cells.

- Describe the classifications, causes, and the commonly observed manifestations of each type of anemia and how anemia affects the other body systems.

- Outline the circulatory events that occur in platelet and coagulation disorders.

- Discuss the various medications that may interfere with platelet function.

- Describe the clinical manifestations of leukemia. Describe what makes each type of leukemia unique.

■ ■ ■ Overview of Red Blood Cells

1. The two primary systems that compromise the hematopoietic system are:

   (a) _____

   (b) _____

2. Immature red blood cells are called:

   a. hemoglobin.

   b. erythrocytes.

   c. reticulocytes.

   d. corpuscles.

3. Red blood cells that are smaller than normal cells are called:

   a. microcytic.

   b. normocytic.

   c. hypochromic.

   d. macrocytic.

4. The body's response to the stimulation of erythropoiesis occurs in which nursing diagnosis?

   a. *Decreased Cardiac Output* related to myocardial infarction

   b. *Pain* related to hepatosplenomegaly

   c. *Risk for Bleeding* related to anticoagulated state

   d. *Impaired Tissue Perfusion* related to hypoxia

5. Which failed organs would contribute to impaired erythropoiesis?

   a. lungs

   b. kidneys

   c. heart

   d. spleen

6. The life span of an RBC is (a) _____ days. The process of RBC destruction is called (b) _____.

7. When increased hemolysis occurs, or when liver function is suppressed, (a) _____ may occur. When this condition occurs, the nurse may observe (b) _____.

▪ ▪ ▪ **The Client with Anemia**

For each of the following types of anemias, identify (a) characteristics of the red blood cells seen in this type of anemia, (b) a clinical manifestation of this type of anemia, and (c) treatment options.

The Nutritional Anemias

8. iron-deficiency anemia
   (a) _____
   (b) _____
   (c) _____

9. vitamin B_{12}–deficiency anemia
   (a) _____
   (b) _____
   (c) _____

10. folic acid–deficiency anemia
    (a) _____
    (b) _____
    (c) _____

11. sickle cell anemia
    (a) _____
    (b) _____
    (c) _____

12. thalassemia
    (a) _____
    (b) _____
    (c) _____

13. acquired hemolytic anemia
    (a) _____
    (b) _____
    (c) _____

14. G_6PD anemia
    (a) _____
    (b) _____
    (c) _____

15. aplastic anemia
    (a) _____
    (b) _____
    (c) _____

16. Regardless of the cause or type of anemia, the characteristic common to all anemias is:
    a. the size of the red blood cells is always the same.
    b. the life span of the red blood cells is always the same.
    c. all anemias reduce the oxygen-carrying capacity of the blood.
    d. iron supplementation is beneficial in all types of anemias.

17. The characteristic which most distinguishes vitamin B_{12}–deficiency anemia from folate-deficiency anemia is the presence of:
    a. pallor.
    b. fatigue.
    c. neurologic impairment.
    d. cardiac arrhythmias.

18. In which of the following cultural groups is sickle cell anemia most prevalent?
    a. African American
    b. European American
    c. Asian American
    d. Native American

19. When caring for a hospitalized client with the sickle cell trait, it is important the nurse ensures:
    a. the client avoids episodes of hypoxia.
    b. the client is placed in a private room.
    c. the client's body fluids are disposed of properly.
    d. the client's creatinine remains within normal limits.

20. In which of the following areas is thalassemia more prevalent?
    a. North American countries
    b. Eastern European countries
    c. Far Eastern countries
    d. Mediterranean countries

Match the tests commonly used to diagnose anemia (a–e) with the correct descriptions listed in questions 21–25.

_____ 21. confirms a diagnosis of glucose-6-phosphate dehydrogenase deficiency

_____ 22. confirms the presence of hemoglobin S

_____ 23. determines the cause of vitamin B_{12} deficiency

_____ 24. indicates the amount of iron the body has on reserve

_____ 25. elevates if the serum iron concentration is low

a. sickle cell screening test
b. total iron binding capacity
c. assay of G_6PD
d. Schilling's test
e. serum ferritin

26. Identify four nursing actions appropriate when administering oral iron preparations to a client.
    (a) _____
    (b) _____
    (c) _____
    (d) _____

27. Clients taking oral iron preparations should be instructed:
    a. that stools may be dark black or green in color.
    b. to limit their fluid intake to 1000 mL daily.
    c. to never mix anything with the medications.
    d. that urine may be orange in color.

28. When teaching a client with folic acid–deficiency anemia about dietary changes, the nurse should instruct the client to consume:
    a. turkey.
    b. seafood.
    c. leafy green vegetables.
    d. all types of cheeses.

29. A client with a nursing diagnosis of *Altered Oral Mucous Membranes* should be instructed to avoid which of the following solutions when performing oral care?
    a. saline solutions
    b. salt water solutions
    c. half-strength hydrogen peroxide
    d. alcohol-based solutions

30. For a client with altered mucous membranes, the nurse should encourage which of the following foods?
    a. spaghetti   b. chicken with broccoli   c. oranges and grapefruits   d. tomatoes

31. Explain why each of the findings listed below is seen in the client with anemia.
    (a) tachycardia _____
    (b) pallor _____
       _____
    (c) fatigue _____
       _____

32. List two possible causes of iron-deficiency anemia in older adults.
    (a) _____
    (b) _____

33. Common assessment findings in iron-deficiency anemia include:
    a. cheilosis, spoon-shaped nails, and pica.
    b. paresthesias and problems with proprioception.
    c. hematuria and jaundice.
    d. pancytopenia and infections.

34. If a person lacks intrinsic factor and suffers from pernicious anemia, the nurse should advise the client to:
    a. take an oral supplement with B vitamins.
    b. eat meats, eggs, and dairy products.
    c. take an iron supplement 3 times per day.
    d. take injections of B_{12} on a regular schedule.

35. A priority nursing intervention when caring for a client in sickle cell crisis includes providing:
    a. fluids and folic acid supplements.
    b. oxygen and analgesics.
    c. rest and blood transfusions.
    d. electrophoresis and dialysis.

36. Which statement by the client undergoing a bone marrow biopsy indicates a need for further teaching?
    a. "I will have to lie still during the procedure."
    b. "I should report any unusual bleeding."
    c. "I may experience some pain during the procedure."
    d. "I won't experience any pain after the procedure."

37. List three food sources of iron.
    (a) _____   (c) _____
    (b) _____

38. List three food sources of folic acid.
    (a) _____   (c) _____
    (b) _____

39. List three food sources of vitamin B$_{12}$.

    (a) _____   (c) _____

    (b) _____

40. A client suffers from anemia. He complains of chronic fatigue and activity intolerance. When the client asks if he should continue activity when he gets short of breath, the most appropriate response by the nurse is:

    a. "You will never gain strength unless you increase your activity each day."

    b. "You should take it easier and try not to do so much."

    c. "You must accept your limitations and try not to get frustrated."

    d. "You should stop activity when short of breath and assess your pulse rate."

▪ ▪ ▪ The Client with Polycythemia

41. The clinical finding that most clearly distinguishes primary polycythemia vera from secondary polycythemia vera is:

    a. hepatomegaly.   b. gastritis.   c. splenomegaly.   d. brittle bone mass.

42. Identify five symptoms associated with the client with polycythemia.

    (a) _____   (d) _____

    (b) _____   (e) _____

    (c) _____

43. List four teaching topics that the nurse should teach the client with polycythemia.

    (a) _____

    (b) _____

    (c) _____

    (d) _____

▪ ▪ ▪ The Client with Thrombocytopenia

44. Which of the following elements, released by platelets, contributes to vessel spasms when injury occurs?

    a. megakaryocytes   c. thromboxane A2

    b. adenosine diphosphate   d. thrombopoietin

45. Von Willebrand's factor is essential in that it:

    a. helps to form platelet plugs.   c. is essential to platelet synthesis.

    b. increases the number of platelets. d. decreases platelet adherence.

46. Thrombocytopenia occurs when the platelet count is less than:

    a. 100,000.   b. 200,000.   c. 300,000.   d. 400,000.

47. Which of the following is an autoimmune disorder of platelet destruction?

    a. platelet transfusion reaction   c. idiopathic thrombocytopenia purpura

    b. aplastic anemia   d. acquired immune deficiency syndrome

48. Which of the following client platelet counts would suggest a risk for fatal bleeding secondary to thrombocytopenia?

    a. 100,000   b. 10,000   c. 50,000   d. 20,000

49. Identify the cutaneous manifestation of thrombocytopenia suggested by the descriptions below.
    (a) The term used to describe a flat or raised area of discoloration caused by subcutaneous bleeding. _____
    (b) Small, flat purple or red spots caused by minute hemorrhages into the dermis. _____
    (c) Hemorrhages into the tissue evidenced by bruising. _____

▪ ▪ ▪ **The Client with Disseminated Intravascular Coagulation**

50. When disseminated intravascular coagulation occurs, two processes are taking place in the circulatory system. One is (a) _____ and the other is (b) _____.

Identify whether each of the following laboratory tests used to diagnose disseminated intravascular coagulation (DIC) is increased or decreased in the client with actual DIC, and explain why each finding occurs.

51. bleeding time

52. platelet count

53. plasma fibrinogen level

54. fibrin degradation products

55. Following a gastrointestinal hemorrhage, a client develops symptoms consistent with DIC. The client complains of severe pain in his right hand. An appropriate intervention by the nurse is to:
    a. recognize that this is part of the disease process.
    b. assess the distal circulation, sensation, and motion.
    c. elevate the hand to promote venous return.
    d. medicate the client for pain and keep him comfortable.

56. The above client's oxygen saturation drops from 92 to 84%. The most appropriate action by the nurse is to:
    a. apply oxygen and reassess his O_2 saturation.
    b. recognize respiratory problems as part of the disorder.
    c. encourage him to cough and deep breathe, and recheck his O_2 saturation.
    d. notify the physician of this finding.

▪ ▪ ▪ The Client with Hemophilia

57. Hemophilia is more likely to be found in which gender? _____

58. Which of the following medication prescriptions would the nurse discuss with the physician when written for a client with hemophilia B?
    a. Propolex 150 units IVP
    b. 2 units of fresh frozen plasma over 30 minutes
    c. Konyne-80 150 units IVP
    d. 20 units of cryoprecipitate

59. Which of the following nursing orders is contraindicated for a client with hemophilia?
    a. administer IM analgesia to deep muscle only
    b. encourage client to use an electric razor
    c. guaiac all stools for occult blood
    d. assess client's understanding of disease process

60. Which statement by the client with hemophilia indicates the need for further teaching?
    a. "I should report any signs of bleeding."   c. "I should wear a medical alert bracelet."
    b. "If I have pain I can take aspirin."   d. "I should brush my teeth regularly."

▪ ▪ ▪ Lymphoproliferative Disorders

61. (a) _____ make up 60 to 70% of the total number of WBCs. They increase in number during an inflammation. Immature forms of these cells are called (b) _____ or (c) _____ cells. These cells have a life span of about (d) _____ hours.

62. Name these alterations in WBC counts.
    (a) A reduction in the number of circulating neutrophils: _____
    (b) Fewer than normal lymphocytes: _____
    (c) A decrease in granulocytes and neutrophils: _____

▪ ▪ ▪ The Client with Acute Infectious Mononucleosis

63. Transmission of the Epstein-Barr virus in infectious mononucleosis is thought to occur:
    a. during intercourse.   c. through kissing.
    b. through blood transfusions.   d. through superficial skin tears.

Read the following statements and determine if they are true or false. Correct any false statements.

_____ 64. The incubation period for infectious mononucleosis is 7 to 10 days.

_____ 65. The most common manifestations of infectious mononucleosis include headache, malaise, fatigue, fever, sore throat, and enlargement and pain in the cervical lymph nodes.

_____ 66. Full recovery from infectious mononucleosis is anticipated in 2 to 3 weeks.

_____ 67. Splenic enlargement rarely occurs in infectious mononucleosis.

▪ ▪ ▪ The Client with Multiple Myeloma

68. Multiple myeloma is characterized by abnormality in which cell type?

    a. erythrocytes   b. CD4   c. monocytes   d. plasma

69. An early clinical manifestation of multiple myeloma is:

    a. back pain.
    b. head and neck abnormalities.
    c. impaired gait.
    d. paresthesia.

70. A client with advanced multiple myeloma is at high risk for:

    a. skin abnormalities.
    b. pathologic fractures.
    c. cardiac arrhythmias.
    d. cerebral dysfunction.

71. A man is taking his mother, who has advanced multiple myeloma, home today. He states, "I am so nervous about cooking for her. Do you have any advice?" The nurse should tell him:

    a. "There are no dietary restrictions."
    b. "Be careful with raw vegetables and fruits. Be certain they are washed and cooked thoroughly."
    c. "Cook foods high in fat to help build muscle."
    d. "Cook foods low in protein because it is hard to digest."

72. The urinalysis of an individual with multiple myeloma would be positive for:

    a. blood.
    b. white blood cells.
    c. Bence-Jones protein.
    d. phosphates.

73. The client with multiple myeloma has a neutrophil count under 500 mm³. The most appropriate response by the nurse is to:

    a. notify the physician to obtain an order for antibiotics.
    b. place the client in protective isolation.
    c. limit visitors with infections.
    d. institute medical and surgical asepsis.

74. A client has multiple myeloma and a neutrophil count under 500 mm³. She has been depressed and crying about the severity of her illness. She receives flowers and asks if she can have a vase. What is the most appropriate response by the nurse?

▪ ▪ ▪ The Client with Leukemia

75. When a client has acute leukemia, this means that:

    a. the disease appeared following a viral infection.
    b. there is no treatment available.
    c. leukemic cells are poorly differentiated.
    d. the duration of the disease is no longer than 4 months.

76. In which type of leukemia is there an abnormality in the Philadelphia chromosome?

    a. acute myelogenous
    b. chronic myelogenous
    c. acute lymphocytic
    d. chronic lymphocytic

77. The most common form of childhood leukemia is:
    a. acute myelogenous leukemia.
    c. acute lymphocytic leukemia.
    b. chronic myelogenous leukemia.
    d. chronic lymphocytic leukemia.

78. Identify three rationales for administering a combination of agents to treat leukemia.
    (a) _____
    (b) _____
    (c) _____

79. When a client receiving chemotherapy reaches nadir, the nurse should:
    a. notify the physician STAT.
    c. restrict the client's visitors.
    b. prepare the family for the client's death.
    d. prepare the client for discharge.

80. The most common cause of death in a client with any type of leukemia is:
    a. infection.   b. thromboemboli.   c. hyponatremia.   d. cancer metastasis.

81. Nursing documentation on a client with neutropenia reads, "there are several diffuse red, raised, fluid-filled lesions on the throat, tongue, and buccal region." This finding may indicate the client has:
    a. candidiasis.
    c. infectious mononucleosis.
    b. a normal response to chemotherapy.
    d. a herpes infection.

82. A client has leukemia and is receiving chemotherapy. Her platelet count is 40,000. She is having pain and has been prescribed Tylenol (acetaminophen) 650 mg PR. An appropriate action by the nurse is to:
    a. administer the drug as prescribed.
    b. have the medication prescription changed to IM Demerol (meperidine).
    c. request that the client be placed on a morphine drip.
    d. have the medication prescription changed to a PO route.

83. In an allogenic bone marrow transplant (BMT), bone marrow comes from a (a) _____.
    In an autologous BMT, bone marrow comes from the (b) _____.

84. What type of procedures should be avoided with the client with leukemia?
    (a) _____

85. List four dietary strategies to increase food tolerance in the client with leukemia.
    (a) _____
    (b) _____
    (c) _____
    (d) _____

Read the following statements and determine if they are true or false. Correct any false statements.

_____ 86. The client with a platelet count between 20,000 and 50,000 mm^3 is at severe risk for bleeding.

_____ 87. The client with leukemia may expect to experience headaches and seizures.

_____ 88. Using an alcohol-based mouthwash will minimize the risk of oral infections in clients with leukemia.

_____ 89. The client with a WBC of 500 to 1000 mm^3 is at moderate risk for infection.

_____ 90. Chronic lymphocytic leukemia is primarily a disorder of young adults.

91. A client has leukemia. She wants her school-age children to visit her on a regular basis. The most appropriate advice by the nurse is:
   a "You are too sick to have any visitors."
   b. "You should ask your doctor about that."
   c. "No one with a cold, flu, or infection should visit,"
   d. "School-age children will bring you an infection."

92. Which statement by the above client indicates a need for further teaching about infection prevention?
   a. "I should report any fevers, chills, or sore throats."
   b. "I should avoid crowds and those who are ill."
   c. "I should take all my immunizations on a regular basis."
   d. "I should avoid raw fruits and vegetables."

93. Which statement by the above client indicates a need for further teaching about preventing bleeding?
   a. "I should not blow my nose forcefully."
   b. "I should avoid straining to have a bowel movement."
   c. "I should avoid coughing and sneezing forcefully."
   d. "I should use tampons instead of peri-pads."

94. List at least three nursing interventions to assist the client with leukemia and her family cope with anticipatory grief.
   (a) _____
   (b) _____
   (c) _____

▪ ▪ ▪ The Client with Malignant Lymphoma

95. Hodgkin's lymphoma and nonHodgkin's lymphoma are most clearly distinguished from each other by:
   a. the initial presentation.
   b. the specific cell type.
   c. the Ann Arbor classification system.
   d. the extra nodal site of involvement.

96. The oncology nurse finds a client in tears in his room. He is upset about losing his hair after chemotherapy. Which response by the nurse will enable the client to cope with his alopecia?
   a. "When you are discharged you can get a wig."
   b. "There's no need to cry. Everyone's hair grows back."
   c. "I'll have a psychiatrist come to see you."
   d. "Your hair loss is only temporary, although the texture of new hair might change."

97. A client has just been diagnosed with Stage 2 Hodgkin's disease. Her family asks the nurse about the client's prognosis. The most appropriate response by the nurse is that:
    a. "Most people with Hodgkin's eventually die from their disease."
    b. "Chemotherapy is a sure cure for this illness."
    c. "60 to 90% of individuals with early Hodgkin's disease survive."
    d. "Only time will tell."

98. A junior in high school complains to the school nurse about a swollen lymph node in his neck. He says that it has been present for over 6 weeks and does not seem to go away. The most appropriate response by the nurse is to:
    a. refer him for evaluation.
    b. reassure him that it is not a problem.
    c. assess the lymph node for pain.
    d. refer him for evaluation, should other symptoms appear.

99. A client with Hodgkin's disease is scheduled for a splenectomy. He asks why it must be done. The most appropriate response by the nurse is:
    a. "to lower the chance of infection."
    b. "to remove tumor cells."
    c. "to prevent the spread of disease."
    d. "to make it easier to give radiation and/or chemotherapy."

100. A client is receiving chemotherapy for Hodgkin's disease. She is experiencing nausea and vomiting. List three nursing interventions to minimize these symptoms.
    (a) _____
    (b) _____
    (c) _____

101. The above client is on a MOPP regimen. This means she is receiving:
    (a) _____
    (b) _____
    (c) _____
    (d) _____

■ ■ ■ Critical Thinking Exercises

102. The nurse is caring for a client with widespread frostbite. The client appears to be developing DIC. What are the most appropriate actions by the nurse?

103. Develop a plan of care for a client with leukemia who has recently developed peripheral vascular disease and requires vascular surgery.

■ ■ ■ Additional Learning Experiences

- Learn more about blood donation facilities in your community.
- Consult with your instructor about attending a sickle cell clinic.
- Consider working with a dietician to learn more about the dietary management of clients with anemias.

Assessing Clients with Respiratory Disorders

■ ■ ■ **Focused Study Tips**

- Identify the components of the respiratory system. Describe each component and identify its purpose.

- Compare and contrast normal and abnormal lung sounds.

- Describe factors affecting respiration.

- List the steps of a respiratory assessment.

■ ■ ■ **Anatomy and Physiology**

1. Identify the four main events in the process of respiration.
   (a) _____
   (b) _____
   (c) _____
   (d) _____

2. Explain the purpose of the upper respiratory system and describe what occurs as air passes through the upper respiratory system.

3. Explain the purpose of the surfactant-containing fluid in the lower respiratory system. _____
   _____
   _____

4. Gas exchange across the respiratory membrane occurs by _____.

5. Describe the two functions of the pleura.
   (a) _____
   (b) _____

6. The main purpose of inspiration is to:
   a. increase intrapulmonary volume.
   b. compress the alveoli.
   c. prevent the collapse of the lungs.
   d. equalize the pressures within the lungs.

7. In addition to volume changes within the thoracic cavity, respiration is dependent upon (a)_____
   _____, (b) _____
   and (c) _____.

Match the descriptions of physiologic function (a–r) with the anatomical structures listed in questions 8–25.

_____ 8. trachea

_____ 9. paranasal sinuses system

_____ 10. hilus

_____ 11. intercostal spaces

_____ 12. epiglottis

_____ 13. pharynx

_____ 14. pleura

_____ 15. nostrils

_____ 16. turbinates

_____ 17. angle of Louis

_____ 18. stroma

_____ 19. alveoli

_____ 20. larynx

_____ 21. mediastinum

_____ 22. ribs

_____ 23. suprasternal notch

_____ 24. bronchial tree

_____ 25. vocal folds

a. collective name for branching passageways of lower respiratory tract

b. components of larynx necessary for voice production

c. two cavities that comprise the external opening of the respiratory system

d. center of the thoracic cavity

e. air cavities that lighten skull, assist in speech, and help trap respiratory debris

f. depression above the manubrium

g. passageway for air extending from larynx to primary bronchi

h. spaces separating ribs

i. mediastinal area where pulmonary and circulatory blood vessels enter and exit the lungs

j. cartilage that covers larynx during swallowing

k. funnel-shaped passageway for food and air

l. pits that increase surface area of air entering nose and filter out heavier particles of debris

m. junction between manubrium and body of the sternum

n. an airway and the site of vocal production

o. smallest structural unit of respiration

p. double-layered membrane covering the lungs

q. bony structures that protect lungs

r. elastic connective tissue of the lungs

Match the descriptions (a–f) with the correct respiratory volume capacities listed in questions 26–31.

_____ 26. expiratory reserve volume (ERV)

_____ 27. tidal volume (TV)

_____ 28. vital capacity

_____ 29. residual volume

_____ 30. inspiratory reserve volume (IRV)

_____ 31. anatomical dead space volume

a. sum of TV + IRV + ERV

b. amount of air that can be forcibly inhaled over the tidal volume

c. amount of air moved in and out of lungs with a quiet, normal breath

d. air left in lungs after forced expiration

e. air never reaching alveoli

f. amount of air that can be forced out of the lungs over tidal volume

32. Briefly describe the purpose of oxyhemoglobin.

▪ ▪ ▪ Assessment of Respiratory Function

33. Identify four abnormal findings that may be observed during the health assessment interview of the respiratory system.

(a) _____

(b) _____

(c) _____

(d) _____

34. Identify three normal age-related variations within the lungs that may be found in the older adult.

(a) _____

(b) _____

(c) _____

35. Two risk factors other than smoking and exposure to environmental chemicals that significantly contribute to respiratory disorders are (a) _____ and

(b) _____ .

36. The physical assessment of the respiratory system is best conducted in which of the following positions?

    a. supine   b. semi-Fowler's   c. sitting   d. standing

37. Lung sounds that are equal in duration between inhalation and exhalation and are heard anteriorly over the primary bronchus on each side of the sternum are:

    a. vesicular.   b. basilar.   c. bronchial.   d. bronchovesicular.

38. On inspection of the turbinates, a pale color or the presence of polyps may denote _____ .

39. List the sequence of the physical assessment of the respiratory system.

40. The term used to describe the lung sound that is short, discrete, and bubbling in nature is:

    a. crackle.   b. friction rub.   c. wheeze.   d. egophony.

41. An abnormally low respiratory rate is called:

    a. apnea.   b. bradypnea.   c. tachypnea.   d. atelectasis.

42. Two weeks ago, a client developed a cold and cough that he cannot seem to shake. He has been admitted today for complaints of difficulty breathing, shortness of breath, fever, persistent coughing, and expectoration of rusty-colored sputum. Auscultation of the client's lung sounds reveals crackles in the right lower lobe, and auscultation of voice sounds are increased over the entire right lower lobe. These findings are consistent with:

    a. a viral bronchitis.   b. asthma.   c. pneumonia.   d. lung cancer.

Match the definitions (a–d) with the abnormal breathing patterns listed in questions 43–46.

_____ 43. dyspnea

_____ 44. apnea

_____ 45. tachypnea

_____ 46. atelectasis

a. abnormally high respiratory rate

b. difficult or labored breathing

c. collapse of lung tissue

d. cessation of breathing

Case Study

David Chan is an 89-year-old independent-living adult who stops by the nurse's office in his senior living complex. The nurse observes that he has kyphosis. He is complaining of increasing shortness of breath on exertion when he climbs the stairs. He is a nonsmoker currently, but smoked 2 packs per day for 25 years before quitting. He does report having more frequent colds and respiratory infections. He also tells the nurse he knows he is not eating well because food just doesn't smell and taste the same.

47. Explain kyphosis to Mr. Chan and the effects of aging on his respiratory system.

48. Describe the subjective and objective data the nurse should collect.

49. Develop a teaching plan to help Mr. Chan avoid respiratory infections.

50. Explain to Mr. Chan why food doesn't smell the same, and develop a plan to increase his caloric intake and interest in food and eating.

▪ ▪ ▪ Critical Thinking Exercises

51. Differentiate among vesicular, bronchovesicular, and bronchial breath sounds.

52. Describe how respiratory volume and capacity are affected by sex, age, weight, and health status.

▪ ▪ ▪ Additional Learning Experiences

- Practice listening to normal and abnormal lung sounds by asking family members or friends for the opportunity to listen.

- Practice the sequence of the physical assessment of the respiratory system with family, friends, and classmates. Familiarity with the process will increase your confidence in clinical settings.

- When listening to lung sounds, close your eyes and try to visualize the movement of air in and out of the lungs for each type of sound.

CHAPTER 33

Nursing Care of Clients with Upper Respiratory Disorders

■ ■ ■ Focused Study Tips

- Describe procedures to establish and maintain a patent airway.

- Identify a nursing intervention to decrease or manage a client's anxiety related to hypoxia.

- Compare and contrast the various methods of providing alternate means of communication.

- Compare and contrast the manifestations of partial and complete obstruction within the upper respiratory tract and the appropriate interventions.

- Review the pharmacologic agents that are used to treat disorders of the upper respiratory tract, concentrating on the actions, side effects, and client teaching required for each category of drug.

- Explain the procedures for suctioning, tracheostomy care, the Heimlich maneuver, and cardiopulmonary resuscitation.

■ ■ ■ The Client with Rhinitis

1. The most important teaching action for the client experiencing viral rhinitis is:
   a. discussing allergies the client may have before giving antibiotics.
   b. instructing the client to rest in bed for about a week and take vitamin C.
   c. teaching the client about prevention of the spread of infection and the importance of increasing fluid intake.
   d. teaching the client to avoid going outside in damp, chilly weather in the future.

2. One of the conditions that is a contraindication for the use of nasal decongestants such as phenylephrine (Neo-Synephrine) and pseudoephedrine (Sudafed) is:
   a. ulcer disease.   c. hypothyroidism.
   b. hypertension.   d. allergic dermatitis.

3. Which of the following statements regarding the client with rhinitis is false?
   a. Because rhinitis may be treated by the client, teaching is a vital part of nursing care.
   b. Frequent hand washing, especially after coughing or sneezing, is an important measure to limit viral transmission.
   c. The client should be taught to limit use of nasal decongestants to every 4 hours for only a few days at a time so as to prevent a rebound effect.
   d. Aspirin or acetaminophen taken regularly will prevent progression of the illness..

■ ■ ■ The Client with Influenza

4. Teaching clients and families about influenza must include:
   a. avoiding persons who are sick, and receiving an annual influenza immunization.
   b. staying in bed for at least 3 days at the onset of the infection.
   c. taking a multivitamin and dressing warmly when going outside.
   d. avoiding taking antibiotics for influenza symptoms.

5. Which of the following statements is false?
   a. Influenza is a highly contagious viral respiratory disease.
   b. Those at increased risk of influenza include children under 5 years of age and adults over age 65.
   c. Although yearly outbreaks of influenza affect many Americans each winter, few hospitalizations and deaths result from this disease.
   d. Influenza is transmitted by airborne droplet and direct contact.

6. The ineffective breathing pattern most commonly observed in the person with influenza is:
   a. slow, shallow respirations.
   b. tachypnea with shallow respirations.
   c. Cheyne-Stokes respirations.
   d. bradypnea with deep respirations.

7. For a client with a nursing diagnosis of *Ineffective Airway Clearance*, an appropriate nursing intervention is:
   a. withholding pain medication.
   b. administering cough suppressants every 4–6 hours around the clock.
   c. administering antibiotics on a round-the-clock schedule.
   d. maintaining adequate hydration and providing increased humidity.

▪ ▪ ▪ The Client with Sinusitis

8. Sinusitis results from _____ of the sinus openings.

Match the locations of sinus pain (a–d) with the sinuses listed in questions 9–12.

_____ 9. maxillary

_____ 10. frontal

_____ 11. ethmoid

_____ 12. sphenoid

a. occiput, vertex, or middle of the head
b. over the cheek and into the upper teeth
c. behind the eye and high on the nose
d. lower forehead

13. Which of the following statements regarding sinusitis is true?
    a. Sinusitis is an acute condition.
    b. Sinusitis is uncommon in clients who have AIDS.
    c. Complications of sinusitis are generally the result of local spread of infection.
    d. Sinusitis has many serious, life-threatening complications.

14. Nursing interventions for pain relief following sinus surgery should include:
    a. keeping the client in a flat position.
    b. administering mild analgesics as ordered.
    c. applying warm compresses over the nose.
    d. changing nasal packing every 4 hours.

▪ ▪ ▪ The Client with Pharyngitis/Tonsillitis

15. The most common organism causing bacterial pharyngitis is _____
    _____.

16. Which of the following statements is false?
    a. Pharyngitis and tonsillitis are contagious and spread by droplet nuclei.
    b. Viral infections are communicable for 7–10 days.
    c. Acute pharyngitis causes throat pain and fever.
    d. Peritonsillar abscess is a potential complication.

17. Client teaching for a person receiving antibiotic therapy for bacterial pharyngitis includes which of the following instructions?
    a. Medication must be taken on a regular schedule for at least 10 days.
    b. The client will be contagious for 1 week after antibiotic therapy is initiated.
    c. Medications such as aspirin and acetaminophen must be avoided.
    d. Tetracycline is the drug of choice for group A streptococci.

18. The diet for a client for the first several days following a tonsillectomy should be:
    a. a bland diet.   c. full liquids.
    b. clear liquids.   d. a regular diet.

19. A client complains of a sore throat and difficulty swallowing. On examination the nurse notes that there is marked swelling and asymmetric deviation of the uvula. The most appropriate action by the nurse is to:
    a. advise warm gargles every 2 hours.   c. encourage warm liquids every hour.
    b. refer him to the emergency room.   d. refer the client for a monospot test.

20. List the priority assessments following a tonsillectomy.
    (a) _____
    (b) _____
    (c) _____

▪ ▪ ▪ The Client with Acute Epiglottitis

21. A client with acute epiglottitis is admitted to an emergency room. The nurse's primary concern for care of this client is related to _____
    _____.

22. Manifestations of airway obstruction for which the nurse must monitor while caring for a client with acute epiglottitis include:
    (a) _____
    (b _____
    (c) _____
    (d) _____
    (e) _____

▪ ▪ ▪ The Client with Laryngitis

23. The primary manifestation of laryngitis is _____.

24. Which of the following is a priority nursing diagnosis when working with a client with laryngitis?
    a. *Anxiety*   c. *Ineffective Breathing Pattern*
    b. *Impaired Verbal Communication*   d. *Risk for Infection*

▪ ▪ ▪ The Client with Diphtheria

25. The most distinguishing manifestation of diphtheria is the presence of a _____ covering the posterior pharynx.

26. Prior to administering diphtheria antitoxin, the nurse should:
    a. perform a skin test for sensitivity to horse serum.
    b. question the client about allergy to penicillin.
    c. give the first dose of the prescribed antibiotic.
    d. question the client about allergy to iodine or seafood.

▪ ▪ ▪ The Client with Epistaxis

27. Anterior epistaxis is most often the result of (a) _____, whereas posterior epistaxis is more often secondary to (b) _____ disorders.

28. Identify four nursing responsibilities when caring for the client with a nasal packing.
    (a) _____
    (b) _____
    (c) _____
    (d) _____

29. A client who has required medical care for epistaxis should be taught before discharge that he/she should:
    a. avoid strenuous exercise until the nasal packing is removed.
    b. blow the nose gently every 2–3 hours while awake.
    c. avoid bending and heavy lifting.
    d. avoid sneezing unless the mouth is kept closed during the sneeze.

30. A client is experiencing a severe nosebleed. She is anxious and asks the nurse, "Am I going to bleed to death?" The most appropriate action by the nurse is to:
    a. tell her not to swallow the blood.
    b. assist her with progressive deep-breathing.
    c. instruct her to pinch her nares.
    d. maintain a calm attitude and approach.

31. The above client continues to bleed. The nurse is concerned about aspiration. The most appropriate action by the nurse is to:
    a. place the client in an upright position with her head forward.
    b. continue working with progressive deep relaxation.
    c. place her in the side-lying position with an emesis basin.
    d. obtain suction equipment and suction her as needed.

▪ ▪ ▪ The Client with Nasal Trauma

32. Which of the following conditions is not a typical manifestation of a nasal fracture?
    a. periorbital edema and ecchymosis
    b. deformity or displacement to one side
    c. cerebrospinal fluid (CSF) rhinorrhea
    d. epistaxis

33. The formation of a hematoma of the septum following a fractured nose predisposes the client to abscess formation as the result of what type of bacteria? _____

34. If rhinorrhea is suspected following a nasal fracture, the drainage should be tested for _____ _____, which is found in CSF but is not present in nasal mucus.

35. The purpose of the ice pack to the nose of a person who has experienced nasal trauma is to decrease (a) _____ and (b) _____.

36. A primary nursing responsibility for a client with nasal trauma is to _____ _____.

37. The nurse is providing discharge teaching for the client with nasal trauma. Which of the following statements is false?
    a. "Elevate the head of the bed with blocks to promote drainage."
    b. "Apply ice or cold packs to the nose for 20 minutes 4 times each day."
    c. "Swelling may persist for several weeks."
    d. "Bruising may persist for several weeks."

■ ■ ■ **The Client with a Deviated Nasal Septum**

38. Deviation of the nasal septum is generally the result of:
    a. a congenital condition.
    b. trauma.
    c. infection.
    d. frequent nosebleeds.

39. Following surgery for a septal deviation, the client should be taught to:
    a. frequently perform vigorous deep breathing exercises, turning and coughing.
    b. avoid blowing the nose for 48 hours following the packing removal.
    c. apply warm, moist compresses to the nose 4 times daily.
    d. avoid mouth care until 24 hours following the packing removal.

■ ■ ■ **The Client with Laryngeal Obstruction**

40. The most frequent cause of laryngeal obstruction in the adult is _____ _____.

41. Describe the Heimlich maneuver.

42. When a hospitalized client develops anaphylaxis and a complete laryngeal obstruction occurs while the client is receiving an intravenous antibiotic, the nurse should stop medication and:
    a. call a code.
    b. give epinephrine subcutaneously.
    c. administer Benadryl (diphenhydramine) intravenously.
    d. give mouth-to-mouth breathing.

▪ ▪ ▪ The Client with Laryngeal Trauma

43. Manifestations of laryngeal trauma may include:

   (a) _____

   (b) _____

   (c) _____

   (d) _____

   (e) _____

44. Conservative treatment may be used to treat laryngeal trauma if the injury is limited to _____
   _____.

45. When developing a plan of care for a client who has sustained trauma to the larynx, the primary objective of nursing care is _____.

▪ ▪ ▪ The Client with Sleep Apnea/Hypopnea Syndrome (SAHS)

46. Sleep apnea is defined as absence of airflow through the upper airways for at least _____
   _____.

47. Three forms of sleep apnea are recognized: obstructive, central, and mixed. Of these, _____
   _____ is the most common form.

48. The clinical manifestations of sleep apnea include:
   a. snoring, afternoon headache, and psychoses.
   b. insomnia, paresthesias, and hypotension.
   c. snoring, depression, and hypertension.
   d. fatigue, seizures, and nighttime headache.

49. Which of the following factors contributes to sleep apnea?
   a. anorexia
   b. female gender
   c. caffeine intake
   d. advanced age

50. Which of the following actions is inappropriate to teach a client with sleep apnea?
   a. Encourage participation in a group for weight reduction if the client is obese.
   b. Suggest the use of wine as a safe sedative to be taken at bedtime.
   c. Use a humidifier in the bedroom to increase humidity in the atmosphere.
   d. Encourage participation in a support group for persons with sleep apnea.

▪ ▪ ▪ The Client with Nasal Polyps

51. Which of the following statements is true regarding nasal polyps?
   a. Nasal polyps are benign growths.
   b. Nasal polyps are neoplastic growths.
   c. Nasal polyps are considered premalignant.
   d. Nasal polyps are not seen in clients who have asthma.

52. Identify three recommendations the nurse should include when teaching the client following a polypectomy.

(a) _____

(b) _____

(c) _____

53. A client had a nasal polypectomy performed in the surgeon's office early in the morning. By the afternoon she feels nauseated, and she notices frequent swallowing and observes blood at the back of her throat. What is an appropriate response by the surgeon's nurse to the client's inquiry about her symptoms?

a. "Pace your activities and the bleeding will subside."

b. "You should breathe through your mouth instead of your nose."

c. "You should see the doctor right away. You could be experiencing posterior bleeding."

d. "Drink plenty of fluids to keep yourself properly hydrated, and the bleeding will subside."

▪ ▪ ▪ The Client with Benign Laryngeal Tumor

54. Benign tumors of the larynx include: (a) _____,
(b) _____, and (c) _____.

55. Which of the following statements is false?

a. The client with chronic hoarseness of recent onset should seek treatment immediately.

b. Benign laryngeal tumors may resolve with correction of the underlying problem.

c. Nodules or polyps that do not resolve with conservative therapy may require surgical excision.

d. Yelling or screaming will not affect the client with benign laryngeal tumors.

56. For a professional singer who has been treated for a benign laryngeal lesion, the nurse should suggest:

a. a change of occupation.

b. voice training with a speech therapist.

c. taking low-dose corticosteroids to reduce inflammation.

d. using inhalation therapy prior to singing engagements.

▪ ▪ ▪ The Client with Laryngeal Carcinoma

57. Cancer of the larynx accounts for (a) _____ percent of all cancers. The two major risk factors for developing laryngeal cancer are prolonged use of (b) _____ and (c) _____.

58. Premalignant changes that may occur in the larynx prior to the development of frank malignant lesions are white patches called (a) _____ and red patches called (b) _____.

59. The most common site for cancer of the larynx is the:

a. glottis.

b. supraglottis.

c. subglottis.

d. epiglottis.

60. The earliest manifestation of cancer of the glottis is usually:
    a. sore throat.
    b. painful swallowing.
    c. sensation of a lump in the throat.
    d. hoarseness.

61. Clients with complaints of persistent hoarseness, a change in voice quality, painful or difficult swallowing, or a lump in the throat should be promptly evaluated using which test?
    a. direct or indirect laryngoscopy
    b. bronchoscopy
    c. gastroscopy
    d. esophagoscopy

62. Which statement regarding the client with laryngeal cancer is false?
    a. The type of surgical approach is based on the site, size, and degree of tumor invasion.
    b. Chemotherapy is the treatment of choice.
    c. A tracheostomy is usually required after surgery.
    d. Precise therapy is determined by the staging guidelines.

63. Collaborative care for a client having a total laryngectomy requires that the nurse work closely both preoperatively and postoperatively with a(n):
    a. psychiatrist.
    b. physical therapist.
    c. speech therapist.
    d. occupational therapist.

64. A client is scheduled for a laryngectomy tomorrow. He states, "I can't wait for this to be over; I am craving a thick, juicy steak." The best response by the nurse is to _____
    _____
    _____.

65. The postoperative total laryngectomy client usually has a nursing diagnosis of *Anxiety*. The nursing intervention that would best address this diagnosis is:
    a. encourage client independence by teaching self-care within the first of couple days after surgery.
    b. complete all of the client's care as quickly and efficiently as possible to demonstrate competence, thus enhancing trust.
    c. enforce visiting hours to allow the client to become increasingly self-reliant instead of depending on the family for care.
    d. keep the call bell within easy reach of the client and answer it immediately when it is on.

66. Identify three nursing interventions appropriate for the client undergoing a laryngectomy with a nursing diagnosis of *Altered Nutrition: Less than Body Requirements*.
    (a) _____
    (b) _____
    (c) _____

Read the statements below and determine if they are true or false. Correct any false statements.

_____ 67. Prior to providing tracheostomy care, the client should be placed in semi-Fowler's or Fowler's position.

_____ 68. Hydrogen peroxide may be used to remove crusted secretions around the incision.

_____ 69. The outer cannula of the tracheostomy tube may be suctioned using clean technique.

_____ 70. Assess the client's breathing after providing tracheostomy care.

71. The client who is being discharged with a tracheostomy following a total laryngectomy requires extensive teaching. Name four major topics the nurse should include in the teaching plan for this client.

    (a) _____

    (b) _____

    (c) _____

    (d) _____

72. A client recently underwent a procedure for laryngeal cancer. Since surgery she has been crying and writes the nurse a message asking, "What is the point of going forward?" The most appropriate intervention by the nurse is to:

    a. encourage her to express her feelings.

    b. tell her that things will get better soon.

    c. tell her that the nurses understand how difficult it is.

    d. refer her to a cancer support group.

73. A client is transferred to the ICU following a laryngectomy. The priority nursing assessment is to assess:

    a. respiratory rate and rhythm.

    b. vital signs and oxygen saturation.

    c. patency of the airway.

    d. dressing for hemorrhage.

74. Develop a plan of care for a client who will experience impaired verbal communication following a laryngectomy.

▪ ▪ ▪ **Critical Thinking Exercises**

75. The nurse is caring for a client with sinusitis and a questionable brain abscess. The client reports a worsening headache and seems a bit confused. What actions, if any, should the nurse take?

76. After undergoing a laryngectomy, a client tells you he cannot wait until he can go boating and water skiing. What advice should you give the client?

▪ ▪ ▪ **Additional Learning Experiences**

▪   Develop a teaching program for school-aged children on preventing the spread of common respiratory infections.

▪   Visit your local pharmacy and become more familiar with the wide variety of cold and cough products.

Nursing Care of Clients with Lower Respiratory Disorders

■ ■ ■ Focused Study Tips

- Review the scientific principles involved in respiration.

- Discuss the strategies for preventing respiratory disease.

- Describe nursing interventions associated with care of the client with a lower respiratory disorder who is anxious.

- Discuss the basic components of blood gases and how the lungs and kidneys work together to maintain normal blood pH.

- Review the procedures for suctioning endotracheal tubes and tracheostomies, and for management of common types of mechanical ventilators.

- Compare and contrast the various categories of drugs that are specific for respiratory disorders. Review the autonomic nervous system and the effects and side effects of drugs used in respiratory system disorders.

■ ■ ■ The Client with Acute Bronchitis

1. Clients with acute bronchitis are rarely hospitalized, and so most nursing interventions are directed toward (a) _____. If the client is a smoker, the nurse should provide information about (b) _____.

■ ■ ■ The Client with Pneumonia

Match the descriptions (a–e) with the organisms listed in questions 2–6.

_____ 2. *Staphylococcus aureus*

_____ 3. *Streptococcus pneumoniae*

_____ 4. *Pneumocystis carinii*

_____ 5. *Mycoplasma pneumoniae*

_____ 6. *Legionella pneumophilia*

a. most common cause of pneumonia

b. associated with nosocomial pneumonia

c. associated with contaminated water-cooled air conditioning units

d. causes pneumonia in young adults

e. associated with persons with HIV infection

7. Persons who are most susceptible to aspiration pneumonia are those who have:
   a. a primary bacterial pneumonia.
   b. a depressed cough or gag reflex.
   c. undergone surgery of the head or neck.
   d. had nothing by mouth for the previous 8–10 hours.

8. A nurse is administering a vaccine for the prevention of pneumococcal pneumonia to an older adult client. The client asks how often the vaccine should be repeated. The appropriate answer is:
   a. "This vaccine needs to be given every year, usually in the early fall."
   b. "You will need this vaccine every other year."
   c. "This vaccine is good for 5 years."
   d. "This vaccine will give you protection for the rest of your life."

9. In obtaining a sputum specimen for the diagnosis of pneumonia, the nurse will:
   a. withhold fluid intake for 8 hours prior to administering the specimen.
   b. administer the ordered antibiotic prior to collecting the specimen.
   c. have the client cough deeply 3 times and expectorate into a sterile sputum container.
   d. postpone mouth care until after the specimen is collected.

10. A client has had a bronchoscopy. Several hours after the procedure, she coughs up a moderate amount of blood-tinged sputum. The nurse knows that this finding:
   a. should be reported to the physician immediately.
   b. is normal. Secretions may be blood-tinged for several hours following bronchoscopy.
   c. indicates that a STAT hemoglobin and hematocrit should be obtained.
   d. indicates that a cough suppressant should be prescribed to allow the inflamed area to heal.

Match the descriptions (a–d) with the methods of oxygen delivery listed in questions 11–14.

_____ 11. nasal cannula

_____ 12. simple face mask

_____ 13. non-rebreathing mask

_____ 14. venturi mask

a. can deliver 40–60% oxygen concentration with flow rates of 5–8 L/min
b. most common high-flow system for adults who do not need mechanical ventilation
c. does not interfere with eating or talking
d. up to 100% O_2 can be delivered

15. *Ineffective Airway Clearance* is a frequent nursing diagnosis for the client with pneumonia. An assessment finding that does not support this diagnosis is:
   a. adventitious breath sounds.
   b. bradypnea with dyspnea.
   c. apprehension/anxiety.
   d. cyanosis.

16. When caring for the client with pneumonia, it is important to:
   a. encourage a fluid intake of 3000 mL/day.
   b. establish discharge goals on the fourth day of hospitalization.
   c. encourage the client to stay as physically active as is possible in the inpatient setting.
   d. encourage a high-calorie diet with at least three substantial meals per day.

▪ ▪ ▪ The Client with a Lung Abscess

17. The drug of choice for treating a lung abscess is
   a. clindamycin (Cleocin).
   b. cefazolin (Ancef).
   c. tobramycin (Nebcin).
   d. chloramphenicol (Chloramycetin).

Read the following statements and indicate if they are true or false. Correct any false statements.

_____ 18. The manifestations of a lung abscess typically occur 3 to 4 weeks after an aspiration or pneumonia.

_____ 19. Manifestations of a lung abscess include productive cough, chills, fever, and pleuritic chest pain.

_____ 20. When a lung abscess ruptures, the client will experience immedate relief of pain and discomfort.

▪ ▪ ▪ The Client with Tuberculosis (TB)

21. The causative organism for tuberculosis is _____.

22. Which of the following clients is at the least risk for developing tuberculosis?
    a. a person living in an economically disadvantaged urban area
    b. a client living with AIDS
    c. a college freshman living in a dormitory
    d. a person living in an inner-city homeless shelter

23. Symptoms of TB that are often mistaken for normal age-related changes in the older adult are (a) _____, (b) _____, (c) _____, and (d) _____.

24. To limit the spread of the disease, the nurse should teach the client with TB to _____ _____ _____.

Match the adverse effects (a–c) with the correct drugs listed in questions 25–27.

_____ 25. isoniazid (INH)

_____ 26. rifampin (Rifadin)

_____ 27. ethambutol (Myambutal)

a. optic neuritis
b. peripheral neuropathy
c. causes red-colored body fluids

28. Why is ineffective individual therapeutic regimen management a problem for those people at highest risk for developing active TB?

29. List four groups at risk for TB.
    (a) _____
    (b) _____
    (c) _____
    (d) _____

30. Describe the procedure for performing an intradermal PPD (Mantoux) test.

31. The physician orders sputums for acid-fast bacillus. The nurse should instruct the client to collect how many specimens and with what frequency?
    a. the next three consecutive specimens that can be obtained
    b. specimens collected early each morning, 3 mornings in a row
    c. three specimens collected over the course of a week
    d. a specimen collected once every week for 3 weeks

32. A client has an indurated area of 4 mm following a tuberculin skin test. This indicates that he has:
    a. an active TB infection.
    b. no evidence of tuberculosis.
    c. a history of tuberculosis.
    d. a chance of being infected.

Read the following statements and determine if they are true or false. Correct any false statements.

_____ 33. Surgical removal of lung tissue infected with tuberculosis is commonly used when the client is noncompliant with his medication regime.

_____ 34. Common manifestations of pulmonary TB include fatigue, weight loss, anorexia, low-grade fever, and night sweats.

_____ 35. A positive tuberculin skin test indicates active disease.

_____ 36. The sputum culture reports for TB will be reported in 48 to 72 hours.

_____ 37. In the U.S., the client newly diagnosed with TB would be prescribed two antitubercular medications for a period of 3 months.

_____ 38. Hospitalized clients with TB should wear masks at all times to prevent the spread of infection.

_____ 39. TB is primarily spread by contact.

_____ 40. Single drug therapy may be indicated for prophylactic treatment.

41. List four components of collaborative health care for clients with tuberculosis.
    (a) _____
    (b) _____
    (c) _____
    (d) _____

▪ ▪ ▪ The Client with a Fungal Infection

42. Which of the following statements is false regarding the client with a fungal infection?
    a. Normal respiratory defense mechanisms allow few fungal spores to ever reach the lungs.
    b. Most fungi are opportunistic, able to cause infection only in an immunocompromised host.
    c. In the United States, clients with fungal lung diseases are rarely seen.
    d. Clients with renal failure, leukemia, or burns are particularly susceptible to fungal diseases.

43. The most common fungal infection in the United States is _____.

44. A priority intervention for most clients with histoplasmosis is _____.

Match the following statements (45–47) with the correct type of fungus (a–c).

_____ 45. The primary acute form may be self-limiting.

_____ 46. This fungus causes pulmonary symptoms, including fever and bloody or purulent sputum.

_____ 47. This fungus causes symptoms similar to influenza and arthritis.

a. blastomycosis
b. histoplasmosis
c. coccidioidomycosis

▪ ▪ ▪ The Client with Asthma

48. Identify four clinical manifestations of an acute asthmatic attack.
    (a) _____   (c) _____
    (b) _____   (d) _____

49. Extrinsic triggers for asthma include:
    a. cold air.
    b. emotional upset.
    c. allergens.
    d. bronchial irritants.

50. Drugs commonly used as bronchodilators for the client with asthma must be used with great caution for the person with:
    a. hypotension.
    b. bradycardia.
    c. hypothyroidism.
    d. dysrhythmias.

51. Because of the significant role played by the anxiety and fear associated with asthma, it is vitally important that the client and nurse have a trusting relationship. The most effective way for the nurse to establish such a trusting relationship is to:
    a. give frequent verbal reassurance to the client.
    b. use active listening related to the client's concerns.
    c. teach the client about self-care related to the prescribed medications.
    d. help family members understand the relationship between anxiety and hypoxia.

52. Identify the two treatment concerns when treating the client with asthma.
    (a) _____
    (b) _____

53. A client with asthma asks the nurse, "What is eosinophilia, and what does it mean?" How should the nurse respond?

54. The nurse is caring for a client with an acute asthma. The client has been experiencing tachypnea, diffuse wheezing, and complaints of dyspnea. On auscultation, the nurse notes decreased wheezing. This finding is consistent with:
    a. resolution of the acute episode.
    b. impending respiratory failure.
    c. worsening emotional distress.
    d. the expected therapeutic outcome.

55. Which statement by the client indicates a need for further teaching regarding the use of a metered-dose inhaler?
    a. "I should rinse my mouth before using the inhaler."
    b. "I should shake the container for 3 to 5 seconds before using it."
    c. "Before using the inhaler, I should exhale fully."
    d. "I should wait 30 seconds to 2 minutes between puffs."

56. A client is taking Theo-Dur for long-term treatment of her respiratory problems. List four nursing implications for this medication.
    (a) _____
    (b) _____
    (c) _____
    (d) _____

57. Develop a teaching plan for a client taking a leukotriene modifier.

58. The client's theophylline level is reported as 32 ug/mL. The nurse should recognize that this:
    a. is within normal limits.
    b. is too low to be therapeutic.
    c. may result in drug toxicity.
    d. is elevated in older adults.

▪ ▪ ▪ The Client with Chronic Obstructive Pulmonary Disease (COPD)

59. List three disorders that may co-exist in chronic obstructive pulmonary disease.
    (a) _____
    (b) _____
    (c) _____

60. The major contributing factor to the development of chronic bronchitis is:
    a. allergies.
    b. smoking.
    c. frequent respiratory infections.
    d. heredity.

61. In teaching a client to use a metered dose inhaler, the nurse instructs the client to:
    a. hold the canister in an upright position before placing the mouthpiece in the mouth.
    b. expel as much air as possible from the lungs prior to pressing the canister down and inhaling deeply.
    c. exhale completely and as rapidly as possible after inhaling the medication.
    d. take the second inhalation immediately if a second dose is prescribed.

62. Which of the following statements regarding the client with emphysema is true?
    a. The onset is after age 35 and there is history of recurrent respiratory infections.
    b. There is a persistent cough productive of copious amounts of mucopurulent sputum.
    c. In performing physical examination of the chest, the nurse notes distant or diminished breath sounds.
    d. When blood gases are obtained, respiratory acidosis is noted.

Match the descriptions (a–d) with the correct terms for lung capacity listed in questions 63–66.

_____ 63. total lung capacity (TLC)

_____ 64. total volume (TV)

_____ 65. minute volume (MV)

_____ 66. vital capacity (VC)

a. the volume inhaled and exhaled with normal quiet breathing

b. total amount of air that can be exhaled to a maximal inspiration

c. total volume of the lungs at their maximum inflation

d. total amount or volume of air breathed in 1 minute

67. Oxygen therapy needs to be administered with great caution to clients with COPD because these persons are _____
_____.

68. Clients with COPD should be taught that they should:
   a. have an influenza vaccine at least twice each year.
   b. limit their fluid intake to 1500 mL/day.
   c. remain on complete bed rest to decrease fatigue.
   d. try to prevent exposure to infection, especially upper respiratory infections.

Match the following statements (69–74) with the correct terms (a–c).

_____ 69. Cigarette smoking is the major causative agent.

_____ 70. Deficiency of this enzyme can result to an early onset of emphysema.

_____ 71. This is characterized by the destruction of the walls of the alveoli.

_____ 72. Dyspnea is the initial presenting symptom.

_____ 73. This is characterized by a productive cough.

_____ 74. This is associated with normal or decreased total lung capacity.

a. chronic bronchitis

b. alpha-1 antitrypsin

c. emphysema

75. Develop a teaching plan for a client with COPD who is still smoking.

▪ ▪ ▪ The Client with Cystic Fibrosis (CF)

76. Which of the following statements about cystic fibrosis (CF) is false?
   a. It is the most common lethal genetic disease found in European Americans, affecting about 1 in 2500 live births.
   b. The inheritance pattern for cystic fibrosis is an autosomal-dominant type, and the trait is carried by about 5% of the European American population in the United States.
   c. CF is particularly damaging to the lungs, resulting in COPD in childhood and early adulthood.
   d. Respiratory manifestations of CF are the most common cause of morbidity and death from this disease.

Read the following statements and determine if they are true or false. Correct any false statements.

_____ 77. Cystic fibrosis is always identified in infancy or early childhood.

_____ 78. When a client with CF undergoes a lung transplant, the transplanted lung will eventually demonstrate evidence of pathophysiologic changes of CF.

_____ 79. For the client with CF, chest physiotherapy with percussion, vibration, postural drainage, and coughing are essential components of care.

_____ 80. In CF, the pancreas is overactive.

▪ ▪ ▪ The Client with Atelectasis

81. Which nursing intervention is contraindicated for the client with atelectasis?
   a. turning the client at frequent intervals
   b. positioning with the affected side in a dependent position
   c. encouraging coughing and deep breathing exercises
   d. increasing the fluid intake

82. The primary therapy for atelectasis is _____.

▪ ▪ ▪ The Client with Bronchiectasis

Read the following statements and indicate if they are true or false. Correct any false statements.

_____ 83. About half of all cases of bronchiectasis are related to cystic fibrosis.

_____ 84. A chronic cough productive of large amounts of mucopurulent sputum is characteristic of bronchiectasis.

_____ 85 Collaborative care for the client with bronchiectasis focuses on maintaining optimal pulmonary function and preventing the disorder from progressing.

_____ 86. Bronchiectasis is characterized by the permanent abnormal dilation of one or more large bronchi and the destruction of bronchial walls, usually accompanied by infection.

▪ ▪ ▪ The Client with Occupational Lung Disease

87. A high-priority nursing diagnosis for clients who have a symptomatic occupational lung disease is:
   a. *Activity Intolerance* related to severe dyspnea
   b. *Ineffective Breathing Pattern* related to restrictive lung disease
   c. *Anticipatory Grieving* related to potential loss of employment and income
   d. *Situational Low Self-Esteem* related to change of occupation

Match the following statements (88–91) with the correct conditions (a–d).

_____ 88. may be observed in foundry workers, sandblasters, and pottery makers

_____ 89. an allergic pulmonary disease, such as farmer's lung

_____ 90. a diffuse fibrotic disease of the terminal airways, alveoli, and pleurae

_____ 91. has a higher incidence in the eastern United States

a. hypersensitivity pneumonia
b. silicosis
c. coal worker's pneumoconiosis
d. asbestosis

▪ ▪ ▪ The Client with Sarcoidosis

92. Treatment for sarcoidosis is reserved for clients with severe or disabling symptoms, because sarcoidosis _____.

93. List at least five symptoms of sarcoidosis.

▪ ▪ ▪ The Client with Pulmonary Embolism

94. Most pulmonary emboli are the result of clot formation in the _____.

95. List at least six risk factors for the development of pulmonary embolus.

(a) _____

(b) _____

(c) _____

(d) _____

(e) _____

(f) _____

96. Which of the following statements by the nurse does not represent a clinical manifestation of pulmonary embolism?

a. "The client's chest pain had an abrupt onset."

b. "The client is dyspneic and short of breath."

c. "The client appeared anxious and apprehensive and she coughed quite a bit."

d. "The client's pulse is 50 and respirations are 12–14."

97. Which of the following statements is true concerning anticoagulant therapy as it relates to pulmonary emboli?

a. Anticoagulant therapy is initiated only when a venous thrombus is diagnosed.

b. Low doses of heparin will affect the partial thromboplastin time and the nurse should be aware of the increased risk of bleeding.

c. The purpose of giving heparin to the client with a pulmonary embolus is to dissolve the blood clot in the lung.

d. The antidote for heparin is protamine, whereas vitamin K is the antidote for warfarin.

98. Which of the following nursing interventions is contraindicated in the care of the client with pulmonary embolism?
    a. frequently conduct and document respiratory assessment
    b. maintain bed rest
    c. place the client in a supine position
    d. frequently assess client for signs of bleeding

▪ ▪ ▪ The Client with Pulmonary Hypertension

99. Right ventricular hypertrophy and failure that results from long-standing pulmonary hypertension is termed _____.

Read the following statements and determine whether they are true or false. Correct any false statements.

_____100. For the client with pulmonary hypertension, it is important to monitor for activity intolerance and plan rest periods.

_____101. Treatment of pulmonary hypertension will assist to reverse the course of the illness.

_____102. The manifestations of pulmonary hypertension are productive cough, progressive dyspnea, wheezing, peripheral edema, and distended neck veins.

▪ ▪ ▪ The Client with Cancer of the Lung

103. The most important cause of lung cancer is _____.

104. Which of the following statements about tobacco and smoking is false?
    a. Cigarette smoke contains about 4000 chemicals, including 43 known carcinogens and cancer promoters.
    b. Smoke activates the cilia of the respiratory tract, thus blocking removal of inhaled tar.
    c. Cessation of smoking reduces many of the risks associated with tobacco use.
    d. The link between tobacco use and cancer was first reported in 1912.

105. Which of the following statements is false?
    a. Manifestations of cancer of the lung include chronic cough and hemoptysis.
    b. Manifestations of cancer of the lung are related to the location and spread of the tumor.
    c. Manifestations of cancer of the lung include severe, sharp chest pain early in the disease.
    d. Manifestations of cancer of the lung include weight loss, anorexia, fever, and fatigue.

106. The primary teaching need of the client with lung cancer and the client's family is information about (a) _____, (b) _____ and (c) _____.

Read the following statement and determine if it is true or false. Correct the statement if it is false.

_____107. Although radiation therapy is well controlled and specifically directed toward the tumor cells, some normal cells are also damaged in the process of treatment.

108. Identify four interventions the nurse can use to manage the pain experienced by the terminally ill client with cancer.

    (a) _____

    (b) _____

    (c) _____

    (d) _____

109. To address the problems that a client with advanced cancer of the lung must face, the nurse makes a diagnosis of *Anticipatory Grieving*. Appropriate interventions for this diagnosis would include:

    a. answering questions with honesty, without promoting false hope.

    b. encouraging stoic acceptance of the inevitable losses.

    c. discouraging the client's family from discussing the prognosis for the illness with the client.

    d. taking control of the decisions for treatment and care to relieve the client and family of this added burden.

▪ ▪ ▪ Disorders of the Pleura

110. The pain associated with pleuritis is:

    a. usually dull and bilateral, occuring mainly with expiration.

    b. often referred into the upper abdomen.

    c. often confused with angina pectoris due to the pressure.

    d. well-localized, sharp, and unilateral.

111. Describe the technique used to perform a thoracentesis.

112. A client who is being treated for pneumothorax with chest tubes and a water-seal system will require which of the following nursing interventions?

    a. assessing and documenting the respiratory status every 8 hours

    b. changing the water-seal apparatus every 24 hours to prevent infection

    c. placing the drainage container on the bedside stand to prevent breakage

    d. maintaining a closed system at all times to prevent collapse of the lung

113. The highest priority of care for the client with pneumothorax is maintaining or restoring adequate (a) _____ and (b) _____.

114. Hemothorax is (a) _____. It usually occurs as a result of (b) _____ or (c) _____.

▪ ▪ ▪ The Client with a Chest Wall Injury

115. Multiple rib fractures with resultant chest wall instability is called a (a) _____. It causes the wall to be drawn inward during inspiration and pushed outward with expirations, a condition called (b) _____ movement.

116. The primary intervention for simple rib fractures is:
    a. providing adequate analgesia to allow breathing, coughing, and movement.
    b. teaching the client to splint the chest when coughing or sneezing.
    c. performing assessments every 4 hours for a pneumothorax.
    d. limiting cigarette smoking during the acute stage of the injury.

▪ ▪ ▪ The Client with Inhalation Injury

117. Smoke inhalation can affect normal respirations through which three mechanisms?
    (a) _____
    (b) _____
    (c) _____

118. A client who has carbon monoxide poisoning will have _____ coloring of the skin and mucous membranes.

119. Identify three clinical manifestations of near drowning.
    (a) _____
    (b) _____
    (c) _____

▪ ▪ ▪ The Client with Acute Respiratory Failure

120. In the person without pre-existing lung disease (such as COPD), respiratory failure exists when arterial blood gases show the PaO_2 to be < _____ mm Hg and the $PaCO_2$ to be > _____ mm Hg.

121. A client was placed on a mechanical ventilator due to acute respiratory failure. He has been given Pavulon (pancuronium bromide), a nondepolarizing neuromuscular blocker, to achieve complete muscle paralysis. The physician has also ordered morphine sulfate to be given along with the Pavulon. Explain why the physician ordered the morphine sulfate.

122. Which of the following statements regarding oxygen therapy is false?
    a. Concentrations of 40–60% oxygen are used only for short periods to avoid oxygen toxicity.
    b. With continued high levels of oxygen delivery, surfactant synthesis is impaired.
    c. The lungs become more compliant with continued high levels of oxygen delivery.
    d. The development of oxygen toxicity depends on both the concentration of oxygen delivered and the duration of therapy.

123. The purpose of the inflated cuff on an endotracheal or tracheostomy tube is to:
    a. maintain positive pressure ventilation.
    b. prevent the swallowing of mouth secretions.
    c. allow the client to talk.
    d. make the tube more comfortable for the client.

124. A client sustained a serious head injury in a skiing accident. In the ICU, he was placed on a mechanical ventilator which was set on the control mode. Control mode means:
    a. all breaths are delivered by the ventilator at a preset frequency, volume or pressure, and inspiratory flow rate.
    b. the client can trigger breaths to be delivered by initiating respiratory effort.
    c. machine-controlled breaths are delivered at a set frequency and volume or pressure. Between these breaths, the client can breathe spontaneously with no ventilator assistance.
    d. positive pressure is applied to the airways of this spontaneously breathing client.

125. Nursing care for a client with a nursing diagnosis of *Inability to Sustain Spontaneous Ventilation* will include:
    a. positioning in a high-Fowler's position to promote lung expansion.
    b. administering sedation to decrease anxiety.
    c. providing high concentrations of oxygen to treat hypoxia.
    d. encouraging activity to maintain muscle tone.

126. In caring for a client who is receiving neuromuscular blocking agents while having mechanical ventilation, the nurse must:
    a. avoid giving narcotics and antianxiety agents, which depress the central nervous system.
    b. administer the blocking agent as an intravenous bolus.
    c. turn off the ventilator alarms while in the room to allow the client to rest.
    d. keep neostigmine or a similar drug at the bedside at all times.

127. The ventilator weaning mode that allows gradual transition from 100% mechanical ventilation to 100% spontaneous ventilation is:
    a. continuous positive airway pressure.
    b. T-piece trial.
    c. pressure support.
    d. intermittent mandatory ventilation.

128. Regarding care of the client who requires endotracheal suctioning, research findings suggest that:
    a. hyperoxgenation should be part of standard endotracheal suctioning technique.
    b. hyperoxgenation should not be part of standard endotracheal suctioning technique.
    c. transcutaneous oxygen measurement is not an accurate indicator of blood oxygen levels.
    d. pulse oximetry readings readily indicate the extent of a fall in arterial oxygen levels.

▪ ▪ ▪ The Client with Adult Respiratory Distress Syndrome (ARDS)

129. The initial manifestations of ARDS are usually:
    a. crackles (rales) and rhonchi.
    b. tissue hypoxia and metabolic acidosis.
    c. dyspnea and tachypnea.
    d. agitation and confusion.

130. In caring for a client with a new diagnosis of ARDS, the nurse would first prepare for:
    a. intubation and mechanical ventilation.
    b. intravenous antibiotic therapy.
    c. placement of a Swan-Ganz line.
    d. insertion of a nasogastric tube for feeding.

131. While caring for a client with ARDS, the nurse would suspect a decreased cardiac output if assessment showed:
    a. a decreasing pulse rate.
    b. a rising arterial pressure.
    c. a urinary output of less than 30 mL/hour.
    d. regular sinus rhythm on the cardiac monitor.

132. Teaching for the client with ARDS should include reassurance that:
    a. intubation and mechanical ventilation is a temporary measure.
    b. recurrence of ARDS is preventable by lifestyle alterations.
    c. long-term aftereffects of ARDS may require several minor alterations in lifestyle.
    d. the avoidance of cigarette smoking during the acute phase of the syndrome will preserve lung function.

▪ ▪ ▪ Critical Thinking Exercises

133. The client has undergone a pneumonectomy and has a chest tube. Develop a teaching plan to explain the purpose and care of chest tubes to the client and visitors.

134. If a chest tube becomes disconnected from the drainage system, what is the most appropriate action by the nurse? What actions should be taken to prevent this in the future?

135. The nurse is at the beach when there is a near-drowning and provides first aid. Discuss the care the nurse should provide until the EMTs arrive.

▪ ▪ ▪ Additional Learning Experiences

- Visit the local office of the American Lung Association and become more familiar with the resources they provide for individuals interested in quitting smoking.
- Contact the state public health office and become more familiar with the incidence of tuberculosis in your community and state.
- Identify Internet resources for clients with respiratory disorders.
- Contact the National Cancer Institute and find out what resources they provide for individuals with lung cancer.

Assessing Clients with Musculoskeletal Disorders

■ ■ ■ **Focused Study Tips**

- Match the assessment of bones and joints with the assessment of the nerves and blood vessels.

- Describe procedures for comparing affected and unaffected sides of the client's body when performing an assessment of musculoskeletal function.

- Describe the movements that the client will be asked to perform during the physical assessment of the musculoskeletal system.

- List the components of a musculoskeletal assessment.

■ ■ ■ **Anatomy and Physiology**

Match the anatomical structures (a–j) with the descriptions of physiologic function listed in questions 1–10.

_____ 1. a double-layered connective tissue covering bone

_____ 2. regions where two or more bones meet

_____ 3. the basic structural unit of compact bone

_____ 4. concentric layers of meshwork forming spongy bone

_____ 5. cells that form bone

_____ 6. thick filaments of protein that make up myofibrils

_____ 7. fibrous connective tissue bands that connect muscles to the periosteum

_____ 8. dense bands of tissue that connect bone to bone

_____ 9. small sacs of synovial fluid that cushion bony areas

_____ 10. structures that make up a single muscle fiber

a. tendons
b. sarcomeres
c. articulations
d. myofibrils
e. periosteum
f. Haversian system
g. trabeculae
h. bursae
i. osteoblasts
j. ligaments

11. Identify four functions of bone.

(a) _____

(b) _____

(c) _____

(d) _____

12. Discuss three factors that influence the process of bone remodeling.

    (a) _____
    _____

    (b) _____
    _____

    (c) _____
    _____

13. Identify the four main functional properties of skeletal muscle.

    (a) _____

    (b) _____

    (c) _____

    (d) _____

14. Describe the effects of the following types of exercise on skeletal muscle.

    a. strenuous exercise:

    b. regular exercise:

    c. lack of exercise:

15. Muscle movement is triggered by the release of the neurotransmitter (a) _____
    _____, which alters muscle cell–fiber permeability. (b) _____
    enter the fiber and cause an action potential that results in muscle contraction.

■ ■ ■ **Assessment of Musculoskeletal Function**

16. The primary manifestations of altered function in the musculoskeletal system are:

    a. stiffness and swelling.   c. fever and fatigue.

    b. pain and limited mobility.   d. rash and unexplained weight loss.

17. A 46-year-old client arrives at the emergency department after a fall during a tennis game. He complains of pain and weakness in his right leg. Prepare a list of assessment interview questions that specifically address the client's chief complaint.

18. List three techniques used to assess the musculoskeletal system.

    (a) _____

    (b) _____

    (c) _____

19. A goniometer is used to measure:
    a. degree of spinal curvature.   c. joint range of motion.
    b. muscle strength.   d. tendon contractility.

20. List the general sequence of the physical assessment of the musculoskeletal system.

Match the terms (a–j) with the definitions listed in questions 21–30.

_____ 21. a general term meaning inflammation of a joint

_____ 22. an increased lumbar curve

_____ 23. break in a bone due to trauma

_____ 24. exaggerated thoracic curvature of the spine

_____ 25. inflammation of the synovial lining of a joint

_____ 26. a grating noise with joint movement

_____ 27. irreversible shortening of muscles and tendons

_____ 28. excessively abducted great toe

_____ 29. hard, nontender nodules on interphalangeal joints

_____ 30. lateral curvature of the spine

a. crepitation
b. lordosis
c. hallux valgus
d. Heberden's nodules
e. contractures
f. scoliosis
g. synovitis
h. fracture
i. kyphosis
j. arthritis

Case Study

Larissa Destone is a 45-year-old home health aide who has been admitted for complaints of chronic low back pain. During the health assessment interview, Ms. Destone tells the nurse that she has had two previous bouts of back pain, but none as severe as this current episode. For her previous back problems, she received anti-inflammatory medications, physical therapy, and diathermy, which she states worked effectively. Ms. Destone tells the nurse she first noticed the pain when transferring an older client from his wheelchair to his living room couch during a recent home visit. Ms. Destone is 5' 4", weighs 168 lbs, and her right leg is ¼ inch longer than her left leg. She is unable to touch her toes and has a 25-degree lateral bending capability. Her back extension and shoulder rotation abilities are each within 2–3 degrees of normal. Ms. Destone's gait is slow, and there is an obvious limp on her left side when she walks. Ms. Destone states she is not taking any medications regularly but did take two Advil last night to try to ease the pain. She also used a heating pad on her back last night with no relief.

31. Explain the possible significance of the assessment data provided above and the impact Ms. Destone's employment has on her back.

32. Which assessment would the nurse perform to detect carpal tunnel syndrome?
   a. Thomas test   b. McMurray's test   c. Phalen's test   d. ballottement test

33. Decreased bone mass and the thinning of intervertebral discs with loss of normal spinal curves result in which variation of assessment findings in the older adult?
   a. muscle wasting, osteoporosis   c. osteoarthritis, decreased height
   b. muscle wasting, osteoarthritis   d. kyphosis, decreased height

Read the following statements and determine if they are true or false. Correct any false statements.

_____ 34. Osteoporosis is more common in European American women with small bones.

_____ 35. Height remains stable as adults age.

_____ 36. Bone remodeling stops as adults grow older.

_____ 37. Joint cartilage becomes more rigid as adults age.

_____ 38. Joint stiffness, pain, and crepitation commonly occur in osteoarthritis.

▪ ▪ ▪ Critical Thinking Exercises

39. Identify common activities or movements that might be helpful in assessing a young adult's mobility without placing them on an examination table.

40. Develop a teaching plan to assist adults in modifying their risk factors for osteoporosis.

▪ ▪ ▪ Additional Learning Experiences

- Practice musculoskeletal assessment procedures on willing family members, friends, and assigned clients.
- Practice performing the motions that the client will be asked to perform during the physical assessment of the musculoskeletal system.

CHAPTER
36

Nursing Care of Clients
with Musculoskeletal Disorders

■ ■ ■ **Focused Study Tips**

- Describe the normal physiology of bone resorption and bone formation and the patho-physiology of osteoporosis, osteomalacia, and Paget's disease.

- Discuss the basic recommendations for an exercise program.

- List key nursing interventions when caring for clients with osteomyelitis, bone tumors, muscular dystrophy, and foot disorders.

- Identify the current recommendations for managing back pain, particularly recommendations related to conservative treatment.

■ ■ ■ **The Client with Osteoporosis**

1. Osteoporosis is a metabolic bone disorder in which there is an imbalance of the processes that influence bone (a) _____ and (b) _____.

2. What percent of individuals affected by osteoporosis are women? _____

3. The primary reason a woman is at greater risk for osteoporosis than a man is because:
   a. a woman's total bone mass is less than that of a man.
   b. a woman's estrogen level increases with age.
   c. a man is more physically active than a woman.
   d. a man's subcutaneous tissue is more evenly distributed than a woman's.

4. During a routine health examination, a client is told by her physician that she has early osteo-porotic changes and that she should exercise. She tells the nurse, "I thought exercise builds mus-cle. What does it have to do with my bones?" The best response by the nurse is that exercise:
   a. encourages a positive mental attitude and promotes healthy aging.
   b. increases the amount of circulating estrogen in the body.
   c. lowers the amount of body fat, reducing the stress on the bones.
   d. increases the blood flow and thus helps create new bone matter.

5. Identify four clinical manifestations of osteoporosis.
   (a) _____
   (b) _____
   (c) _____
   (d) _____

6. _____ percent of bone mass must be lost before it is demonstrated on x-rays.

7. Pharmacologic therapy for the client with osteoporosis focuses on:
   a. osteocalcin therapy to slow bone "turnover."
   b. calcium supplementation to restore lost bone mass.
   c. hormone-replacement therapy to preserve existing bone mass.
   d. fluoride therapy to reduce urinary hydroxyproline.

278   ■

8. A 75-year-old client taking estrogen for osteoporosis comes to the clinic complaining of vaginal bleeding. When obtaining her health history, the nurse should ask:
   a. whether the client has had a tubal ligation.
   b. if the client has stopped taking the prescribed estrogen for any period of time.
   c. the age at which the client experienced menarche.
   d. whether the client smokes.

9. A client with Type 2 diabetes is starting estrogen-replacement therapy for osteoporosis. Regarding oral hypoglycemic medication, what information should the nurse provide her?
   a. The dosage of oral hypoglycemic medication she takes may need to be adjusted.
   b. The dosage of oral hypoglycemic medication she takes will likely decrease.
   c. She should stop taking oral hypoglycemic medication.
   d. She should only take oral hypoglycemic medication if she feels tired.

10. A client with osteoporosis is instructed to increase his intake of dietary calcium. The client states, "I don't like milk." List other sources of dietary calcium that the nurse might suggest.

Read the following statement and determine if it is true or false. Correct it if it is false.

_____ 11. Estrogen therapy is safe for a 35-year-old client with a family history of osteoporosis.

Read the following statements and complete them.

12. A 69-year-old client asks, "Why must I learn about foods that contain calcium when my friend just takes a vitamin pill?" The best response by the nurse would be that _____
    _____.

13. It is recommended that calcium supplements be taken in combination with _____ in order to enhance absorption.

14. Activities such as walking and jogging have a beneficial effect on _____.

15. Most adults should ingest (a) _____ mg of calcium each day. Postmenopausal women not on ERT should ingest (b) _____ mg.

16. How can a client test how well a brand of calcium supplement will be absorbed in the stomach?

17. Older clients with osteoporosis are at risk for which nursing diagnosis related to *Impaired Physical Mobility?* _____

▪ ▪ ▪ The Client with Osteomalacia

18. Which of the following nursing diagnoses most accurately reflects the pathophysiologic basis of osteomalacia?
    a. *Altered Nutrition: Less than Body Requirements*
    b. *Impaired Physical Mobility* related to limited range of motion
    c. *Fear* related to a chronic condition
    d. *Pain* secondary to pathologic fractures

19. State the two main factors that may cause osteomalacia.
    (a) _____
    (b) _____

20. Which of the following clients is most at risk for the development of osteomalacia?
    a. a pregnant client   c. a fair-skinned client
    b. a client with diabetes   d. a client in renal failure

21. A retired 65-year-old male develops osteomalacia following a gastrectomy. He is readmitted to the hospital and will begin taking oral vitamin D supplements. Which symptom will the client most likely report during his physical assessment?
    a. muscle cramps   c. pain in the pelvis or long bones
    b. lack of coordination   d. nausea and anorexia

22. Which of the following complications would necessitate discontinuing the above client's vitamin D supplements?
    a. an elevated serum calcium level   c. premature ventricular contractions
    b. a seizure   d. elevated urinary hydroxyproline

23. Identify four steps to maintaining safety in the home of a client with osteomalacia.
    (a) _____
    (b) _____
    (c) _____
    (d) _____

24. Identify three dietary sources of vitamin D.
    (a) _____
    (b) _____
    (c) _____

▪ ▪ ▪ The Client with Paget's Disease

25. Paget's disease is a disorder characterized by:
    a. excessive osteoblastic wasting.
    b. diminished osteoblastic activity.
    c. excessive osteoclastic bone resorption.
    d. diminished osteoclastic activity.

26. During the initial stage of Paget's disease, the bones actually (a) _____ in size. As the disease progresses bone remodeling is (b) _____ or (c) _____.

27. Which statement by the client taking alendronate (Fosamax) indicates a need for further teaching?
    a. "I should take this with a full glass of water upon arising, 30 minutes before food or other medication."
    b. "My doctor told me I could not take this medication if I develop renal insufficiency or renal failure."
    c. "I can take this medication with milk or an antacid if this medication upsets my stomach or results in heartburn."
    d. "This medication may prevent and treat osteoporosis as well as relieve the bone pain I experience from Paget's disease."

28. Which of the following statements by the client taking alendronate (Fosamax) is correct?
    a. "I have eaten breakfast, I should not lie down."
    b. "This medication should bring quick relief of my symptoms."
    c. "Tingling around the mouth is an expected side effect."
    d. "Heartburn and indigestion are expected side effects."

29. Identify key components when teaching clients with Paget's disease about impaired physical mobility.

30. Prior to discharging the client with Paget's disease, the nurse should teach the client that pain typically occurs:
    a. at night.
    b. continuously.
    c. only when walking.
    d. only with heavy activity.

31. Clients with untreated Paget's disease will have:
    a. increasing acid phosphatase.
    b. increasing alkaline phosphatase.
    c. abnormal liver function tests.
    d. decreasing calcium levels.

▪ ▪ ▪ The Client with Osteomyelitis

Match the microorganism's mode of entry (a–c) with the correct cause of osteomyelitis listed in questions 32–37. Modes of entry may be used more than once.

_____ 32. endocarditis

_____ 33. an open leg fracture

_____ 34. a bullet wound

_____ 35. venous stasis ulcers

_____ 36. a urinary tract infection

_____ 37. an animal bite

a. secondary to local infection
b. hematogenous infection
c. via extension

38. Which of the following clinical manifestations is associated with early osteomyelitis?
    a. warmth at involved site
    b. tachycardia
    c. high temperature
    d. skin ulceration

39. Which diagnostic test has high affinity for soft tissue abscesses?
    a. plain radiographs
    b. differential WBC
    c. ESR
    d. bone scan or gallium scan

40. In the older client with osteomyelitis, the nurse should remember that:
    a. osteomyelitis causes pressure ulcers.
    b. warm, flushed skin is an early clinical manifestation of infection.
    c. typical signs and symptoms of infection and inflammation may not be present.
    d. a pathologic fracture may be the first clinical manifestation of infection.

41. The most common infectious organism in osteomyelitis is:
    a. *Escherichia coli.*   b. *Pseudomonas.*   c. *Proteus.*   d. *Staphylococcus aureus.*

42. Which statement by the client undergoing a bone scan indicates a need for further teaching?
    a. "I will remove my jewelry and any metal before the procedure."
    b. "I will not eat or drink before the procedure."
    c. "My family shouldn't worry about having contact with me."
    d. "The bone scan may take 30 to 60 minutes to complete."

▪ ▪ ▪ The Client with Common Spinal Deformities

43. Scoliosis is usually first noted by asymmetry of the (a) _____
    (b) _____, and (c) _____.

44. Which one of the following conditions poses a risk for the development of kyphosis?
    a. diabetes   b. renal failure   c. Paget's disease   d. Cushing's syndrome

▪ ▪ ▪ The Client with Common Foot Deformities

45. A client with hallux valgus should be taught to:
    a. exercise at least three times daily.
    b. select and wear corrective shoes.
    c. choose foods high in calcium and vitamin D.
    d. wear elastic stockings.

46. Which of the following statements best describes hammertoe?
    a. a dorsiflexion of the first phalanx with plantar flexion of the second and third phalanges
    b. a hyperextension of the second and third phalanges and extension of the first phalanx
    c. an extension of the first phalanx and plantar flexion of the second and third phalanges
    d. a lateral displacement of the first metatarsal

47. Prevention of a Morton's neuroma involves:
    a. wearing corrective footwear.
    b. obtaining pads to relieve pressure.
    c. wearing shoes that fit correctly.
    d. not wearing high heels.

▪ ▪ ▪ The Client with Low Back Pain

48. Which of the following physical findings would indicate that a client with low back pain might need to be hospitalized?
    a. fever and chills
    b. unrelieved pain
    c. limited range of motion
    d. numbness in a lower extremity

49. Which of the following clients would be at most risk for acute back pain?
    a. a pregnant client
    b. a person shoveling snow
    c. a secretary
    d. a client who takes birth control pills

50. The nurse should teach the client with low back pain to:
    a. maintain bed rest until the pain subsides.
    b. begin a program of prescribed exercises.
    c. purchase a back brace.
    d. apply heat or an ice pack over the affected area for 1 hour.

51. Which of the following statements describes appropriate body mechanics when lifting an object?
    a. place the object away from the body's center of gravity
    b. never lift an object above knee level
    c. keep the object close to the body
    d. rotate the spine slightly during the lift

52. List two psychosocial risk factors for low back pain.
    (a) _____
    (b) _____

53. A client who has injured his back tells the nurse that he would like to have surgery so that he can return to work as soon as possible. The most appropriate response by the nurse is:
    a. "Surgery may make things worse and you may never return to work."
    b. "You will have to miss 6 weeks of work before the doctor will consider surgery."
    c. "Surgery helps only 1 out of 100 individuals with acute back pain."
    d. "Surgery is no guarantee that you will return to work."

54. The most appropriate position for the client with back pain is:
    a. side-lying, with hips and knees flexed.
    b. lying flat on back with bedboard.
    c. sitting in a straight-back chair.
    d. reclining in a firm recliner.

55. The rationale for maintaining ice for no longer than 15 minutes and heat no longer than 30 minutes is to prevent:
    a. skin injury.
    b. vasoconstriction.
    c. vasodilation.
    d. rebound phenomenon.

56. Identify five lifestyle changes that may lessen back pain.
    (a) _____
    (b) _____
    (c) _____
    (d) _____
    (e) _____

▪ ▪ ▪ The Client with Bone Tumors

57. The most commonly occurring type of malignant bone tumor is:
    a. chondrosarcoma.   b. fibrosarcoma.   c. giant cell tumors.   d. osteosarcoma.

58. Which test will determine the exact type of bone tumor?
    a. x-ray   c. MRI
    b. CT scan   d. percutaneous needle biopsy

59. Signs and symptoms of a pelvic neoplasm may include:
    (a) _____
    (b) _____
    (c) _____
    (d) _____

60. Clients with a malignant bone tumor will have a(n) _____ alkaline phosphatase.

▪ ▪ ▪ The Client with Muscular Dystrophy

61. The most common form of muscular dystrophy is:
    a. Duchenne's.   b. myotonic.   c. Lewis's.   d. Becker's.

62. A client is pregnant. Her sister has muscular dystrophy, and the client is concerned that her child may also develop muscular dystrophy. The nurse should advise the client that:
    a. she should seek genetic counseling.
    b. she should have an ultrasound.
    c. there is no way to detect the underlying genetic defect.
    d. she is unlikely to pass this condition to her child.

63. The three main goals of nursing care for a client with muscular dystrophy include:
    (a) _____
    (b) _____
    (c) _____

▪ ▪ ▪ Critical Thinking Exercises

64. Develop a teaching plan for a client who will be discharged on home intravenous antibiotic therapy for osteomyelitis.

65. Develop a nursing care plan for a client who is on prednisone and is also suffering from osteomyelitis.

▪ ▪ ▪ Additional Learning Experiences

- Consult with your instructor about observing bone density testing or a bone scan.
- Develop a teaching program for elderly women about increasing their dietary intake of calcium.
- Consult with your instructor about attending a scoliosis clinic.

CHAPTER
37

Nursing Care of Clients with Musculoskeletal Trauma

▪ ▪ ▪ Focused Study Tips

- Describe the different types of fractures and the nursing care associated with each type.

- Explain the different types of traction and the nursing care of the client in traction.

- Identify the principles associated with cast care.

- Compare and contrast the clinical manifestations of the seven major types of fracture

complications: compartment syndrome, shock, fat embolism, deep vein thrombosis (DVT), infection, delayed union, and reflex sympathetic dystrophy.

- Describe the nursing care for the client with a hip fracture and for the client following an amputation.

▪ ▪ ▪ Overview of Musculoskeletal Trauma

1. Which factor has the most effect on the severity of a traumatic injury?
   a. the client's age
   b. the amount of force applied to the impact point
   c. the client's height and weight
   d. the location of the impact point

2. Describe the two types of force that cause trauma.
   (a) _____
   (b) _____

3. The older client is at higher risk for musculoskeletal trauma because of:
   a. brittle bones.
   b. decreased muscle mass.
   c. poor vision.
   d. increased falls.

4. Nursing care of clients with musculoskeletal trauma focuses on:
   a. preventing injuring.
   b. providing pain control.
   c. promoting rehabilitation.
   d. restoring homeostasis.

▪ ▪ ▪ The Client with a Fracture

Match the types of fractures (a–f) with the correct definitions listed in questions 5–10.

_____ 5. The fractured bone moves out of anatomical alignment.

_____ 6. A jagged break due to twisting force applied to the bone.

_____ 7. A fracture occurring along the lengthwise plane of the bone.

_____ 8. The broken ends of bone protrude through soft tissue and skin.

_____ 9. The bone fragments into many pieces.

_____ 10. The bone breaks cleanly and does not interrupt the skin integrity.

a. open (compound) fracture
b. greenstick fracture
c. unstable (displaced) fracture
d. simple (closed) fracture
e. comminuted fracture
f. spiral fracture

11. Prehospital care of fractured extremities includes:
    a. wrapping the affected extremity with a towel.
    b. application of a tourniquet.
    c. immobilization.
    d. applying pressure to the pulse proximal to the fracture.

12. Identify three types of traction.
    (a) _____   (c) _____
    (b) _____

13. Pharmacologic interventions for a client with a complex fractured femur focus on:
    a. minimizing histamine response.   c. reducing blood pressure.
    b. promoting bone healing.   d. alleviating pain.

14. When caring for a client with skeletal traction of the leg, the nurse should:
    a. maintain the client's position and traction.
    b. not remove the weight without an order.
    c. always keep the client's foot flush with the footboard.
    d. reposition the traction as per patient comfort.

15. A 34-year-old client sustains a fracture of the left tibia while skiing. He is admitted to an orthopedic unit after having the fracture reduced and a long leg cast applied. A priority nursing intervention is to assess:
    a. neurovascular status.   c. respiratory status.
    b. skin integrity.   d. joint range of motion.

16. Which of the following is the priority nursing assessment for detecting compartment syndrome?
    a. auscultating the pulse   c. assessing skin color
    b. palpating the client's pulses   d. monitoring oxygen saturation

17. Clients are most at risk for developing compartment syndrome (a) _____
    after a musculoskeletal injury, when (b) _____ is at its peak.

18. The best treatment for deep vein thrombosis is _____.

19. Which assessment finding might suggest the presence of fat embolism?
    a. ecchymosis   b. hematoma   c. petechiae   d. edema

20. Name the "five Ps" for neurovascular assessment for clients with fractures.

    (a) _____   (d) _____

    (b) _____   (e) _____

    (c) _____

21. Identify four key symptoms of fractures.

    (a) _____   (c) _____

    (b) _____   (d) _____

22. When caring for the client in skeletal traction, the nurse should:

    a. place the client's feet flush with the footboard.

    b. provide frequent analgesics.

    c. remove weights when assessing pin sites.

    d. turn the pins daily to prevent crusting.

23. Which statement by the client with a short leg cast indicates a need for further teaching?

    a. "I should not place anything in my cast."

    b. "I should report any changes in circulation and sensation or increase in pain."

    c. "I can dry my plaster cast with a blow dryer if it becomes wet when I shower."

    d. "Using a blow dryer on cool may relieve itching under the cast."

24. An early sign of compartment syndrome is:

    a. cyanosis.   c. tingling.

    b. loss of sensation.   d. worsening pain.

25. Identify seven topics to discuss with older adults when teaching them about fall prevention.

    (a) _____

    (b) _____

    (c) _____

    (d) _____

    (e) _____

    (f) _____

    (g) _____

26. Identify three risk factors for deep vein thrombosis.

    (a) _____

    (b) _____

    (c) _____

Read the following statements and determine if they are true or false. Correct any false statements.

_____ 27. Bivalving a cast allows the client to bend the proximal joint.

_____ 28. Immediately following a fracture, elevate the injured extremity 2 inches above the heart.

_____ 29. Distraction is of little value in orthopedic-related pain.

_____ 30. Delayed union is related to limited calcium ingestion.

_____ 31. Unique manifestations of fat embolism are pin-sized purple or red spots on the skin.

_____ 32. A fracture of the pelvis is considered the most serious type of fracture.

▪ ▪ ▪ The Client with Fractures of Specific Sites

33. Which fracture is usually immobilized by a splint, not a cast?
    a. a fracture of the clavicle
    c. a fracture of the elbow
    b. a fracture of the humerus
    d. a fracture of the radius

34. Which fracture generally requires the lengthiest rehabilitation?
    a. a fracture of the wrist
    c. a fracture of the tibia
    b. a fracture of the femur
    d. a fracture of the spine

35. The client with rib fracture(s) should be encouraged to:
    a. breathe deeply even if pain occurs.
    b. breathe as deeply as possible as long as no pain occurs.
    c. expect a certain degree of shortness of breath.
    d. avoid regular use of a spirometer.

36. The priority nursing assessment following facial fractures is to assess:
    a. respiratory rate.
    c. airway.
    b. heart rate.
    d. level of pain.

37. The nurse is attending a country fair and there is a ferris wheel accident. The nurse suspects one of the victims has a spinal cord fracture. The most appropriate action is to: _____
    _____
    _____

38. The priority assessments to be performed on this individual with suspected spinal cord injury include: _____
    _____
    _____

39. What is the treatment for a nondisplaced spinal fracture?

40. The EMTs arrive and ask the nurse to stay with a person with a compound fracture of the femur. What should the nurse do until the EMTs can take over the care of this individual?

41. The nurse is caring for an elderly, independent-living woman who recently fractured her ribs. Develop a plan of care for her.

42. A 42-year-old hairdresser fractures his tibia and fibula ice skating. He tells the nurse he is planning to return to work in 1 week. What is the most appropriate advice for the nurse to provide the client?

▪ ▪ ▪ The Client with a Hip Fracture

43. An extracapsular hip fracture involves the:
   a. femoral periosteum.
   b. femoral head.
   c. femoral neck.
   d. inter- and subtrochanteric regions of the femur.

44. The optimal positioning for a client following a total hip arthroplasty is:
   a. high-Fowler's.
   b. legs abducted.
   c. legs adducted.
   d. legs externally rotated.

45. Which of the following discharge instructions would the nurse provide to the client returning home after a right hip replacement surgery?
   a. avoid vigorous activity
   b. use a cane at all times for walking
   c. sit only on high chairs
   d. keep the legs straight at all times

46. A client is hospitalized following surgery for a fractured hip. She asks the nurse why a pillow is kept between her legs. The rationale for this nursing intervention is that it:
   a. prevents external rotation.
   b. prevents excessive extension.
   c. prevents adduction.
   d. promotes comfort.

47. The client using a cane should use it :
   a. on the affected side.
   b. on the unaffected side.
   c. in the dominant hand.
   d. wherever it seems comfortable.

48. Which statement by the client being prepared for hip surgery indicates a need for further teaching?
   a. "I will start getting out of bed 2–3 days postoperatively."
   b. "I will be able to have pain medication if I need it."
   c. "I must perform my exercises to strengthen my legs."
   d. "I will have to sit in a high, straight-back chair."

▪ ▪ ▪ The Client with an Amputation

49. What is the major cause for amputation of a lower extremity?
   a. trauma
   b. aneurysm
   c. peripheral vascular disease
   d. infection

50. Which position should the client with a below-the-knee amputation maintain postoperatively?
   a. knee extended, stump elevated
   b. knee flexed, stump prone
   c. knee hyperextended, stump prone
   d. knee hyperflexed, stump elevated

51. Which statement is true about phantom pain?
   a. Phantom pain is present at the suture line.
   b. Phantom pain results from edema formation.
   c. Phantom pain results from trauma to the nerves at the amputation site.
   d. Phantom pain results from muscle spasms.

52. A client with an above-the-knee amputation should lie:
    a. supine with the stump elevated.
    b. prone for periods throughout the day.
    c. in the position of comfort if no rehabilitation is planned.
    d. supine with the stump in a neutral position.

53. The correct way to wrap a stump dressing is from:
    a. the proximal to the distal aspect.
    b. the waist to the stump.
    c. the distal to the proximal aspect.
    d. around the wound dressing.

54. Describe components of care to assist a recent amputee in coping with body image disturbance.

55. Develop a plan of care for a client with acute surgical pain and phantom pain following an amputation.

56. Develop a teaching plan to assist a client in preventing contractures following a below-the-knee amputation.

■ ■ ■ **The Client with Soft Tissue Trauma**

Identify the type of soft tissue injury described.

57. A microscopic tear in a muscle. _____

58. Injury to a ligament. _____

59. The rupture and bleeding of small blood vessels into soft tissue. _____

60. Soft tissue injuries benefit from care that follows the acronym RICE. Define each letter.
    R: _____
    I: _____
    C: _____
    E: _____

61. Four days after a sprain, a client continues to complain of pain. The most appropriate intervention is to:
    a. continue to apply ice.
    b. apply heat.
    c. try more pain medication.
    d. see an orthopedic physician.

▪ ▪ ▪ The Client with Joint Dislocation, Subluxation, or a Repetitive Use Injury

62. List the two most common sites for a dislocation.

(a) _____

(b) _____

63. Carpal tunnel syndrome results from:
    a. compression of the median nerve.
    b. sprains to hand ligaments.
    c. injury to the radial and ulnar nerve.
    d. contusion to the hand.

64. Following a reduction of a dislocation, a priority nursing intervention is:
    a. applying a splinting device and stabilizing the joint.
    b. assessing distal circulation, motion, and sensation.
    c. monitoring vital signs and oximeter.
    d. providing pain medication and comfort measures.

▪ ▪ ▪ Critical Thinking Exercises

65. The nurse is driving on a rural road and comes to the scene of an automobile accident. The nurse does not have a first aid kit in the car. The victims all appear to be suffering from fractures. What materials could the nurse use to immobilize the fractures until the EMTs arrive?

66. The nurse is caring for an elderly woman about to be discharged home following the repair of a fractured hip. She starts complaining of increasing pain and discomfort in the fracture site. What should the nurse do?

▪ ▪ ▪ Additional Learning Experiences

- Interview friends and family members who have suffered from fractures, and ask them to describe their experiences.

- Practice walking and stair-climbing with crutches. Describe your experience.

CHAPTER 38

Nursing Care of Clients with Arthritic and Connective Tissue Disorders

■ ■ ■ Focused Study Tips

- Compare and contrast the treatments for osteoarthritis and rheumatoid arthritis. Review all pharmacologic, nonpharmacologic, and surgical therapies associated with these disorders.

- Describe the postoperative nursing care for the client with total hip replacement.

- Summarize the short-term and long-term pharmacologic therapies for the client with gout.

- Identify the characteristic joint deformities seen in rheumatoid arthritis.

- Explain the cutaneous manifestations of systemic lupus erythematosus (SLE) and teaching points for the client with SLE.

- Discuss the key nursing interventions for clients with scleroderma and other connective tissue disorders.

■ ■ ■ Overview

1. Which of the following statements about rheumatic disorders is correct?
   a. Rheumatic disorders are part of the normal aging process.
   b. Rheumatic disorders always occur secondary to another disease process.
   c. Although debilitating, rheumatic disorders are never fatal.
   d. Rheumatic disorders can cause problems with mobility, deformity, and disability.

2. Define arthritis.

■ ■ ■ The Client with Osteoarthritis

3. Osteoarthritis differs from other rheumatic disorders because it is not associated with an (a) ___ _____ process. Osteoarthritis is characterized by a loss of (b) _____ in the synovial joints.

4. While examining a client with osteoarthritis, the nurse notes swollen, tender, bony enlargements of the distal interphalangeal joints. The nurse recognizes these signs as:
   a. tophi.
   b. swan-neck deformity.
   c. Heberden's nodules.
   d. Bouchard's nodes.

5. A continuous, passive range of motion (CPM) device is used in the early postoperative period following:
   a. total hip replacement.
   b. total knee replacement.
   c. osteotomy.
   d. arthroscopy.

6. The most crucial information the nurse can provide a client before a total hip replacement is:
   a. the signs and symptoms of infection.
   b. the average lifespan of a prosthetic joint.
   c. that there will be a non–weight-bearing period for at least 6–10 weeks following the procedure.
   d. the importance of turning, positioning, and early mobility.

7. The client with a total hip replacement is allowed out of bed and into a chair:
   a. on the day of surgery.
   b. on the first postoperative day.
   c. on the fifth postoperative day.
   d. after the implant is secured by new bone growth.

8. Postoperatively, the client with a total hip replacement should be taught to:
   a. maintain hip flexion of 90 degrees.
   b. use an abduction pillow while supine and turning.
   c. remain in bed until pain subsides.
   d. distribute weight evenly between both legs.

9. A client who suffers from osteoarthritis asks what he can do to relieve pain. The nurse should suggest:
   a. application of cold.
   b. vigorous exercise.
   c. application of heat.
   d. obtaining a prescription for prednisone.

10. A primary prevention strategy for osteoarthritis is:
   a. weight loss.
   b. non–weight-bearing exercise.
   c. administering vitamin E.
   d. resting the joints.

11. List the possible complications of total joint replacements.
   (a) _____
   (b) _____
   (c) _____
   (d) _____
   (e) _____
   (f) _____

12. Following a total hip replacement, the hip of the affected leg should not be flexed more than _____ degrees.

13. A client is recovering from a total hip replacement. She will be discharged home tomorrow. The client complains of worsening pain in the affected hip. An appropriate action by the nurse is to:
   a. encourage the client to rest, and medicate her for pain.
   b. recognize the pain as a sign of discharge anxiety.
   c. assess the wound and her neurovascular status.
   d. caution her about dependency on pain medication.

14. Identify six steps to slow joint destruction and preserve function in osteoarthritis.
   (a) _____
   (b) _____
   (c) _____
   (d) _____
   (e) _____
   (f) _____

▪ ▪ ▪ The Client with Gout

15. Gout is a metabolic disorder characterized by:
    a. polyarticular deformities.
    b. an immunologic reaction.
    c. decreased purine metabolism.
    d. elevated serum uric acid levels.

16. Hyperuricemia that occurs as a result of another disorder or treatment is known as _____ _____ gout.

17. A priority nursing diagnosis for the client with acute gout is:
    a. *Altered Nutrition.*
    b. *Activity Intolerance.*
    c. *Pain.*
    d. *Body Image Disturbance.*

18. An acute attack of gout is least likely to occur:
    a. in the middle of the night.
    b. in the metatarsophalangeal joint of the great toe.
    c. after vigorous activity.
    d. after ingesting a heavy meal.

19. Which three laboratory tests are elevated during gout?
    (a) _____   (c) _____
    (b) _____

▪ ▪ ▪ The Client with Rheumatoid Arthritis (RA)

Match the medications used to treat rheumatoid arthritis (a–e) with the descriptions listed in questions 20–28. Medications may be used more than once.

_____ 20. These medications are the treatment of choice for clients with severe RA who do not respond to NSAID.

_____ 21. Inexpensive and effective, this medication is usually prescribed first.

_____ 22. This class of medication includes gold salts, antimalarial agents, sulfasalazine, and D-penicillamine.

_____ 23. This medication is prescribed when the development of tinnitus indicates toxicity.

_____ 24. These medications are prescribed when hypertension and weight gain may result from salt and water retention.

_____ 25. These medications work by inhibiting prostaglandin synthesis.

_____ 26. When the client is taking a medication in this class, the nurse should monitor glucose level for hyperglycemia.

_____ 27. This type of medication may not produce full benefit until after several weeks or months of therapy.

_____ 28. Long-term use of this type of medication may cause fat deposits in the face and trunk.

a. aspirin
b. nonsteroidal anti-inflammatory agents
c. corticosteroids
d. disease-modifying drugs
e. immunosuppressants

29. The hallmark of rheumatoid arthritis is the production of autoantibodies known as _____ _____.

30. Rheumatoid arthritis destroys joints by means of an extensive network of vascular granulation tissue known as _____ in the synovial membrane.

31. Laboratory testing of a client with active RA will nearly always show:
    a. elevated serum creatinine.
    b. decreased erythrocyte sedimentation rate.
    c. autoantibodies to IgG.
    d. hyperproteinemia.

32. When synovial fluid is aspirated in the client with severe RA, the fluid is likely to be:
    a. yellow.
    b. bloody.
    c. clear.
    d. cloudy.

33. Rheumatoid arthritis is a (a) _____ disease. It is characterized by
    (b) _____.

34. A client is being evaluated for rheumatoid arthritis (RA). His rheumatoid factor (RF) is negative. He asks the nurse if that means he doesn't have RA. The most appropriate response by the nurse is:
    a. "You do not have RA."
    b. "You only have RA if you have an elevated RF."
    c. "This test is not always conclusive."
    d. "If you don't have RA, you probably have osteoarthritis."

35. Identify five strategies that will minimize fatigue in clients with RA.
    (a) _____
    (b) _____
    (c) _____
    (d) _____
    (e) _____

▪ ▪ ▪ The Client with Systemic Lupus Erythematosus (SLE)

Read the statements below and determine if they are true or false. Correct any false statements.

_____ 36. Males are more commonly affected by SLE.

_____ 37. Genetic, environmental, and hormonal factors play a role in the development of SLE.

_____ 38. The onset of SLE is usually during young adulthood.

_____ 39. Typical early manifestations of SLE mimic those of acute gouty arthritis.

40. At some point, most clients with SLE exhibit what distinctive clinical manifestation of the disease?
    a. alopecia
    b. butterfly rash across the cheeks and nose
    c. discrete, fluid-filled vesicles on the arms and legs
    d. intense pruritus

41. Which laboratory test is the most specific for SLE?
    a. antinuclear antibody
    b. anti-DNA antibody
    c. eosinophil sedimentation
    d. serum complement levels

42. The client taking hydroxychloroquine sulfate (Plaquenil) should be taught that this medication may:
    a. improve renal function.
    b. worsen cutaneous manifestations.
    c. cause retinal toxicity and blindness.
    d. cause hypertension and sodium retention.

43. A priority nursing diagnosis for the client receiving immunosuppressive agents for the treatment of SLE is:
    a. *Impaired Physical Mobility.*   c. *Impaired Skin Integrity.*
    b. *Risk for Infection.*   d. *Body Image Disturbance.*

44. Although fever, anorexia, and weight loss are features of SLE, the predominant symptom is:
    a. arrhythmias.   c. diarrhea.
    b. joint pain.   d. palpitations.

45. An 18-year-old client with SLE shows the school nurse a reddened, tender, warm, swollen area on her forearm. The client remembers that she recently bumped and scratched her arm. The most appropriate intervention by the nurse is to:
    a. cover the area with Bacitracin and a dry, sterile dressing.
    b. tell the client to use warm compresses 4 times each day.
    c. refer the client to her physician as soon as possible.
    d. cleanse the area with hydrogen peroxide and continue to monitor the area.

46. Which statement by the client with lupus indicates the need for further teaching?
    a. "I must be careful of skin and protect it from drying."
    b. "I should avoid crowds and those with infection."
    c. "I should avoid pregnancy and should use oral contraceptives."
    d. "I should wear a medical alert bracelet."

▪ ▪ ▪ The Client with Systemic Sclerosis (Scleroderma)

47. List the five disorders that make up the CREST syndrome associated with scleroderma.
    (a) _____
    (b) _____
    (c) _____
    (d _____
    (e) _____

48. Which combination of characteristics best describes the skin of a client with scleroderma?
    a. easily bruised, edematous, ulcerated
    b. tight, shiny, hyperpigmented
    c. covered with discrete, fluid-filled vesicles on the arms and legs
    d. dry, brittle, easily broken

49. List two priority nursing diagnoses for the client with systemic sclerosis.
    (a) _____
    (b) _____

▪ ▪ ▪ The Client with Other Connective Tissue Disorders

Match the connective tissue disorders (a–g) with the conditions listed in questions 50–56.

_____ 50. connective tissue disorder associated with skeletal muscle weakness and atrophy

_____ 51. autoimmune disorder associated with dysfunction of the salivary and lacrimal glands

_____ 52. inflammatory arthritis primarily affecting the axial skeleton

_____ 53. inflammatory disorder caused by a spirochete

_____ 54. may be precipitated by a sexually transmitted or dysenteric infection

_____ 55. characterized by small, localized trigger points of muscle tightness and spasm

_____ 56. results when joint space is invaded by a pathogen

a. Lyme disease
b. polymyositis
c. Sjögren's syndrome
d. ankylosing spondylitis
e. fibromyalgia
f. reactive arthritis
g. septic arthritis

57. The correct technique for removing a tick is to:
   a. cover the tick with Vaseline so it will suffocate.
   b. use the head of a match to burn out the tick.
   c. scratch out the tick using a fingernail.
   d. use tweezers to grasp the mouth of the tick and pull it out.

58. Following a tick bite, a hiker experiences flulike symptoms and notices a reddened rash around the bite. She calls her HMO advice nurse. The appropriate response by the nurse is:
   a. "Rest, drink plenty of fluids, and monitor your fever. Call back if you are not feeling better in a few days."
   b. "A rash is not uncommon after a tick bite and is of no concern. You probably have the flu."
   c. "You should see a physician immediately."
   d. "Apply Benadryl (diphenhydramine) cream to the rash and it should go away; the flulike symptoms will go away in a couple of days."

59. A worker tells the employee health nurse that she has fibromyalgia. Based on the nurse's understanding of this condition, the most appropriate nursing action is to _____ .

▪ ▪ ▪ Critical Thinking Exercises

60. Develop a teaching plan for a client about to be discharged following total hip surgery.

61. Develop a rehabilitation program for a client following total knee replacement.

62. What is the major complication of total joint replacement? If this complication occurs, what are its sequelae?

▪ ▪ ▪ Additional Learning Experiences

▪ Visit the local department store and identify items that might assist someone with arthritis in meeting their self-care needs.

▪ Consult with your instructor about observing total hip surgery.

CHAPTER 39

Assessing Clients with Neurologic Disorders

■ ■ ■ **Focused Study Tips**

- Describe the structures and functions of the neurologic system. Subdivide sections of the system into smaller parts, diagramming and defining structures as you go.

- Explain the spinal nerves in terms of the areas of the body that they affect.

- Discuss the autonomic nervous system and how target organs and tissues are affected by sympathetic or parasympathetic stimulation.

■ ■ ■ **Anatomy and Physiology**

1. The nervous system is divided into two regions. Name these regions and their parts.

2. Which of the following structures is part of a neuron?
   a. astrocytes
   b. dendrite
   c. microglia
   d. ependyma

3. The white lipid substance covering neural axons is known as the _____.

4. Briefly describe the role of the afferent and efferent neurons.

5. The chief regulators of membrane potential are (a) _____ and (b) _____.

6. Nerves that transmit impulses through the release of norepinephrine are known as:
   a. cholinergic.
   b. sensory.
   c. adrenergic.
   d. excitator.

7. Nerves that transmit impulses through the release of acetylcholine are known as:
   a. cholinergic.
   b. sensory.
   c. adrenergic.
   d. excitator.

Match the descriptions (a–k) with the correct anatomical structures of the brain system listed in questions 8–18.

_____ 8. cerebrum

_____ 9. hypothalamus

_____ 10. basilar artery

_____ 11. blood-brain barrier

_____ 12. medulla oblongata

_____ 13. midbrain

_____ 14. reticular activating system

_____ 15. cerebral cortex

_____ 16. cerebellum

_____ 17. pons

_____ 18. thalamus

a. stimulating system for the cerebral cortex

b. vessel supplying brain stem and cerebellum

c. mechanism for preventing harmful substances from entering the brain

d. responsible for coordination, balance, and control of fine movements

e. outer surface of cerebrum

f. center for auditory and visual reflexes in the brain

g. plays an important role in regulating heart rate, blood pressure, and respiration

h. contains nuclei that control respiration

i. regulates temperature, water metabolism, and emotional expressions

j. most superior and heaviest part of brain

k. serves as the station for sorting, processing, and relaying sensory input

Match the descriptions (a–f) with the correct anatomical structures of the spinal cord listed in questions 19–24.

_____ 19. spinal cord

_____ 20. corticospinal tracts

_____ 21. spinothalamic tracts

_____ 22. upper motor neurons

_____ 23. lower motor neurons

_____ 24. nucleus pulposa

a. spinal pathways carrying sensations for pain, temperature, and crude touch

b. center for conducting messages to and from brain

c. spinal passageways that mediate voluntary purposeful movements

d. gelatinous core component of intravertebral disc

e. pathways carrying impulses from cerebral cortex to anterior grey column

f. "final common pathways" for nervous impulses

25. The role of the peripheral nervous system is to (a) _____ and

(b) _____ ;
while the role of the autonomic nervous system is to (c) _____
_____ .

26. The effects of stimulation of the sympathetic division of the autonomic nervous system include:
   a. decreased metabolic rates.
   b. decreased digestion.
   c. decreased mental alertness.
   d. increased urine output.

27. The effects of stimulation of the parasympathetic division of the autonomic nervous system include:
   a. dilated pupils.
   b. dilated bronchioles.
   c. increased heart rate.
   d. increased peristalsis.

▪ ▪ ▪ Assessment of Neurologic Function

28. Assessment of the client's level of consciousness is determined using the _____ _____.

29. How can a nurse gather subjective information if the client has an altered level of consciousness?

_____

30. List the six major portions of the physical assessment of the neurologic system.

(a) _____   (d) _____

(b) _____   (e) _____

(c) _____   (f) _____

31. The term used to describe difficulty speaking is:

   a. dysphonia.
   b. dysarthria.
   c. dysphagia.
   d. dyskinesia.

32. Define the term *receptive aphasia*.

33. Assessment of cognitive functioning includes:

   a. recalling seven items after 10 minutes.
   b. repeating nine numbers.
   c. orientation to place.
   d. recalling birth dates of parent.

Match the neurologic function (a–i) with the correct cranial nerve listed in questions 34–42.

_____ 34. facial

_____ 35. oculomotor, trochlear, abducens

_____ 36. olfactory

_____ 37. spinal accessory

_____ 38. trigeminal

_____ 39. hypoglossal

_____ 40. optic

_____ 41. acoustic

_____ 42. glossopharyngeal

   a. ability to smell
   b. ability to feel light, deep, and dull facial sensations
   c. ability to project and move tongue side-to-side
   d. ability to hear ticking of a watch
   e. ability to shrug shoulders, turn head against force
   f. gag reflex and swallowing ability
   g. PERRLA and extraocular movements
   h. ability to frown, show teeth, raise eyebrows
   i. ability to see

43. Assessment of the client's ability to discriminate fine touch is part of which component of the physical assessment of the neurologic system?

   a. sensory exam
   b. cranial nerve exam
   c. motor exam
   d. reflex exam

Case Study

Loraine Larue is an 82-year-old widow admitted for testing related to progressive muscle weakness on her left side, difficulty speaking, visual difficulties, and lack of coordination. Mrs. Larue lives alone in a first-floor, one-story apartment where she has resided since the death of her husband 12 years ago. Mrs. Larue's two children, John and Marie, are both married and live out of state. Until the death of her husband, Mrs. Larue worked as a full-time customer service representative in a local bank. She tells the nurse that she loved her work and especially enjoyed meeting and talking with so many different kinds of people. During the health assessment interview, the nurse notes that Mrs. Larue's speech is occasionally slurred, and that Mrs. Larue has difficulty pronouncing words with many syllables. Mrs. Larue tells the nurse she smoked between 1 and 1½ packs of cigarettes daily for about 50 years. Following the death of her husband, she quit smoking. Mrs. Larue is 5'6" and 180 lbs. Her vital signs are: temperature 98.8F, pulse 94, respirations 18, and B/P 168/94. Additional physical examination findings reveal homonymous hemianopsia, Horner's syndrome of the left eye, decreased sensation of the left face, drooping of the left facial muscles, dysphagia, and ataxic episodes. Mrs. Larue's deep-tendon reflexes are slightly hyperactive, and both Brudzinski's and Kernig's tests are negative.

44. Identify the abnormal assessment findings and the contributing factors of Mrs. Larue's condition.
    (a) abnormal assessment findings:

    (b) contributing factors:

45. List five variations the nurse would expect to observe when completing a neurologic examination of an older client.
    (a) _____
    (b) _____
    (c) _____
    (d) _____
    (e) _____

46. A positive Brudzinski's or Kernig's sign indicates:
    a. a ruptured disc.
    b. meningeal irritation.
    c. lesions of the pons.
    d. lesions of the corticospinal tracts.

47. When performing a Romberg's test, the nurse should:
    a. have a reflex hammer available.
    b. ensure the client's safety.
    c. have the client heel-toe walk.
    d. have the client run each heel down each shin.

Match the descriptions (a–c) with the terms listed in questions 48–50.

_____ 48. kinesthesia

_____ 49. stereognosis

_____ 50. graphesthesia

a. one uses numbers written on the hand to test for this ability

b. one uses a coin or key to test for this ability

c. sense of position

51. Explain the Glasgow Coma Scale to a family member who is going to monitor a client with a recent head injury.

Read the following statements and indicate if they are true or false. Correct any false statements.

_____ 52. In older adults, all reflexes may be diminished.

_____ 53. The older adult walks at the same rate as the younger adult.

_____ 54. Motor strength is maintained as one ages.

_____ 55. An older adult's intellectual function is maintained despite a decrease in brain mass.

▪ ▪ ▪ Critical Thinking Exercise

56. Compare and contrast the sympathetic and parasympathetic divisions of the autonomic nervous system.

57. The nurse is caring for a client who does not speak. How might the nurse assess cognitive function and complete the neurologic exam?

▪ ▪ ▪ Additional Learning Experiences

- Practice performing neurologic assessments on family, friends, and all assigned clients, regardless of whether they have neurologic problems.

- Review the neurologic system using your anatomy and physiology book.

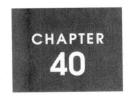

CHAPTER 40

Nursing Care of Clients with Intracranial Disorders

■ ■ ■ **Focused Study Tips**

- Describe the anatomy and physiology of the brain and its functioning, and relate this knowledge to the various diagnostic tests that are used to identify brain disorders.

- Explain the principles and procedures for diagnostic testing, especially the nursing responsibilities and client teaching.

- Compare and contrast the various classes of medications used to treat the various intracranial disorders. List the modes of action of the drug categories, their side effects, adverse effects, and toxic effects.

- Recognize risk factors for various disorders that affect the brain and its functioning.

- Summarize the types of nursing interventions that are required to perform the ongoing monitoring required of clients with intracranial disorders.

- Describe the teaching needs of the client and family for each of the intracranial disorders.

- Compare and contrast specific nursing interventions required for persons with increased intracranial pressure, seizures, meningeal irritation, headaches, and neurologic deficits (both sensory and motor).

■ ■ ■ **The Client with an Altered Level of Consciousness**

Match the definitions (a–f) with the states of consciousness listed in questions 1–6.

_____ 1. full consciousness

_____ 2. confusion

_____ 3. disorientation

_____ 4. semicomatose

_____ 5. deep coma

_____ 6. obtunded

a. not aware of time, place, or person

b. unresponsive to pain; no reflexes present

c. poor memory and judgment; inability to think clearly

d. responds to vigorous, painful stimulation by stirring or withdrawing without arousal

e. alert, oriented, and comprehends spoken and written word

f. dull or blunt sensitivity to pain

7. Full consciousness implies that a person demonstrates both normal (a) _____ and full (b) _____.

8. While the nurse must understand and use terms related to level of consciousness (LOC) accurately, professional communication can be enhanced by describing a client's _____ _____ rather than using the LOC labels.

9. Any state or condition that alters the normal delivery of (a) _____, (b) _____, or (c) _____ to the brain is likely to decrease the client's LOC.

10. The altered LOC associated with seizure activity is most likely related to:
    a. apnea that occurs with seizures.
    b. the exhaustion of energy sources and the production of toxic substances within the brain.
    c. extensive disruption and distortion of sensory input during and after the seizure.
    d. the occurrence of an absolute refractory period following the disorganized firing of neurons in the brain.

11. Number the following abnormal responses in the order in which they occur as brain function deteriorates.

    _____ breathing

    _____ LOC

    _____ motor responses

    _____ oculomotor responses

    _____ pupillary responses

12. Reflexive movement of the eyes in the opposite direction of head rotation is called (a) _____
    _____ movements. Absence of this reflex indicates damage to the
    (b) _____.

13. When a client presents with coma of unknown etiology, one of the first laboratory tests to be done is the blood glucose level. Ascertaining glucose is of vital importance because _____
    _____
    _____.

14. If a coma has been determined to be the result of a narcotic overdose, the most likely treatment will be:
    a. diuretics and increased fluids.   c. naloxone (Narcan).
    b. peritoneal or hemodialysis.   d. methadone (Dolophine).

15. The proper turning and positioning of a client in a coma involves:
    a. changing of position every 4 hours using both sides, the back, and abdomen.
    b. using the Trendelenburg position to facilitate drainage of oral secretions.
    c. keeping the head of the bed flat to decrease intracranial pressure.
    d. elevating the head of the bed and turning side-to-side every 2 hours, avoiding the back-lying position.

16. A priority nursing intervention for an unconscious client is an assessment of the:
    a. rate and rhythm of respirations.   c. intracranial pressure.
    b. blood pressure and pulse.   d. patency of airway.

17. A client is admitted unconscious with basilar skull fracture and spinal fluid draining from her nares. The physician has ordered suctioning on a PRN basis. The correct procedure is to perform an (a) _____ suction for no more than (b) _____ seconds.

18. The client in question 17 has absent corneal reflexes. The correct nursing action is to:
    a. tape the eyelids closed.   c. keep the lights dim.
    b. apply cool compresses.   d. apply sunglasses.

19. An indicator of altered nutrition in an unconscious adult is:
    a. increased transferrin level.
    b. increased serum albumin.
    c. weight loss.
    d. improved healing.

■ ■ ■   **The Client with Increased Intracranial Pressure**

20. The most frequent cause of sustained increase in intracranial pressure (ICP) is _____.

21. The term autoregulation, when applied to the brain, refers to the ability of the brain to:
    a. control its amount of electrical activity.
    b. maintain the appropriate blood flow by relaxing and contracting cerebral arterioles.
    c. produce a hormone that is released by the posterior pituitary to decrease the cerebral fluid content as ICP increases.
    d. decrease the amount of oxygen and glucose it needs when cerebral blood flow is compromised.

22. Because the neurons in the cerebral cortex are the most sensitive to hypoxia, the earliest manifestations of increased ICP will most likely be:
    a. visual disturbances.
    b. auditory hallucinations.
    c. rising temperature and pulse rate.
    d. behavior and personality alterations.

23. A client's initial vital signs were: BP = 120/70; T = 98.6F; P = 80; and R = 20. Which of the following assessment findings would indicate a rising ICP?
    a. BP = 90/40, T = 97.2F, P =96, R = 38
    b. BP = 130/90, T = 100F, P = 84, R = 28
    c. BP = 160/94, T = 103.2F, P = 60, R = 12
    d. BP = 40/0, T = 105F, P = 120, R = 10

24. Cerebral edema peaks within _____ hours after an injury has occurred.

25. If increased ICP progresses until cerebral tissue is displaced downward, a lethal complication called brain _____ is likely to occur.

26. The main categories of medications used to treat increased ICP are:
    a. loop diuretics and narcotics.
    b. osmotic diuretics and corticosteroids.
    c. thiazide diuretics and anticonvulsants.
    d. potassium-sparing diuretics and barbiturates.

27. The most common position used when caring for clients who are experiencing increased ICP is:
    a. with the head of bed elevated and neck kept in a neutral position.
    b. lateral Sims', with the neck in extension.
    c. flat, propped to one side with pillows, with neck flexed.
    d. any position of comfort that the client desires.

28. Which of the following value(s) is indicative of a normal ICP? (More than one may be correct.)
    a. 14 mm Hg   b. 18 mm Hg   c. 190 mm H_2O d. 160 mm H_2O

29. A client is being monitored for increased ICP. Which of her complaints is most indicative of increasing ICP?
    a. hearing problems
    b. shortness of breath
    c. blurred vision
    d. nausea

Match the descriptions (30–33) with the correct terms (a–d).

_____ 30. most common type of cerebral edema causing intracranial hypertension

_____ 31. an increase in volume of CSF within and dilation of the ventricular system

_____ 32. changes of the functional or structural integrity of cell membranes due to intracranial hypoxia and ischemia

_____ 33. an increase in interstitial fluids in the brain

a. interstitial cerebral edema
b. hydrocephalus
c. vasogenic edema
d. cytotoxic edema

34. List four nursing responsibilities when caring for a client receiving mannitol.

(a) _____

(b) _____

(c) _____

(d) _____

35. A client is being monitored for ICP. The physician orders an IV of D5W. The most appropriate action by the nurse is to:

a. initiate therapy and utilize an IV pump to control the rate.
b. utilize microdrip tubing and infuse the IV at a KVO rate.
c. contact the physician regarding using a hypoosmolar solution.
d. initiate therapy if the client is unable to take oral fluids.

36. Which of the following will exacerbate increased ICP?

a. use of a ventilator
b. emotional upsets
c. dehydration
d. elevation of head

■ ■ ■ The Client with Seizure Disorders

37. An episode of excessive, abnormal electrical discharge within the brain causes a (a) _____ _____. When this condition is chronic and a person has a tendency to have recurrent episodes of excessive electrical discharge, the client is diagnosed as having (b) _____.

38. Complex partial seizures are characterized by:

a. a loss of consciousness, but no motor abnormalities.
b. altered consciousness, often with nonpurposeful activities called automatisms.
c. a sudden, brief interruption of all motor activity, and brief unresponsiveness.
d. sudden loss of consciousness, muscle rigidity, and apnea.

39. The clonic phase of a tonic-clonic seizure is characterized by:

a. automatisms.
b. urinary incontinence.
c. an aura.
d. alternating contraction and relaxation of muscles.

40. For status epilepticus, the drug of choice and its route of administration is:

a. phenytoin (Dilantin) intramuscularly.
b. phenobarbital (Luminal) intravenously.
c. diazepam (Valium) intravenously.
d. valproic acid (Depakane) by inhaler.

41. In teaching a client who is having an electroencephalogram as an outpatient, the nurse should tell the client:
   a. to fast for 12 hours prior to the test.
   b. to wash the hair prior to the test.
   c. that the test causes only mild discomfort.
   d. that the client must avoid going to sleep during the test.

42. A female client who has been diagnosed with a seizure disorder is prescribed phenytoin (Dilantin). The nurse instructs her to tell her dentist that she has epilepsy and is taking phenytoin because:
   a. the stress of dental work is likely to trigger seizure activity.
   b. the dentist must obtain special equipment to manage possible seizure activity should it occur in the dentist's office.
   c. seizure activity may cause dental problems such as chipped or broken teeth.
   d. gingival changes are a frequent side effect of phenytoin.

43. Which nursing intervention is contraindicated when caring for a client during a grand mal seizure?
   a. turning the client on the side
   b. placing a padded tongue blade in the client's mouth
   c. loosening clothing around the neck
   d. protecting from injury

44. The nurse is teaching a client and family about preventing injury from seizures. Which statement by the client indicates a need for further teaching?
   a. "I should avoid excessive intake of alcohol."
   b. "I should avoid excessive fatigue."
   c. "I should not lock the bedroom or bathroom doors."
   d. "I should avoid excessive intake of caffeine."

45. A client recently had a grand mal seizure and was started on medications to control the seizures. He is a traveling salesman and drives over 1000 miles each week. He asks the nurse about driving. The most appropriate response by the nurse is:
   a. "You should not drive because you might have another seizure and cause an accident."
   b. "You can continue driving as long as you take your medication."
   c. "You will have to check with local and state laws and your physician."
   d. "You'll be able to drive in 2 months if you do not experience another seizure."

▪ ▪ ▪ The Client with Headaches

46. The type of headache that may be associated with the menstrual cycle and has a strong familial component is:
   a. cluster headaches.
   b. tension headaches.
   c. migraine headaches.
   d. sinus headaches.

47. Cluster headaches are typically characterized by:
   a. occurring more often in females than in males.
   b. beginning in the infraorbital region, with unilateral spread to the head and neck.
   c. a feeling of tight, vise-like pressure associated with sustained contraction of the neck muscles.
   d. being closely associated with stress.

48. A female client is prescribed ergotamine therapy for migraine headaches. The nurse should teach her to:
    a. take the medication daily at bedtime.
    b. avoid taking the medication during menses.
    c. be certain to take the medication at regular intervals around the clock.
    d. take the medication immediately at the onset of a migraine headache.

49. Name and describe the three stages of a migraine headache.
    (a) _____
    (b) _____
    (c) _____

50. Name at least five trigger factors for migraine headaches.

51. A client suffers from migraine headaches. Her health care provider has given her a prescription for atenolol. Which statement by the client indicates a need for further teaching?
    a. "I should take this as needed for headaches."
    b. "I should carefully rise from a sitting or lying position."
    c. "I should avoid an excessive intake of alcohol."
    d. "I should report cough, nasal stuffiness, or depression."

52. List two nursing responsibilites related to the administration of sumatriptan succinate injection.
    (a) _____
    (b) _____

53. Develop a teaching plan for a client who will be taking sumatriptan succinate injections for migraine headaches.

▪ ▪ ▪ The Client with a Skull Fracture

54. A client who has sustained a skull fracture and is having rhinorrhea or otorrhea most likely has a:
    a. linear fracture.
    b. comminuted fracture.
    c. depressed fracture.
    d. basilar fracture.

55. The presence of rhinorrhea or otorrhea places the client at increased risk for:
    a. infection.
    b. seizures.
    c. cerebral edema.
    d. decreased LOC.

▪ ▪ ▪ The Client with a Brain Injury

56. When a client has had a brain contusion, the nurse should expect the edema resulting from this injury to peak how many hours following the injury?
    a. 6–12   b. 12–24   c. 24–48   d. 48–72

57. Diffuse axonal injury (DAI) results in a poor prognosis and is usually associated with injuries that are the result of a _____.

Read the following statements and determine if they are true or false. Correct any false statements.

_____ 58. A cerebral concussion results in some degree of permanent neurogenic dysfunction.

_____ 59. With a severe cerebral concussion, seizures and respiratory arrest may occur.

_____ 60. Postconcussion syndrome is characterized by drowsiness, confusion, and seizures.

_____ 61. A contusion is typically accompanied by small, diffuse, venous hemorrhages.

_____ 62. A client with a concussion or contusion requires close observation for increased cerebral edema.

▪ ▪ ▪ The Client with an Intracranial Hemorrhage

Match the types of hematoma (a–c) with the correct locations of a brain injury listed in questions 63–71. Hematoma types may be used more than once.

_____ 63. located within the brain tissue

_____ 64. located between the dura and arachnoid

_____ 65. located between the skull and dura

_____ 66. usually over the temporal bone

_____ 67. occurs in the frontal or temporal region

_____ 68. symptoms may appear long after injury

_____ 69. contralateral hemiplegia with deep coma

_____ 70. associated with long history of hypertension

_____ 71. more frequent in children and young adults

a. epidural
b. subdural
c. intracerebral

72. Epidural hematomas tend to demonstrate rapid progression because they:
    a. often result from anticoagulation therapy.
    b. are associated with hypertension.
    c. are arterial bleeds.
    d. occur mainly in older, debilitated persons.

73. A male client's family brings him to the emergency department following major motor seizure activity. They report that he fell on ice 5 weeks previously, hitting his head. If this seizure is the result of a hematoma, it is most likely a(n):
    a. epidural hematoma.
    b. intracerebral hematoma.
    c. subacute subdural hematoma.
    d. chronic subdural hematoma.

74. Persons who are at greatest risk for intracerebral hematomas are:
    a. alcohol abusers and older adults.
    b. children and the malnourished.
    c. clients with diabetes and clients on dialysis.
    d. young adults and drug abusers.

75. The primary focus of nursing care of persons with craniocerebral trauma is:
    a. identification of the cause of the trauma.
    b. neurologic assessment and monitoring.
    c. establishment and maintenance of a patent airway and effective ventilation.
    d. prevention of complications and long-term sequelae.

▪ ▪ ▪ The Client with Meningitis, Encephalitis, or a Brain Abscess

76. Organisms causing meningitis can gain access to the CNS by (a) _____ _____ or via the (b) _____.

77. The proper positioning of a client for having a lumbar puncture performed is:
    a. on the abdomen with no pillows.
    b. sitting on a stool with feet firmly on the floor.
    c. lateral Sims'.
    d. on the side, with head and knees flexed.

78. Pharmacologic treatment of meningitis usually involves administering high doses of:
    a. oral antibiotics.
    b. corticosteroids.
    c. intravenous antibiotics.
    d. antipyretic and anticonvulsant agents.

79. The most common causative organism for encephalitis is a:
    a. virus.   b. bacteria.   c. fungus.   d. protozoa.

80. Infections of which of the body areas places a client at the highest risk for developing a brain abscess?
    a. pharynx   b. skin   c. middle ear   d. pericardium

Read the following statements and determine if they are true or false. Correct any false statements.

_____ 81. Viral meningitis is a medical emergency.

_____ 82. Individuals with bacterial meningitis should be placed on strict or respiratory isolation until the organism has been identified.

83. List at least four symptoms of bacterial meningitis.

84. Define Brudzinski's sign.

85. Define Kernig's sign.

▪ ▪ ▪ The Client with Brain Tumors

Brain tumors in particular areas of the brain often result in specific manifestations. Match the regions of the brain where a tumor would most likely result (a–e) with the correct manifestations of brain tumor listed in questions 86–90.

_____ 86. impaired judgment/concentration

_____ 87. psychomotor seizures

_____ 88. visual disturbance

_____ 89. sensory deficits

_____ 90. coordination/equilibrium disturbance

a. occipital lobe
b. cerebellum
c. frontal lobe
d. parietal lobe
e. temporal

91. The most highly malignant brain tumor is a(n):
   a. astrocytoma.
   b. glioblastoma multiforme.
   c. astroblastoma.
   d. meningioma.

92. Tumors of which organs are most likely to result in metastatic tumors into the brain?
   a. stomach   b. colon   c. lung   d. bone

93. A growing brain tumor is most likely to result in:
   a. meningeal irritation.
   b. cerebral infarction.
   c. respiratory arrest.
   d. cerebral edema.

94. Identify four physical findings the nurse should tell family members to expect when they first see the client following brain surgery in the intensive care unit.
   (a) _____
   (b) _____
   (c) _____
   (d) _____

95. A client with a brain tumor has had surgery that was not curative. Identify six topics for client/family teaching at the time of discharge.
   (a) _____
   (b) _____
   (c) _____
   (d) _____
   (e) _____
   (f) _____

96. Following intracranial surgery for a brain tumor, the client complains of a "runny nose." The most appropriate action by the nurse is to:
   a. insert a soft nasal packing to absorb the drainage
   b. report leakage if it tests positive for glucose
   c. keep the head of the bed flat
   d. provide nasal suctioning

97. Narcotic analgesics are administered cautiously in individuals following brain surgery. The rationale for this practice is that:
    a. brain surgery does not result in much pain or discomfort.
    b. sedation may lead to a paradoxical increase in ICP.
    c. pupillary responses may be impaired and respirations depressed.
    d. psychologic dependence may occur more quickly following brain surgery.

▪ ▪ ▪ Critical Thinking Exercises

98. Develop a nursing care plan for a client in a persistent vegetative state. Describe the ethical issues related to withholding feeding from such an individual.

99. Develop a teaching plan for a young adult recently diagnosed with a seizure disorder.

100. A 19-year-old is diagnosed with a skull fracture. He refuses hospitalization and is about to be discharged to the care of his family. Develop a discharge teaching plan to assist the family in providing necessary care and monitoring of his condition.

▪ ▪ ▪ Additional Learning Experiences

- Consult with your instructor about visiting a facility that provides care to adults who have suffered brain injuries.

- Develop a community education program to teach citizens about the signs and symptoms of equine encephalitis.

- Participate in a safety program that encourages children to wear bike helmets and to use their seat belts.

Nursing Care of Clients with Cerebral Blood Flow Disorders and Spinal Cord Disorders

CHAPTER 41

■ ■ ■ **Focused Study Tips**

- Describe the different types of cerebrovascular accidents (CVAs) that can occur. State the various deficits and disorders associated with each type of CVA, as well as the appropriate nursing care.

- Discuss means of communication for clients who experience altered speech patterns.

- Compare the nursing assessments and interventions for a client with a ruptured intervertebral disk and for the client undergoing a laminectomy.

- Distinguish the client problems associated with each level of spinal cord injury.

- Identify the principles of mental health nursing and note how they apply to nursing of clients with spinal cord disorders.

■ ■ ■ **The Client with a Cerebral Vascular Accident (CVA)**

1. The brain accounts for _____ % of the body's oxygen consumption.

2. Veins of the cerebral system differ from other veins in that:
   a. they contain no valves.
   b. they are the only veins capable of autoregulation.
   c. they are innervated by the sympathetic nervous system.
   d. there is no difference in veins of the cerebral system and other veins.

3. The flow of venous blood depends on (a) _____ or
   (b) _____ differences between the venous sinuses and extracranial veins.

4. List three activities that increase extracranial pressure.
   (a) _____
   (b) _____
   (c) _____

Match the types of CVA (a–d) with the correct descriptions listed in questions 5–8.

_____ 5. This type of CVA commonly occurs when the person is sleeping.

_____ 6. This type of CVA often occurs in older adults who have long-term, poorly controlled hypertension.

_____ 7. This type of CVA often serves as a warning signal of an ischemic thrombotic CVA. The neurologic defects it causes last less than 24 hours.

_____ 8. This type of CVA occurs after of a blood clot or foreign matter travels through cerebral vessels and lodges in small vessels.

a. TIA
b. thrombotic CVA
c. embolic CVA
d. hemorrhagic CVA

9. List five risk factors for developing a CVA.

   (a) _____

   (b) _____

   (c) _____

   (d) _____

   (e) _____

10. A stroke on the right side of the brain results in deficits in:
    a. the left side.
    b. the right side.
    c. both sides.
    d. the affected regions of the brain.

Match the terms (a–e) with the correct descriptions listed in questions 11–15.

_____ 11. increased resistance to stretching (uniform throughout the stretching)   a. hemiplegia

_____ 12. absence of motor tone

b. hemiparesis
c. flaccidity

_____ 13. weakness of the left or right half of the body

d. spasticity

_____ 14. increased resistance to stretching of extremities (resistance
increasing as extremity is stretched)

e. rigidity

_____ 15. paralysis of left or right half of the body

16. A client recently had a stroke. He calls his watch a "clock" and his pen a "writing thing." He is suffering from:
    a. hemianopia.   c. apraxia.
    b. agnosia.   d. unilateral neglect.

17. A client is admitted with a CVA. She follows simple directions, but cannot speak. This condition is:
    a. dysarthria.   c. receptive aphasia.
    b. global aphasia.   d. expressive aphasia.

18. Preparation for a computed tomography (CT) of the head includes:
    a. informing the client that pain will occur.
    b. preparing the client for the administration of general anesthesia.
    c. informing the client that the client's head will be immobilized during the procedure.
    d. informing the client that the exam will last 2 hours.

19. Proper positioning of the client after a lumbar puncture is:
    a. Sims' position.   c. prone.
    b. lateral recumbent.   d. high-Fowler's.

20. Which medication is used as a preventive measure for the client at risk for CVA?
    a. Procardia (nifedipine)   c. nitroglycerin
    b. nimodipine   d. heparin

21. Which of the following medications is contraindicated in the client with hemorrhagic CVA?
    a. Procardia (nifedipine)   c. nitroglycerin
    b. aspirin   d. heparin

22. Which of the following medications can be used to reduce cerebral vasospasms in the client with a CVA?
    a. Procardia (nifedipine)
    b. aspirin
    c. nitroglycerin
    d. heparin

23. A client is admitted to the ICU unconcious following a CVA. The priority nursing diagnosis is:
    a. *Anxiety.*
    b. *Ineffective Airway Clearance.*
    c. *Self-Esteem Disturbance.*
    d. *Impaired Physical Mobility.*

24. The above client should be positioned:
    a. prone, with HOB elevated.
    b. in semi-Fowler's.
    c. on his side.
    d. supine, with HOB flat.

25. A client is admitted following a right carotid endarterectomy. She complains of a "tight dressing." The most appropriate action by the nurse is to:
    a. loosen the dressing.
    b. medicate her for discomfort.
    c. assess the dressing and neck for bleeding.
    d. reposition her head and neck.

26. When assisting the client with a CVA with dressing, the nurse should _____
_____.

▪ ▪ ▪ The Client with an Intracranial Aneurysm

27. The client with an intracranial aneurysm may have prodromal symptoms associated with which body function?
    a. vision   b. hearing   c. muscular   d. gastrointestinal

28. Which clinical manifestation would be found in the client with a ruptured intracranial aneurysm?
    a. arrhythmias
    b. rectal bleeding
    c. explosive headache
    d. hyperactivity

29. A nurse is preparing the client for transfer. If the nurse reports to the receiving nurse that the client has a grade V aneurysm, the receiving nurse knows that the client:
    a. is alert and able to respond.
    b. is awake but unable to respond.
    c. has a meningeal infection.
    d. is in a deep coma with decerebrate posturing.

30. A client with an actual rupture of a cerebral aneurysm should:
    a. receive no nutrition by mouth.
    b. have all visitors restricted.
    c. be placed in a quiet room with the lights dimmed.
    d. maintain the head of the bed in a supine position.

31. Following a rupture of a cerebral aneurysm, the greatest risk for rebleeding is in (a) _____
_____, and again in (b) _____.

32. A client has been on bed rest for 1 week following a ruptured cerebral aneurysm. She complains of "endless boredom." The most appropriate nursing action is to _____
_____
_____.

■ ■ ■ The Client with an Arteriovenous Malformation

33. Which of the following statements most accurately describes an arteriovenous malformation? An arteriovenous malformation occurs when:
    a. a tumor displaces brain tissue.
    b. there is shunting of blood from the arterial to the venous system.
    c. a cerebral tumor encompasses normal brain tissue.
    d. there is shunting of blood from the venous to the arterial system.

34. Identify two methods used to treat inaccessible arteriovenous malformations.
    (a) _____
    (b) _____

■ ■ ■ The Client with a Spinal Cord Injury

35. Which of the following clients has the highest risk of spinal cord injury?
    a. a 2-year-old male   c. a 20-year-old male
    b. a 17-year-old female   d. a 45-year-old male

36. The majority of spinal cord injuries are the result of:
    a. falls.   c. acts of violence.
    b. sports injuries.   d. motor vehicle accidents.

37. "Whiplash" is an example of:
    a. hyperflexion.   b. axial loading.   c. hyperextension.   d. excessive rotation.

Match the terms for response to spinal cord injury (a–e) with the correct descriptions listed in questions 38–45. Terms may be used more than once or not at all.

_____ 38. This response to spinal cord injury is a temporary loss of reflexive function below the level of spinal cord injury.

a. upper motor neuron disease
b. tetraplegia
c. spinal shock
d. paraplegia
e. autonomic dysreflexia

_____ 39. This is an exaggerated sympathetic response that occurs in clients with injuries at or above T6.

_____ 40. This neurologic deficit results in impairment of the arms, trunk, legs, and pelvic organs.

_____ 41. This response to a spinal cord injury is triggered by a stimuli that would normally cause abdominal discomfort.

_____ 42. This response to spinal cord injury results in loss of autonomic function. The parasympathetic system dominates, causing bradycardia and hypotension.

_____ 43. This response to spinal cord injury creates spasticity and hyperreflexia. The client may be unable to carry out skilled movements.

_____ 44. This response to spinal cord injury may occur within 1 hour after the injury.

_____ 45. This neurologic deficit results in paralysis of the client's lower trunk.

46. A nursing diagnosis of *Risk for Ineffective Breathing Pattern* would be supported by damage to the spinal cord at which of the following levels?

    a. L9   b. T3   c. C8   d. C3

47. The most important principle to remember when caring for a client with a suspected spinal cord injury is to:

    a. immobilize the client's neck.
    b. monitor the client's bowel sounds.
    c. reposition the client every 2 hours.
    d. assess the client for hypoglycemia.

48. Which of the following devices allows the client in cervical traction the most flexibility?

    a. Stryker frame   c. CircOlectric bed
    b. Halo traction   d. Gardner-Wells tong

49. A client with spinal cord injury at L4 will have difficulty with:

    a. vision.   c. voiding.
    b. breathing.   d. central syndrome.

50. Nursing interventions for a client with a nursing diagnosis of *Altered Urinary Elimination* secondary to spinal cord injury would include:

    a. maintaining a Foley catheter at all times.
    b. teaching the client self-catheterization.
    c. assisting with insertion of a suprapubic tube.
    d. preparing the client for lifelong diuretic therapy.

51. A client was in a motor vehicle accident and fractured his spine. He tells the nurse that he and his wife have been trying to have a baby. "Now it will never happen," he says. How should the nurse respond?

52. A client is recovering from a spinal cord injury. The nurse notes that his blood pressure is dangerously elevated. The most appropriate action by the nurse is to:

    a. raise the HOB and remove TEDS.
    b. notify the physician.
    c. administer a muscle relaxant.
    d. administer pain medication.

▪ ▪ ▪ The Client with a Herniated Intervertebral Disk

53. The most common site of a herniated disk is in the:

    a. cervical region.   c. lumbar region.
    b. thoracic region.   d. sacral region.

54. The most common cause of a herniated disk is thought to be due to:

    a. pregnancy.   c. trauma.
    b. old age.   d. cardiovascular disease.

Identify whether each of the following symptoms are associated with (a) central cervical herniation or (b) lateral cervical herniation.

_____ 55. hyperactivity of the lower extremities

_____ 56. paresthesia

_____ 57. sexual dysfunction

_____ 58. urinary elimination

_____ 59. absent arm reflexes

60. For a client with acute pain related to an acute ruptured intervertebral disk treated with a conservative approach, the nurse should teach the client to:
    a. remain on bed rest.
    b. exercise to the point of pain.
    c. engage in vigorous activity.
    d. limit exercise to walking.

61. A client is scheduled for a myelogram. Which statement by the client indicates a need for further teaching?
    a. "I won't be able to eat or drink for 6 hours before the procedure."
    b. "The procedure may take 2–3 hours."
    c. "I may experience a feeling of warmth or burning when the dye is injected."
    d. "I might be strapped down during the procedure."

62. The nurse is caring for a client following a laminectomy. The client is incontinent of urine at 3 A.M. This is the first time the client has ever been incontinent. The most appropriate action by the nurse is to:
    a. monitor for further incontinence and report this in the morning.
    b. contact the health care provider immediately.
    c. assess the client for bladder distention.
    d. provide reassurance to the client.

63. The nurse is providing teaching to a 350 lb client with a ruptured intervertebral disk. Which statement by the client indicates a need for further teaching?
    a. "I should sleep on a firm mattress."
    b. "I should avoid twisting motions, bending, and lifting."
    c. "Wearing comfortable slippers will relieve pressure on my back."
    d. "Losing weight will relieve pressure on my back."

▪ ▪ ▪ The Client with a Spinal Cord Tumor

64. The first clinical sign seen with spinal cord tumor is usually:
    a. change in LOC.   b. absent DTR.   c. pain.   d. hematuria.

65. With a spinal cord tumor, neurologic deficits are related to how (a) _____ or (b) _____ the tumor grows, and whether it is a (c) _____ or (d) _____ tumor.

Read the following statements and determine if they are true or false. Correct any false statements.

_____ 66. Spinal cord tumors are always considered malignant.

_____ 67. Most spinal tumors are seen between the ages of 20 and 60.

_____ 68. Tumors of the spinal cord may be primary or secondary.

_____ 69. Syringomyelia always occurs with spinal cord tumors.

70. List important nursing assessments for a client with a spinal cord tumor.

▪ ▪ ▪   Critical Thinking Exercises

71. Develop a teaching program for senior citizens that will help them recognize signs and symptoms of a CVA and the importance of treating it as a "brain attack."

72. The nurse is caring for a 49-year-old telemarketer who is recovering from a CVA. He has impaired verbal communication. Develop a plan of care to address this problem and assist him with rehabilitation.

73. The nurse is at a remote campground and is summoned to a lake where someone has experienced a diving accident. The nurse suspects that the accident victim is suffering from spinal shock. What are the most appropriate actions pending the arrival of the EMTs?

▪ ▪ ▪   Additional Learning Experiences

▪ Wear an eye patch over one eye, and observe how this affects your perception.

▪ Observe a speech therapist working with a client with impaired swallowing or a language disorder.

▪ Observe a client undergoing a CAT scan.

▪ Consult with your instructor regarding an observational experience at a rehabilitation facility.

Nursing Care of Clients with Degenerative Neurologic, Neuromuscular, and Cranial Nerve Disorders

CHAPTER 42

■ ■ ■ **Focused Study Tips**

- Discuss approaches to teach the client's family about protecting the client with Alzheimer's disease from injury.

- Discuss the pathophysiology of multiple sclerosis (MS).

- List the neurotransmitters involved in Parkinson's disease. Identify the common pharmacologic treatments for neurologic and neuromuscular disorders.

- Discuss the various treatment approaches for myasthenia gravis (MG) and focus on the nursing care and client teaching related to MG.

- Compare and contrast the causes of toxic and infectious neurologic disorders. List the key nursing assessments of these disorders and related nursing interventions.

■ ■ ■ **The Client with Alzheimer's Disease**

1. The first sign seen in a client with Alzheimer's disease is often a change in:
   a. vision.   b. memory.   c. affect.   d. weight.

2. Structural characteristics typical of the brain of the client with Alzheimer's will reveal (a) _____ _____ and (b) _____.

3. A client with Alzheimer's disease is found to repeat the same words over and over again. This condition is called:
   a. paraphasia.   b. aphasia.   c. echolalia.   d. monophasia.

4. It is important to teach the client and his family that tacrine hydrochloride (Cognex) is used to:
   a. cure the client of Alzheimer's disease.
   b. sedate the client to prevent injury.
   c. allieviate depression.
   d. improve the memory of the client.

5. A desired outcome for the client with a nursing diagnosis of *Altered Thought Process* is to:
   a. increase client's dependence on nursing staff and others.
   b. structure the client's environment to prevent self-harm.
   c. restrain the client when at risk for self-harm.
   d. medicate the client PRN to prevent self-harm.

6. A client in the second stage of Alzheimer's disease would experience:
   a. disturbed sleeping and wandering.
   b. good physical health and would seem alert.
   c. incontinence and would be unable to communicate.
   d. delusions and would be paranoid.

7. A client experiences "sundowning." In the client's nursing care plan, her home care nurse should include which intervention?
   a. making sure lights are on at all times
   b. providing for restraints when the sun goes down
   c. including increased use of PRN sedation at night
   d. increasing assessments and monitoring in the afternoon and evening

8. A client has been diagnosed with Alzheimer's disease after a complete evaluation. His wife asks, "Are you sure it's Alzheimer's disease?" The most appropriate response by the nurse is:
   a. "He should have a brain biopsy to make certain."
   b. "The doctor has ruled out other possible causes for his illness."
   c. "We will just have to wait and see how his symptoms develop."
   d. "Perhaps you should get a second opinion."

9. A client scores a 19 on the mini-mental status examination. This result indicates:
   a. normal brain function.
   b. dementia, depression, or delirium.
   c. a stuporous or comatose state.
   d. a low IQ.

10. Identify four appropriate nursing interventions for a client with Alzheimer's disease experiencing anxiety and restlessness.
    (a) _____
    (b) _____
    (c) _____
    (d) _____

11. A client with Alzheimer's disease is taking tacrine hydrochloride (Cognex). Which statement by the family indicates a need for further teaching?
    a. "Cognex should not be stopped abruptly."
    b. "I should report any yellow coloring of the skin."
    c. "He can smoke when taking this medication."
    d. "I should monitor for any problems with urination."

▪ ▪ ▪ The Client with Multiple Sclerosis (MS)

12. Which of the following symptoms is most indicative of multiple sclerosis?
    a. weakness following a hot shower or bath
    b. increased energy following a brisk long walk
    c. muscular pain after vigorous exercise
    d. shortness of breath following a long, brisk walk

13. A client with multiple sclerosis would first notice changes in which body system?
    a. cardiovascular
    b. integumentary
    c. visual
    d. gastrointestinal

14. A client is being discharged after an acute attack of multiple sclerosis. Her primary care provider has prescribed Betaseron to be taken every other day. The discharge nurse should teach the client:
    a. to stop taking the medication when she feels better and her symptoms are gone.
    b. that the medication increases bleeding and she should be alert for signs and symptoms associated with bleeding.
    c. that this medication increases fertility and she should be cautious if pregnancy is unwanted.
    d. that this medication may cause depression and she should be alert for the signs associated with depression.

15. Several months later, the above client's condition has worsened. Her health care provider recommends plasmapheresis. This recommendation is given based on the fact that _____ _____ _____.

16. In MS, the _____ of nerve fibers slows conduction of nerve impulses.

17. The most definitive test used in the diagnosis of multiple sclerosis is a(n):
    a. CT scan of the brain.
    b. lumbar puncture.
    c. evoked potential.
    d. MRI of the brain.

18. A client is being treated with azathioprine (Imuran) for her MS. Which statement by the client indicates a need for further teaching?
    a. "I should report infection, bleeding, or anemia immediately."
    b. "I will have to undergo frequent blood tests."
    c. "Jaundice or yellow coloring of the skin should be reported if present for more than 2 weeks."
    d. "I should avoid pregnancy when taking this medication."

▪ ▪ ▪ The Client with Parkinson's Disease

19. List three cardinal neuromuscular findings characteristic of Parkinson's disease.
    (a) _____
    (b) _____
    (c) _____

20. Which of the following statements most clearly defines the physiology found in Parkinson's disease?
    a. insufficient amount of dopamine in the basal ganglia
    b. too much dopamine in the basal ganglia
    c. too little acetylcholine at the neuromuscular junction
    d. an overabundance of serotonin in the brain

21. When are Parkinsonian tremors more frequently observed?
    a. when the client is agitated
    b. at all times
    c. at rest
    d. never, if properly medicated

22. Which of the following laboratory or diagnostic tests most clearly indicates Parkinson's disease?
    a. complete blood count
    b. electroencephalogram
    c. video fluoroscopy
    d. no specific laboratory or diagnostic tests

In questions 23–26, identify how each class of medication affects neurotransmitters, and give an example of a drug in each class.

23. Monoamine oxidase (MAO) inhibitors:

24. Dopaminergics:

25. Dopamine agonists:

26. Anticholinergics:

27. Clients on which class of drugs may develop secondary Parkinsonism or Parkinsonian syndrome?

_____

Match the movements (a–f) with the correct descriptions listed in questions 28–33.

_____ 28. walking backwards

_____ 29. pill rolling of the thumb and finger

_____ 30. slowed movements due to muscle rigidity

_____ 31. involuntary, short, rapid shuffling

_____ 32. voluntary movement is lost

_____ 33. eyes are fixed with lateral and upward gaze

a. festination
b. retropulsion
c. akinesia
d. bradykinesia
e. non-intention tremor
f. oculogyric crisis

34. Which statement by the family caring for a client on levadopa (L-Dopa) indicates a need for further teaching?
    a. "There should be an immediate and dramatic effect from this medication."
    b. "The dosage should not be altered unless directed by the physician."
    c. "Position changes should be slow."
    d. "This medication will cause changes in urine color."

35. A 78-year-old client suffering from Parkinson's disease has severe benign prostatic hypertrophy. The doctor prescribes benztropine mesylate (Cogentin). The most appropriate action by the nurse is to:
    a. administer the medication as prescribed.
    b. withhold the medication, as it may cause side effects.
    c. monitor the client for dry mouth and constipation.
    d. question the physician about the prescription.

■ ■ ■ The Client with Huntington's Disease

36. Huntington's disease is characterized by which two primary neuromuscular abnormalities?

    (a) _____

    (b) _____

37. Which of the following patterns best describes Huntington's chorea?

    a. increased acetylcholine, increased dopamine

    b. decreased acetylcholine, increased dopamine

    c. decreased acetylcholine, decreased dopamine

    d. increased acetylcholine, decreased dopamine

38. To relieve the symptoms associated with Huntington's chorea, nursing interventions should focus on:

    a. frequent client contact.

    b. administration of sedatives.

    c. decreasing environmental stimuli.

    d. decreasing sedation and increasing stimuli.

39. Which nursing diagnosis is related to the most common cause of death in the client with Huntington's chorea?

    a. *Risk for Aspiration*

    b. *Urinary Incontinence*

    c. *Altered Nutrition: Less than Body Requirements*

    d. *Powerlessness* related to disease progression

40. A client is seeing the nurse-midwife in the clinic because she is considering pregnancy. The client tells the nurse-midwife that her father died of Huntington's chorea. She has no signs of the disease but is concerned about transmitting the disease during pregnancy. The best response by the nurse-midwife would be:

    a. "If you have the genetic marker, you could pass the disease to your child."

    b. "If you do get pregnant, we can test the fetus for the disease."

    c. "You are taking a 50–50 chance of transmitting the disease via pregnancy."

    d. "You have no symptoms of the disease, so you cannot pass it on during pregnancy."

■ ■ ■ The Client with Amyotrophic Lateral Sclerosis (ALS)

41. ALS is most clearly distinguishable from other progressive neurologic disorders in that:

    a. weakness is not a key feature of ALS.

    b. there is no cognitive impairment with ALS.

    c. the client's brain remains unaffected in ALS.

    d. the client with ALS remains independent in activities of daily living.

42. The first symptoms of ALS are (a) _____ and (b) _____ in (c) _____.

43. Fasciculations are defined as _____.

44. A client has ALS. The nurse has made a nursing diagnosis of *Ineffective Breathing Pattern*. Which nursing intervention is most appropriate?

    a. reporting an O_2 saturation < 92%

    b. turning the client every 4 hours

    c. elevating the HOB 15–20 degrees

    d. reporting clear lung sounds

▪ ▪ ▪ The Client with Myasthenia Gravis (MG)

45. The primary defect associated with myasthenia gravis is:
    a. destruction of acetylcholine receptor sites.
    b. a deficit in the amount of acetylcholine.
    c. the removal of the thymus gland.
    d. increased production of dopamine.

46. The nurse is examining a client with myasthenia gravis and observes ptosis. Ptosis is defined as:
    a. unilateral vision.
    b. field defects.
    c. drooping of the eyelid.
    d. excessive tearing of the eye.

47. Which of the following assessments would be the best way to confirm the diagnosis of myasthenia gravis?
    a. assessing the client for ptosis
    b. assessing the client for the development of diplopia and other visual complaints
    c. assessing the client for weakness of the intercostal muscles and difficulty breathing
    d. assessing the client for increased muscle strength after administration of an anticholinesterase drug

48. A client has myasthenia gravis. She is admitted with severe muscle weakness and respiratory distress. The physician administers Tensilon (edrophonium) but her condition does not improve. The nurse can anticipate that the next course of action will be to:
    a. discontinue the use of anticholinesterase drugs.
    b. increase the dosage of oral anticholinesterase medications.
    c. determine the level of anti-acetylcholine receptor antibodies.
    d. administer Tensilon (edrophonium) continuously until her symptoms resolve.

49. Clients with myasthenia gravis are at risk for *Ineffective Airway Clearance* because:
    a. the medications used to treat MG increase the client's risk for infection.
    b. MG affects the client's ability to cough effectively.
    c. MG increases mucous production.
    d. the client with MG is on immunosuppressants.

50. List five nursing interventions for the client with myasthenia gravis with impaired swallowing.
    (a) _____
    (b) _____
    (c) _____
    (d) _____
    (e) _____

▪ ▪ ▪ The Client with Guillain-Barré Syndrome

51. Which of the following findings is characteristic of the client with Guillain-Barré syndrome?
    a. symmetric paralysis
    b. tachycardia
    c. increased peristalsis
    d. hyperactivity

52. Plasmapheresis for Guillain-Barré syndrome is most effective if accomplished:
    a. very early, when symptoms appear.
    b. 1 month after symptoms appear.
    c. daily until the client is better.
    d. daily for the rest of the client's life.

53. Clients with Guillain-Barré often experience pain. Which of the following nursing interventions would be most effective in managing a client's pain?
    a. repositioning the client every 2 hours
    b. encouraging coughing and deep breathing every hour
    c. applying heat or cold to the affected area
    d. referring the client to a physical therapist

54. A client has Guillain-Barré syndrome. Her vital capacity drops to 7.0 mL/kg of body weight. The appropriate intervention by the nurse is to:
    a. continue to monitor respiratory status and report any further decreases.
    b. increase nasal O_2 to 5 L and check O_2 saturation.
    c. contact the physician and increase frequency of respiratory assessment.
    d. do nothing. This is a normal finding in a female.

▪ ▪ ▪ The Client with Trigeminal Neuralgia

55. The client with trigeminal neuralgia often has pain in the:
    a. abdomen.   c. legs.
    b. head.   d. face.

56. List four aspects of client teaching regarding eye care for a client with trigeminal neuralgia.
    (a) _____
    (b) _____
    (c) _____
    (d) _____

▪ ▪ ▪ The Client with Bell's Palsy

57. Prior to the observable clinical manifestations of Bell's palsy, the client may complain of:
    a. pain behind the ear.   c. swollen lymph nodes
    b. projectile vomiting.   d. difficulty swallowing.

58. Although the exact cause of Bell's palsy is unknown, it is most commonly associated with:
    a. the AIDS virus.   c. a bacterial infection.
    b. the herpes virus.   d. a fungal infection.

59. The clinical manifestation most associated with Bell's palsy is:
    a. non-productive cough.
    b. prolonged fever.
    c. facial paralysis.
    d. gastrointestinal bleeding.

60. A client with Bell's palsy has a nursing diagnosis of *Risk for Disuse Syndrome*. Identify four nursing actions that would decrease this client's risk.
    (a) _____
    (b) _____
    (c) _____
    (d) _____

▪ ▪ ▪ The Client with Rabies

61. Which of the following clinical findings is most indicative of rabies?
    a. fever   b. pain at the site   c. hydrophobia   d. depression

62. Which nursing intervention is most appropriate for the client who has a nursing diagnosis of *Altered Sensory Perception* due to rabies?
    a. take the client's temperature every 2 hours
    b. place the client in a darkened, quiet room
    c. conduct passive range-of-motion exercises
    d. administer rabies immune globulin to the client

▪ ▪ ▪ The Client with Tetanus

63. The most important intervention for the prevention of infection with tetanus is:
    a. active immunization.   c. antibiotics for a suspected infection.
    b. avoiding contaminated dirt.   d. debridement of an infected wound.

64. The majority of clients with tetanus are over age _____.

65. All adults should have a booster shot every (a) _____ years, or at the time of a major injury if the last booster was given more than (b) _____ years prior to the injury.

▪ ▪ ▪ The Client with Botulism

66. Client teaching for the prevention of botulism includes instructing the client to:
    a. examine the stool for blood.
    b. eat only fresh foods.
    c. induce vomiting if suspected.
    d. examine commercially prepared canned foods.

67. Manifestations of botulism appear (a) _____ hours after ingestion of contaminated food.

68. The most serious clinical manifestation of botulism is _____.

Read the following statements and determine if they are true or false. Correct any false statements.

_____ 69. The risks for botulism can be reduced by observing food safety rules.

_____ 70. Botulism is a self-limiting illness and often resolves without medical intervention.

_____ 71. Diplopia and visual disturbances are common manifestations of botulism.

_____ 72. Botulism antitoxin is administered if botulism is expected.

73. Describe five points to be included when teaching about food safety.
    (a) _____
    (b) _____
    (c) _____
    (d) _____
    (e) _____

▪ ▪ ▪ The Client with Postpolio Syndrome

Read the following statements and determine if they are true or false. Correct any false statements.

_____ 74. Postpolio syndrome occurs in individuals immunized with oral live trivalent virus.

_____ 75. Manifestations of postpolio syndrome include fatigue, muscle and joint weakness, pain, and respiratory difficulty.

_____ 76. A support group may be helpful to a client who is experiencing postpolio syndrome and to the client's family.

▪ ▪ ▪ The Client with Creutzfeldt-Jakob Disease (CJD)

77. CJD is (a) _____ and (b) _____.
The peak age for onset is between ages of (c) _____.

78. The nurse is caring for a client who may have CJD. A family member asks about a definitive diagnosis. What is the most appropriate response by the nurse?

79. The family members ask the nurse if CJD is similar to Alzheimer's disease. What is the most appropriate response by the nurse?

▪ ▪ ▪ Critical Thinking Exercises

80. A 67-year-old woman is newly diagnosed with myasthenia gravis. She has a number of questions about her condition and its treatment. Her physician has told her she will need a thymectomy within the next 6 months. Develop a teaching plan to assist her in managing her illness.

81. A 73-year-old man is admitted with weakness and numbness of the legs. At 1 AM, the nurse notes that he has not voided for 12 hours. His respirations are shallow, but not labored. What are the most appropriate actions by the nurse?

82. Develop a community health program to teach citizens about the importance of preventing tetanus with immunization.

▪ ▪ ▪ Additional Learning Experiences

▪ Attend an Alzheimer's disease caregivers support group. Listen to the concerns and issues of the attendees.

▪ Identify Internet resources for clients with multiple sclerosis.

▪ Check with your state health department about the incidence of rabies in your area. Contact a public health nurse and discuss the latest recommendations for postexposure care.

Assessing Clients with Eye or Ear Disorders

■ ■ ■ **Focused Study Tips**

- Recognize both normal and abnormal findings during the assessment of the eyes.

- Practice using an ophthalmoscope and other instruments used in the physical assessment of the eyes and ears.

- Review anatomical structure and function of the eyes and ears.

■ ■ ■ **Anatomy and Physiology**

1. Identify the two primary functions of the eye.
   (a) _____
   (b) _____

2. The eye is made up of two types of structures known as (a) _____ and
   (b) _____ structures.

3. (a) _____ are those portions of the eye outside the
   eyeball yet vital to its protection. (b) _____ transmit
   visual images and maintain homeostasis of the inner eye.

4. The place where the optic nerves meet that lies anterior to the pituitary gland is known as the
   _____.

5. Nerve impulses that originate in the retina are interpreted in the:
   a. visual cortex.
   b. cell axons.
   c. optic radiations.
   d. optic tracts.

6. Refraction occurs when (a) _____
   _____,
   Accommodation occurs when (b) _____
   _____.

7. Identify the two primary functions of the ear.
   (a) _____
   (b) _____

8. Identify the two main functions of cerumen.
   (a) _____
   (b) _____

Match the functions of the eye (a–v) with the correct structures listed in questions 9–30.

_____ 9. eyebrows

_____ 10. eyelids

_____ 11. eyelashes

_____ 12. conjunctiva

_____ 13. lacrimal apparatus

_____ 14. sclera

_____ 15. cornea

_____ 16. choroid

_____ 17. iris

_____ 18. pupil

_____ 19. anterior cavity

_____ 20. aqueous humor

_____ 21. canal of Schlemm

_____ 22. posterior cavity

_____ 23. lens

_____ 24. uvea

_____ 25. ciliary body

_____ 26. retina

_____ 27. rods

_____ 28. cones

_____ 29. optic disc

_____ 30. macula

a. regulates the amount of light reaching the retina by controlling the shape of the lens

b. lines outside of eyeball that give shape to eyeball

c. clear fluid that fills anterior chamber of eye

d. short, coarse hairs that shade eye and keep perspiration away from eyes

e. drainage system for fluid moving between anterior and posterior chambers

f. dark center of eye through which light enters

g. short hairs that protect eyes from foreign objects

h. area behind the lens filled with vitreous humor

i. area lateral to optic disc with no visible blood vessels

j. allow for vision in bright light and perception of color

k. regulate entry of light into the eye and distribute tears

l. pigmented, vascular area of eye that absorbs light and keeps it from scattering within the eye

m. disc of muscle tissue surrounding pupil

n. middle coat of the eyeball

o. innermost lining of the eyeball

p. point at which optic nerve enters the eye

q. thin, transparent mucous membrane that lubricates eye

r. allow for vision in dim light and for peripheral vision

s. space between the cornea and the lens

t. secretes, distributes, and drains tears to cleanse and moisten eye's surface

u. sensitive covering over iris that allows light to enter eye

v. focuses and refracts light onto the retina

Match the functions of the ear (a–h) with the correct structures listed in questions 31–38.

_____ 31. auricles

_____ 32. external auditory canal

_____ 33. tympanic membrane

_____ 34. middle ear

_____ 35. auditory tube

_____ 36. labyrinth

_____ 37. cochlea

_____ 38. organ of Corti

a. connects with nasopharynx and helps to equalize air pressure in the middle ear (Eustachian tube)

b. direct sound waves into the ear

c. receptor organ for hearing

d. transfers vibrations to middle ear in the form of sound waves

e. contains tiny bony chamber that houses the organ of Corti

f. serves as a resonator for range of sound waves typical of human speech

g. air-filled cavity containing malleus, incus, and stapes

h. also called the inner ear; involved in equilibrium

39. The two main types of equilibrium are called (a) _____ and
   (b) _____.

■ ■ ■ Assessment of Eye and Ear Function

40. Identify two types of nonverbal client behavior that suggest problems with eye function.

    (a) _____

    (b) _____

41. Define tinnitus.

42. The chart used to assess near vision is called the:

    a. E-chart.   c. sensorineural chart.

    b. Snellen chart.   d. Rosenbaum chart.

43. The cover-uncover test is used to detect _____.

44. The term that describes impaired near vision resulting from a loss of elasticity of the lens secondary to aging is:

    a. hyperopia.   b. presbyopia.   c. myopia.   d. anopia.

45. Briefly explain why pupils of unequal size are usually cause for concern.

46. How would the nurse test consensual pupil response?

47. A client comes to the clinic complaining of a "sty" in his right eye. The nurse practitioner notes a localized inflammation of a hair follicle in the client's right eye. He tells the client he is probably suffering from a:

    a. chalazion.   b. pterygium.   c. hordeolum.   d. xanthelasma.

48. Inspection of the internal structures of the eye is accomplished using a(n): _____

    _____.

49. A 70-year-old client presents at the clinic with "vision problems." He tells the nurse, "I just can't see out of my left eye the way I used to." Upon examination, the nurse notes an opacity of the lens of the client's left eye. The opacity is seen as a dark shadow on ophthalmoscopic examination. The nurse can anticipate that the client has a _____.

50. Physical assessment of the ears and hearing is conducted primarily with which of the following assessment techniques?

    a. inspection   b. auscultation   c. percussion   d. palpation

51. A nurse wants to determine if a client's hearing loss is conductive or perceptive. To determine this, she must use a _____.

52. When a tuning fork is placed on the midline vertex of the client's head the test is known as the:

    a. Rinne test.   b. vibratory test.   c. whisper test.   d. Weber test.

53. A nurse is performing an examination of the client's ear. She believes she has the tympanic membrane in view. She knows that the normal tympanic membrane is (a) _____ _____, (b) _____, and (c) _____.

Case Study

Xavier Ramos, an 80-year-old client, comes to the clinic for his annual physical exam. Upon examination, the nurse practitioner notes that Mr. Ramos' eyes appear to be sunken due to loss of fat from the orbits. Mr. Ramos complains that his eyes are "often dry."

54. The nurse practitioner can anticipate that Mr. Ramos:
    a. has bilateral cataracts.
    b. is experiencing normal age-related changes.
    c. may be suffering from a retinal hemorrhage.
    d. is probably suffering from near-sightedness.

55. Mr. Ramos has an increased risk for impaction of cerumen in his auditory canals because
    _____
    _____.

56. The nurse practitioner tells Mr. Ramos he has presbycusis. What does that mean?

57. Which sounds are Mr. Ramos less likely to hear?

58. The nurse practitioner records a finding of arcus senilis. What does that mean? How will it affect Mr. Ramos?

▪ ▪ ▪ Critical Thinking Exercises

59. Develop a teaching program to assist older adults in understanding the changes that occur in the eyes and ears associated with aging.

60. A neighbor calls and tells the nurse she is worried that she has vision problems. What assessment questions should the nurse ask?

▪ ▪ ▪ Additional Learning Experiences

▪ Practice assessment skills by examining the eyes and ears of as many family members and friends as possible.

▪ Consult with your instructor about participating in an eye or ear screening clinic.

▪ Develop flash cards to help you review the anatomy and physiology of the eyes and ears.

Nursing Care of Clients with Eye and Ear Disorders

■ ■ ■ Focused Study Tips

- Compare the clinical factors of open-angle glaucoma and angle-closure glaucoma, and describe the testing used to distinguish these conditions.

- Describe how medications work in the eye to reduce intraocular pressure.

- Discuss the emergency care of the client with a retinal detachment.

- Discuss the nursing care of the client having ear surgery.

■ ■ ■ The Client with Age-Related Changes in Vision

1. A 65-year-old female comes to the walk-in clinic complaining of an irritation of her left eye. She states that 1 week ago she was at the beach with her grandchildren on a windy day, and she thinks sand may have blown into her eyes. She had not noticed a problem until yesterday, when her daughter told her that her left eye was quite red. Which of the following statements best describes the client's condition?
   a. The client has limited peripheral vision due to senile enophthalmos.
   b. The client may have yellowing of the sclera due to fatty deposits.
   c. The client has decreased corneal sensitivity, which increases her potential for damage from a foreign body.
   d. The client has decreased lens elasticity and increased lens density, which causes decreased visual acuity especially affecting close vision.

2. Which of the following findings is a common age-related change of the eye?
   a. increased eye motility
   b. presbycusis
   c. decreased tear secretion
   d. decreased lens density

■ ■ ■ The Client with an Infectious or Inflammatory Eye Disorder

3. The older client is at a higher risk for infection of the external structures due to which age-related change?
   a. increased eyestrain
   b. decrease of tear production
   c. loss of subcutaneous tissue
   d. decreased pupil size

4. The infecting organism most commonly seen with a hordeolum (sty) infection is:
   a. *Staphylococcus.*
   b. herpes simplex A.
   c. *Escherichia coli.*
   d. *Candida albicans.*

5. _____, a chronic conjunctivitis, is a significant preventable cause of blindness worldwide.

6. Corneal infections are difficult to treat due to the fact that:
   a. the surface area of the cornea is small.
   b. the causative organisms cannot be recovered.
   c. corneal infections are painless.
   d. the cornea is an avascular organ.

7. To reduce the risk of corneal ulcerations, a client should be taught to:
   a. cleanse the eyes vigorously on a daily basis.
   b. perform eye exercises at least 3 times daily.
   c. wear contact lenses as recommended.
   d. wear an eyepatch at night.

8. Which of the following client statements indicates that successful client teaching has occurred following corneal transplant surgery?
   a. "I shouldn't cry for 3 months."
   b. "I will return next week to have my sutures removed.
   c. "I will not lift any heavy objects."
   d. "I am wearing the eye patch to prevent light from shining into my eyes."

9. Following corneal transplant surgery, which of the following client positions is most appropriate?
   a. high-Fowler's   b. Sims'   c. prone   d. supine

10. The client who has undergone corneal transplantation has an increased risk for injury. Identify four nursing interventions to decrease risk for injury.
    (a) _____
    (b) _____
    (c) _____
    (d) _____

11. Which of the following instructions is essential for the client with a corneal abrasion?
    a. exercise the eye by reading
    b. do not wear contact lenses
    c. irrigate the eyes with a hydrogen peroxide solution
    d. temporary vision loss is a normal response to the abrasion

▪ ▪ ▪ **The Client with Eye Trauma**

12. The greatest risks for thermal burns of the eye are (a) _____ and (b) _____.

13. Explain the difference between a penetrating injury and a perforating injury.

14. What are the primary roles of the nurse when working with a client in relation to eye trauma?
    (a) _____
    (b) _____

15. List at least three common causes for corneal abrasions.

16. Identify the emergency treatment for the eyes in each of the following situations:
    (a) chemical burns _____
    (b) penetrating wounds _____
    (c) blunt trauma _____

▪ ▪ ▪ The Client with Cataracts

17. An early manifestation of a cataract is:
    a. loss of vision.
    b. opacification of the lens at the periphery.
    c. opacification of the lens centrally.
    d. opacification of the entire lens.

18. A client is having outpatient cataract surgery. Identify four important self-care principles for the immediate postoperative period that the nurse should teach the client prior to discharge.
    (a) _____
    (b) _____
    (c) _____
    (d) _____

Read the following statements and determine if they are true or false. Correct any false statements.

_____ 19. Corticosteroids taken orally can result in cataract formation.

_____ 20. Acquired cataracts are the most common form of cataracts.

_____ 21. Senile cataracts tend to be bilateral.

_____ 22. Surgical removal is the only treatment for cataracts.

▪ ▪ ▪ The Client with Glaucoma

23. Define glaucoma.

24. Which of the following pressure readings is consistent with an increased intraocular pressure?
    a. 12 mm Hg   b. 15 mm Hg   c. 20 mm Hg   d. 25 mm Hg

Match the types of glaucoma (a–b) with the correct descriptions listed in questions 25–28. Glaucoma types may be used more than once.

_____ 25. Of the two types of glaucoma, this form is less common, accounting for only 5–10% of cases.

_____ 26. There is a high incidence of this type of glaucoma in persons of Asian descent.

_____ 27. This type of glaucoma typically affects both eyes.

_____ 28. With this type of glaucoma, teach the client to avoid pupil-dilating medications.

a. open-angle glaucoma
b. angle-closure glaucoma

29. Which of the following diagnostic tests is used to differentiate between open-angle or angle-closure glaucoma?
    a. tonometry
    b. noncontact tonometry
    c. gonioscopy
    d. visual field testing

30. What is the advantage of using beta-adrenergic blocking medications (Timoptic) over the miotic drugs (pilocarpine) in the treatment of glaucoma? Beta-adrenergic blocking medications:
    a. are not systematically absorbed.
    b. increase the amount of aqueous humor in the body.
    c. produce very little, if any, side effects.
    d. have a longer duration of activity.

31. Which of the following classes of drugs can be used as diuretics and as a method to reduce intra-ocular pressure?
    a. miotics
    b. mydriatics
    c. carbonic anhydrase inhibitors
    d. beta-adrenergic receptor blockers

Read the statements below and determine if they are true or false. Correct any false statements.

_____ 32. Surgical management of chronic open-angle glaucoma involves improving the drainage of aqueous humor from the posterior chamber of the eye.

_____ 33. Iridectomy, iridotomy, and gonioplasty are all effective in reducing intraocular pressure for the client with angle-closure glaucoma.

34. Which of the following client statements indicates successful client teaching about glaucoma?
    a. "I should use my eye drops when I feel pain in my eyes."
    b. "I will have to take this medication for the rest of my life."
    c. "Glaucoma can be corrected by wearing special lenses."
    d. "I should not drink excessively. If I do, it can increase the pressure in my eyes."

▪ ▪ ▪ The Client with Retinal Detachment

35. Which of the following client symptoms is most consistent with retinal detachment?
    a. severe pain
    b. blood in the eye
    c. cloudy vision
    d. floaters

36. Prompt intervention by the nurse caring for the client with retinal detachment includes:
    a. reassuring the client that there is nothing to worry about.
    b. keeping the client npo in preparation for emergency surgery.
    c. positioning the client so the area of detachment is inferior.
    d. covering the client's eyes with a dry sterile gauze.

37. Identify at least four points that should be addressed in the teaching plan for a client who has experienced a retinal detachment.

▪ ▪ ▪ The Client with Macular Degeneration

38. A 75-year-old client is being seen by his health care provider. When obtaining his health history, it is noted that the client has some loss of vision. Which of the following complaints by the client is most indicative of macular degeneration?
    a. loss of central vision
    b. loss of peripheral vision
    c. acute vision loss
    d. clouding of the lens

39. Essential nursing activities for the client with macular degeneration include:
    a. administering mydriatics as ordered.
    b. providing visual aids to the client to adapt for loss of vision.
    c. applying warm soaks to the eyes bilaterally.
    d. encouraging the client to minimize light into the eye.

▪ ▪ ▪ The Client with Retinitis Pigmentosa

40. Which of the following is true regarding retinitis pigmentosa?
    a. Retinitis pigmentosa is caused by a virus.
    b. The initial manifestation of retinitis pigmentosa is often noted during the early adult years.
    c. Retinitis pigmentosa never results in total blindness.
    d. Retinitis pigmentosa is corrected through surgery.

▪ ▪ ▪ The Client with Diabetic Retinopathy

41. The severity of disease in the client with diabetic retinopathy is most closely associated with:
    a. the duration of time a client has had diabetes.
    b. the client's unstable glucose levels.
    c. the partial pressure of oxygen.
    d. the variability of insulin metabolism.

42. The client with diabetic retinopathy should have an ophthalmology visit at least:
    a. every 2 months.
    b. every 6 months.
    c. yearly.
    d. biannually.

Read the following statements and determine if they are true or false. Correct any false statements.

_____ 43. Clients with diabetic retinopathy should expect episodes of blurred vision and floaters.

_____ 44. Only 25% of clients with diabetes will develop retinopathy.

_____ 45. Nonproliferative retinopathy is typically the initial form of diabetic retinopathy.

▪ ▪ ▪ The Client with HIV Infection

46. The most serious and frequent ocular infection associated with the HIV infection is:
    a. Kaposi's sarcoma.
    b. non-Hodgkin's lymphoma.
    c. HIV retinopathy.
    d. CMV retinitis.

▪ ▪ ▪ The Client with an Enucleation

47. Identify five reasons surgical removal of the eye may be necessary.

   (a) _____

   (b) _____

   (c) _____

   (d) _____

   (e) _____

▪ ▪ ▪ The Client Who Is Blind

Read the following statements and determine if they are true or false. Correct any false statements.

_____ 48. The adjustment of the person who is born blind and raised to become an independent member of society differs from that of the person who has been sighted and becomes blind.

_____ 49. The legal definition of blindness is visual acuity no better than 20/200 in the better eye with optimal correction.

_____ 50. Only one-third of all causes of blindness are preventable or curable.

_____ 51. Releasing the hope that vision will be regained indicates acceptance of one's blindness.

_____ 52. When assisting a blind person to ambulate, the nurse should hold the client's arm.

53. List at least four major causes of blindness.

▪ ▪ ▪ The Client with External Otitis

54. External otitis (swimmer's ear) is thought to be caused by:
   a. poor ear hygiene.
   b. chlorinated water.
   c. removal of cerumen.
   d. incorrect cleansing of the external ear canal.

55. A client is seeing the occupational health nurse for "a feeling of fullness" in her ear. To determine if the client's fullness is a problem of the internal canal or external canal, the nurse should:
   a. press on the tragus of the ear.
   b. perform the Weber test.
   c. perform the Rinne test.
   d. suction the ear.

56. The most common infecting organism seen in the client with external otitis is:
   a. *Staphylococcus epidermidis.*
   b. *Pseudomonas aeruginosa.*
   c. herpes simplex virus.
   d. *Helicobactor pylori.*

57. Primary prevention of external otitis includes teaching the client to:
   a. cleanse the ear canal with a cotton-tipped applicator and hydrogen peroxide.
   b. cleanse the ear canal with soap and water.
   c. wear ear plugs if the ear is acutely infected when swimming.
   d. not cleanse the ear canals.

▪ ▪ ▪ ▪ The Client with Impacted Cerumen and Foreign Bodies

58. A student is seeing the school nurse because an insect flew into her ear during cheerleading practice. Which nursing intervention is contraindicated?
    a. instilling water into the ear canal
    b. instilling mineral oil into the ear canal
    c. visualizing the ear canal with an otoscope
    d. use of suction in the canal to remove the insect

59. What should clients be taught about cleaning their ears?

▪ ▪ ▪ The Client with Otitis Media

60. Which assessment finding is associated with serous otitis media?
    a. cerumen in the ear
    b. gray, shiny tympanic membrane
    c. bulging of the membrane
    d. a cone of light

61. Which of the following tests is most beneficial in the diagnosis of acute otitis media?
    a. Valsalva maneuver
    b. culture of the ear canal
    c. Rinne or Weber test
    d. pneumatic otoscope

62. The nurse should teach the client with acute otitis media to:
    a. apply cold to the affected side.
    b. avoid air travel, rapid changes in elevation, and diving.
    c. cleanse the ear with a soft cotton-tipped applicator.
    d. discontinue antibiotic therapy when ringing in the ear diminishes.

63. A client with acute otitis media is scheduled for a myringotomy. He asks the nurse if this procedure will help the pain in his ear. The most appropriate response by the nurse is:
    a. "Yes; as soon as the procedure is complete, the pain will subside."
    b. "No; however, we can give you analgesics to help with the pain."
    c. "No; this procedure is done so that cultures can be obtained."
    d. "No, but the pain will subside over time."

64. Which of the following client symptoms is indicative of a complication associated with acute otitis media?
    a. mild fever
    b. abrupt relief of pain
    c. congestion and nasal discharge
    d. feeling of fullness in the ear

▪ ▪ ▪ The Client with Acute Mastoiditis

65. Collaborative care and nursing care related to mastoiditis focuses primarily on _____
_____.

Read the following statements and determine if they are true or false. Correct any false statements.

_____ 66. Symptoms of acute mastoiditis usually develop within 2–3 weeks after an episode of acute otitis media.

_____ 67. Acute mastoiditis is easily treated with the correct oral antibiotics.

_____ 68. There is a risk of meningitis with mastoiditis.

69. List at least five symptoms of mastoiditis.

■ ■ ■ The Client with Chronic Otitis Media or Otosclerosis

70. _____ are benign and slow-growing tumors, which can enlarge to fill the entire middle ear.

71. Would the client with otosclerosis experience anxiety related to concern about transmission of the disorder to his/her children? If so, why?

■ ■ ■ The Client with Inner Ear Disorders

Read the statements below and determine if they are true or false. Correct any false statements.

_____ 72. Labyrinthitis is a common disorder.

_____ 73. Labyrinthitis is an inflammation of the inner ear.

_____ 74. Labyrinthitis is also called otitis interna.

_____ 75. Labyrinthitis typically causes vertigo.

76. The rationale for administering a diuretic to a client with Ménière's disease is to:
    a. reduce the amount of potassium in the serum.
    b. reduce the intravascular fluid compartment.
    c. reduce the fluid pressure in the inner ear.
    d. encourage drainage through the outer ear canal.

■ ■ ■ The Client with an Acoustic Neuroma

Read the statements below and determine if they are true or false. Correct any false statements.

_____ 77. Early manifestations of an acoustic neuroma are similar to disorders of the inner ear.

_____ 78. Acoustic neuromas are easily treated with corticosteroids.

_____ 79. Acoustic neuromas are usually malignant in nature.

▪ ▪ ▪   The Client with Hearing Loss

Identify whether each of the descriptions below is common to (a) conductive hearing loss or (b) sensori-neural hearing loss.

_____ 80. In this type of hearing loss, damaged receptor cells distort the ability to receive sound waves.

_____ 81. Noise exposure is often the cause of this type of hearing loss.

_____ 82. Obstruction of the external ear canal may be the etiology for this type of hearing loss.

_____ 83. Ototoxic drugs may be the cause of this type of hearing loss.

_____ 84. In this type of hearing loss, hearing aids are useful.

85. When a client is fitted with a hearing amplification device, it is important that the nurse teach the client that:
   a. hearing will gradually become restored.
   b. hearing devices do not treat the hearing loss.
   c. only partial hearing will be restored.
   d. relying on the hearing device may lead to further hearing loss.

86. A 65-year-old male is scheduled for a cochlear implant today. He tells his nurse, "I can't wait to hear again like a 20-year-old!" How should the nurse respond?

▪ ▪ ▪   Critical Thinking Exercises

87. Develop a community health program that focuses on strategies for preventing eye injuries and first-aid measures for eye injuries.

88. The nurse is enjoying the day at the beach and suddenly hears loud screaming. Upon investigating, the nurse finds a young man with a dart in his eye. What is the most appropriate action?

89. The nurse is caring for a group of elderly clients with vision and hearing deficits. Identify strategies to enhance their safety and communication.

▪ ▪ ▪   Additional Learning Experiences

▪ Visit a hearing aid center, and identify the services that are offered and determine the fee structure.

▪ Participate in a vision or hearing screening program for older adults.

▪ Identify resources for individuals with hearing or vision impairments.

Assessing Clients with Reproductive Disorders

■ ■ ■ **Focused Study Tips**

- Examine your feelings about asking clients questions related to sensitive topics concerning reproduction.

- Describe the normal findings during the assessment of the reproductive system.

- Discuss with other students the difficult issues they may have encountered when conducting an assessment of the reproductive system.

■ ■ ■ **Anatomy and Physiology**

1. Identify three major functions of the reproductive organs in both men and women.

   (a) _____

   (b) _____

   (c) _____

Match the anatomical structures in the male reproductive system (a–k) with the correct functions listed in questions 2–12.

_____ 2. where sperm are stored until ejaculation

_____ 3. homologous to the female's ovaries

_____ 4. regulates the temperature of the testes

_____ 5. produce testosterone

_____ 6. covering of the glans in uncircumcised men

_____ 7. correctly balanced mixture of sperm and seminal fluid

_____ 8. responsible for sperm production

_____ 9. male genital organ that encloses the urethra

_____ 10. produce 60% of the volume of seminal fluid

_____ 11. produces about 30% of the volume of seminal fluid

_____ 12. final storage and maturation area for sperm

a. testes
b. seminiferous tubules
c. Leydig's cells
d. epididymis
e. ampulla
f. seminal vesicles
g. semen
h. scrotum
i. prostate gland
j. penis
k. prepuce

13. Identify three functions of seminal fluid as it relates to sperm.

   (a) _____

   (b) _____

   (c) _____

14. _____ is the series of physiologic events that generate sperm in the seminiferous tubules.

15. The male sex hormones are called (a) _____, the primary hormone being (b) _____.

Match the anatomical structures of the female reproductive system (a–k) with the correct descriptions listed in questions 16–26.

_____ 16. skin-covered adipose tissue anterior to the symphysis pubis

_____ 17. pear-shaped muscular organ between the bladder and rectum

_____ 18. thin, tubular structures attached to the uterus by broad ligaments

_____ 19. highly sensitive erectile organ; analogous to the male penis

_____ 20. pigmented breast area containing sebaceous glands and nipple

_____ 21. fibromuscular tube that serves as a route for excretion and an organ of sexual response

_____ 22. lateral ends of uterine tubes that capture the ovum after it is released from the ovary

_____ 23. primary purpose is to supply nourishment for the infant

_____ 24. store female germ cells and produce female hormones

_____ 25. secrete lubricating fluid during the sexual response cycle

_____ 26. connects the uterine cavity with the vagina

a. vagina
b. cervix
c. uterus
d. fallopian tubes
e. fimbriae
f. ovaries
g. mons pubis
h. Bartholin's glands
i. clitoris
j. breasts
k. areola

27. _____ is the hormone essential for the development and maintenance of secondary sex characteristics in women.

28. _____ is the hormone that primarily affects the development of breast glandular tissue and the endometrium.

29. _____ are the hormones responsible for normal hair growth patterns at puberty.

30. During the ovarian cycle, the oocyte is expelled from the mature ovarian follicle into the abdominal cavity by the process called:
    a. oogenesis.   b. menstruation.   c. fimbriaeosis.   d. ovulation.

31. If pregnancy does not occur, the corpus luteum:
    a. begins to degenerate.   c. causes decreased secretion of LH and FSH.
    b. causes estrogen levels to increase.   d. is reabsorbed by the ovary.

32. List the three phases of the menstrual cycle.
    (a) _____
    (b) _____
    (c) _____

33. The endometrium is receptive to the implantation of an embryo for:
    a. 14 days.   b. 7 days.   c. 2 days.   d. 28 days.

▪ ▪ ▪ Assessment of Reproductive Function

34. Which method for obtaining subjective data related to assessment of the reproductive system is inappropriate?
    a. The nurse is not embarrassed by the client's terminology.
    b. The nurse uses clinically correct terms to describe anatomical parts.
    c. The interview begins with more general questions then progresses to specific questions.
    d. Questions are asked in a way that gives client permission to report behaviors.

35. Testicular cancer is related to a history of:
    a. an undescended testicle.   c. celibacy.
    b. testicular swelling with chickenpox.   d. use of condoms.

36. List three causes of impotence.
    (a) _____
    (b) _____
    (c) _____

37. Which of the following factors or behaviors increases a woman's risk of developing cervical cancer?
    a. smoking, maternal use of DES
    b. maternal use of DES, use of oral contraceptives
    c. use of oral contraceptives, exposure to asbestos
    d. exposure to asbestos, history of fibrocystic disease

38. Physical assessment of the reproductive system is conducted using which pair of assessment techniques?
    a. inspection and auscultation   c. palpation and percussion
    b. auscultation and percussion   d. inspection and palpation

Case Study

Donald Rimstrom is a 52-year-old divorced client who is complaining of difficulty in starting urination, dribbling, and nocturia over the past 2 months. Mr. Rimstrom works as a construction foreman for a local firm. He tells the nurse he has been divorced for 2 years and decided to begin dating again last year. He states he has no history of sexually transmitted diseases but has had sexual relations with more than one woman over the past 6 months and wears condoms during sexual activity. Mr. Rimstrom states that the color, consistency, and clarity of his urine is unchanged. Physical assessment findings reveal an uncircumcised penis with slight phimosis, normal testicular and scrotal findings, a small bulge in the right inguinal area, and enlargement of the prostate gland without tenderness.

39. List the subjective and objective data and identify possible etiologies.

    subjective findings:

objective findings:

abnormal findings and etiologies:

40. Physical examination of the female client begins with the _____.

41. The nurse assists the female client into the _____ position in order to examine the genitalia and reproductive organs.

42. A _____ is used to inspect the vaginal walls and cervix.

43. In order to palpate the cervix, uterus, and ovaries, the examiner performs a _____ _____.

▪ ▪ ▪   **Critical Thinking Exercises**

44. Identify the key components of a health education curriculum related to reproduction.

45. Develop a community health education program designed to assist parents in providing their children with developmentally appropriate education related to reproductive health.

▪ ▪ ▪   **Additional Learning Experiences**

- Obtain and review a copy of *The New Our Bodies, Ourselves* written by the Boston Women's Health Book Collective. Consider situations in which this reference might be helpful to women with concerns about their reproductive health.

- Determine how your local school system provides reproductive health education to school-aged children. Identify the strengths and weaknesses of the health curriculum.

- Assess an older adult's knowledge regarding reproductive health.

Nursing Care of Male Clients with Reproductive System Disorders

■ ■ ■ Focused Study Tips

- Describe the various laboratory and diagnostic tests used to diagnose problems of the male reproductive system, and know the nursing implications associated with each.

- List the clinical manifestations for prostatic cancer, BPH, and testicular cancer.

- Discuss the risk factors associated with testicular cancer, as well as the treatment options. Describe the emotional, psychologic,

functional, and sexual significance of testicular cancer and its treatment.

- Summarize the nursing care for a client undergoing a prostatectomy.

- Describe the appropriate technique for self-examination of the testicles.

- Review the common causes and treatment approaches for erectile dysfunction.

■ ■ ■ The Client with Benign Prostatic Hypertrophy (BPH)

1. Which of the following factors is most often associated with the development of benign prostatic hypertrophy?
   - a. ethnic origin
   - b. diet
   - c. dihydrotestosterone (DHT)
   - d. sexual activity

2. An early symptom of BPH is (a) _____. If BPH is left untreated it leads to vesicoureteral reflux, which means (b) _____.

3. A client has undergone a transurethral resection of the prostate for BPH. Which of the following nursing actions is contraindicated postoperatively?
   - a. assessing for fluid volume excess
   - b. assessing for hyponatremia
   - c. offering 2 to 3 liters of water
   - d. providing hypertonic fluids as ordered

4. A 53-year-old client tells the nurse he has been experiencing difficulty initiating voiding and diminished force of the urine stream. The most appropriate response by the nurse is:
   - a. "You should have a prostate-specific antigen (PSA) test to check for prostate cancer."
   - b. "Many men experience this as they grow older."
   - c. "You should discuss these changes with your physician."
   - d. "You may need a urinary catheter."

Read the following statements and determine if they are true or false. Correct any false statements.

_____ 5. Prostate cancer is the most common disorder in the aging male client.

_____ 6. A man must be older than 50 years of age and have testes in order to develop BPH.

_____ 7. Finasteride is very effective in relieving symptoms of BPH.

_____ 8. Transuretheral resection of the prostate is the second most common surgery performed in the United States.

▪ ▪ ▪ The Client with Prostatic Cancer

9. Which of the following is an early manifestation of prostate cancer?
   a. hematuria
   b. retroperitoneal lymphadenopathy
   c. suprapubic pain
   d. disturbances in urine flow

10. In a client with prostate cancer, metastasis to the _____ is uncommon due to a tough sheet of tissue that acts as a physical barrier.

11. Which of the following tests is the most specific for the detection of prostate cancer?
    a. prostate-specific antigen (PSA)
    b. digital rectal examination (DRE)
    c. tissue biopsy
    d. transrectal ultrasonography (TRUS)

12. A client is undergoing a transurethral resection of the prostate gland (TURP) for a stage IV prostate cancer. When performing preoperative teaching, it is essential for the client to understand that:
    a. performing prostatic exercises will help prevent recurrence of the tumor.
    b. this surgery is only palliative.
    c. an artificial sphincter is available.
    d. this surgery will require a penile prosthesis.

13. Which of the following nursing interventions would be most appropriate for a client experiencing stress incontinence?
    a. teaching the client Kegel exercises
    b. suggesting the client wear an absorbent pad
    c. inserting an indwelling catheter into the client
    d. recommending surgery to the client

14. Permanent erectile dysfunction occurs in clients treated with which one of the following therapies for prostate cancer?
    a. TURP
    b. orchiectomy
    c. suprapubic prostatectomy
    d. radical prostatectomy

15. Which statement by the client undergoing a transrectal, ultrasound-guided biopsy of the prostate indicates a need for further teaching?
    a. "Blood clots in my urine and stools are common after this procedure."
    b. "I should avoid strenuous activity for the rest of the day."
    c. "I will be monitored for about 1 hour after the procedure."
    d. "I should report rectal pain, painful urination, and urgency."

16. Men at high risk for prostrate cancer should have a digital rectal and an annual prostate-specific antigen test starting at age (a) _____ .

17. Identify three preoperative interventions for the client undergoing a prostatectomy for prostate cancer.
    (a) _____
    (b) _____
    (c) _____

18. Which nursing intervention is contraindicated for the postoperative care of a client with a prostatectomy for prostate cancer?
    a. Maintain the patency of the urinary catheter.
    b. Manage pain through assessment and intervention.
    c. Minimize movement to help control bleeding.
    d. Maintain continuous bladder irrigation.

19. Which statement by the client during discharge teaching following prostate surgery indicates the need for further teaching?
    a. "I should not have intercourse for 6 weeks after surgery."
    b. "I should avoid constipation and straining for a bowel movement."
    c. "I should not expect any bleeding and should report it immediately."
    d. "I should avoid strenuous activity and heavy lifting."

Read the following statements and determine if they are true or false. Correct any false statements.

_____ 20. Prostate cancer is the second leading cause of cancer death in North America.

_____ 21. Once diagnosed, prostate cancer is rarely curable.

_____ 22. An elevated PSA is diagnostic for prostate cancer.

23. List three types of pain a client who has undergone a prostatectomy may experience.
    (a) _____
    (b) _____
    (c) _____

24. Following a transurethral prostatectomy (TURP), the client complains that the tape on his catheter is pulling too tight. The most appropriate action by the nurse is to:
    a. loosen the tape to a position of comfort.
    b. explain to the client the tape must stay in place.
    c. remove the tape and re-tape the catheter.
    d. contact the physician for orders.

25. The purpose of continuous bladder irrigation (CBI) is to:
    a. maintain urine output.
    b. prevent formation of clots.
    c. minimize bleeding.
    d. prevent bladder spasm.

26. Following a transurethral prostatectomy, the client complains of bladder spasms. The nurse should:
    a. tell him this is a normal experience following surgery.
    b. encourage him to deep breathe and relax.
    c. administer oral medications for pain.
    d. provide belladona and opium suppositories.

27. What are the two conditions that comprise TURP syndrome?
    (a) _____
    (b) _____

28. List five symptoms of TURP syndrome.

    (a) _____

    (b) _____

    (c) _____

    (d) _____

    (e) _____

29. A client has undergone a prostatectomy. Which of the following statements indicates a need for further teaching?
    a. "This is the end of my sex life as I know it."
    b. "I may experience some burning on urination."
    c. "I should have regular bowel movements."
    d. "I should drink ten 8-ounce glasses of water each day.

30. Identify key elements of discharge instructions related to activity level following prostate surgery.

■ ■ ■ **The Client with Prostatitis or Protatodynia**

31. When teaching the client with nonbacterial prostatitis about the disorder, the nurse should inform the client:
    a. that he is infectious and should refrain from sexual activity.
    b. that he should massage his prostate.
    c. of the seven warning signs of cancer.
    d. that sexual intercourse may relieve some of the symptoms.

32. Which statement by the client with prostatitis indicates the need for further teaching?
    a. "I should drink 3 liters of fluids each day."
    b. "I should take my antibiotics as ordered."
    c. "I should avoid sitz baths and soaking in the tub."
    d. "I should avoid constipation and straining for a bowel movement."

■ ■ ■ **The Client with Testicular Cancer**

33. The client with testicular cancer often presents with:
    a. painful testicles.
    b. an enlarged scrotum.
    c. a painless nodule.
    d. painful urination.

34. Which form of treatment is used for all stages of testicular cancer?
    a. orchiectomy   b. chemotherapy   c. radiotherapy   d. brachytherapy

35. The nurse is teaching a high school class about testicular self-examination. Which statement by a student indicates a need for further teaching?
    a. "A good time to perform self-examination is during a warm shower or bath."
    b. "In order to detect a problem, I must firmly squeeze each testicle."
    c. "One testicle may be slightly larger than the other."
    d. "I should examine myself once each month."

36. The nurse is providing discharge teaching to a client who just had an orchiectomy for testicular cancer. Which statement by the client indicates a need for further teaching?
    a. "I should report excessive bleeding immediately."
    b. "I should not have any changes in my sexual or reproductive health."
    c. "A scrotal support may help control pain and discomfort."
    d. "In order to have children, I will have to save sperm in a sperm bank."

Read the following statements and determine if they are true or false. Correct any false statements.

_____ 37. Testicular cancer is associated with cryptorchidism.

_____ 38. The majority of young men who develop testicular cancer have one or more risk factors.

_____ 39. Chemotherapy has little effectiveness in testicular cancer.

_____ 40. An orchiectomy results in sterility and sexual dysfunction.

■ ■ ■ The Client with Disorders of the Scrotum and Testes

Match the disorders (a–e) with the correct descriptions listed in questions 41–45.

_____ 41. infection or inflammation of the testicles

_____ 42. fluid-filled mass within the scrotum

_____ 43. a painless mass that forms in the epididymis

_____ 44. failure of the testes to descend during the first 7 months of gestation

_____ 45. dilation of pampiniform venous complex of the spermatic cord

a. spermatocele
b. cryptorchidism
c. hydrocele
d. varicocele
e. orchitis

■ ■ ■ The Client with Cancer of the Penis

46. Cancer of the penis is associated with:
    a. tightening of foreskin.
    b. use of condoms.
    c. heredity.
    d. absence of foreskin.

47. Cancer of the penis spreads to (a) _____, (b) _____, (c) _____, or (d) _____.

■ ■ ■ The Client with Priapism

48. Which of the following best describes the physiologic phenomenon of priapism? Priapism is:
    a. a psychiatric disorder associated with abnormal sexual behavior.
    b. a clinical condition associated with an inability to obtain an adequate erection.
    c. a state of sustained erection due to vascular injury.
    d. a condition associated with a painful ejaculation.

49. Which of the following is an appropriate treatment for priapism?
    a. application of heat
    b. vigorous massage
    c. urinary catheterization
    d. vigorous exercise

■ ■ ■ ■ The Client with Erectile Dysfunction

50. The most common cause for erectile dysfunction for men over age 60 is:
    a. psychologic.
    b. age-related changes.
    c. physiologic.
    d. complications of surgery.

51. Identify the two surgical therapies that can be used to correct a problem of erectile dysfunction.
    (a) _____
    (b) _____

52. Which of the two surgical procedures for erectile dysfunction is considered temporary? _____
    _____

53. Which of the following disorders of ejaculation is the most responsive to medical therapy?
    a. premature ejaculation
    b. delayed ejaculation
    c. retrograde ejaculation
    d. depressed ejaculation

54. A client is taking sildenafil (Viagra). Which statement indicates a need for further client teaching?
    a. "A high-fat meal can delay the onset of the effects."
    b. "I must still practice safe sex."
    c. "I can only take this drug twice a day."
    d. "I need to take it one hour before intercourse."

Read the following statements and determine if they are true or false. Correct any false statements.

_____ 55. Psychologic factors cause over 25% of cases of erectile dysfunction.

_____ 56. Damage to arteries, smooth muscles, and fibrous tissues is the most common cause of impotence.

_____ 57. Sildenafil is contraindicated for men taking nitrates.

_____ 58. Woman can safely take sildenafil.

■ ■ ■ Critical Thinking Exercises

59. Develop a health education program about testicular self-examination.

60. The nurse is caring for a client with prostate cancer. He asks about his ability to return to his normal sexual life. Develop a plan to provide him and his wife counseling regarding his concern.

61. The nurse who is caring for a client following a TURP suspects the client may be developing TURP syndrome. What is the most appropriate action by the nurse? What key assessments should be performed?

■ ■ ■ Additional Learning Experiences

■ Identify Internet resources for men with reproductive health concerns.

■ Contact the school nurse at your local high school and find out more about the health curriculum. Determine whether male students are taught about testicular self-examination.

■ Identify resources for men without health insurance to obtain screening evaluations for prostate cancer.

Nursing Care of Female Clients with Reproductive System Disorders

■ ■ ■ Focused Study Tips

- Define the different terms (amenorrhea, oligomenorrhea, menorrhagia, metrorrhagia, and postmenopausal bleeding) used to describe disorders of dysfunctional uterine bleeding. Compare and contrast the nursing care associated with each disorder.

- Describe the client teaching for the menopausal client and the client with premenstrual syndrome (PMS), dysmenorrhea, and vaginal infections.

- Discuss the risk factors and treatment options for endometrial, cervical, and ovarian cancer. Discuss emotional, psychologic, functional, and sexual significance of these cancers.

- Summarize the client education related to normal anatomy and physiology, perineal hygiene, self-care, and safe sex.

- Discuss the pharmacologic therapies used to treat disorders of the female reproductive system.

- Explain the emotional and functional concerns related to the female reproductive organs.

■ ■ ■ The Client with Premenstrual Syndrome and Dysmenorrhea

1. It is believed that falling levels of (a) _____ and (b) _____ combined with rising levels of (c) _____ contribute to the development of premenstrual syndrome.

2. When instructing a client in self-care measures to relieve the symptoms of PMS, the nurse would suggest:
   a. a diet high in protein.
   b. balancing periods of activity with rest.
   c. practicing Kegel exercises.
   d. applying ice packs to the abdomen.

3. List five clinical manifestations of primary dysmenorrhea.
   (a) _____   (d) _____
   (b) _____   (e) _____
   (c) _____

Read the following statements and determine if they are true or false. Correct any false statements.

_____ 4. A diet low in complex carbohydrates will minimize the symptoms of PMS.

_____ 5. Primary dysmenorrhea is the result of excessive prostaglandins.

_____ 6. Primary dysmenorrhea can be caused by endometriosis or fibroid tumors.

▪ ▪ ▪   The Client with Abnormal Uterine Bleeding

Match the terms used to describe different characteristics of menses (a–d) with the correct definitions listed in questions 7–10.

_____   7. excessive or prolonged menstruation

_____   8. absence of menstruation

_____   9. bleeding between menstrual periods

_____   10. scant menses

a. amenorrhea
b. oligomenorrhea
c. menorrhagia
d. metrorrhagia

11. A 34-year-old female client will undergo a dilation and curettage (D and C) for the treatment of dysfunctional uterine bleeding. While the nurse is performing a preoperative assessment, the client states, "I'm a little nervous. What exactly is a D and C?" The best response by the nurse is:
    a. "The cervical canal will be dilated and the uterine lining will be scraped to remove excess tissue."
    b. "The lining of the uterus will be permanently destroyed in order to stop the bleeding."
    c. "A lighted instrument will be inserted through the vagina to visualize the pelvic cavity."
    d. "The uterus, ovaries, and fallopian tubes will be examined when the cervix is dilated."

12. Which of the following statements by a client following a D and C indicates that discharge teaching has been successful?
    a. "I will call the physician if my next period is delayed."
    b. "Intercourse may decrease postoperative pain."
    c. "I will count the number of tampons I use immediately postoperative."
    d. "I should rest for a few days and avoid straining."

13. The nurse is providing discharge teaching to a client who is going home after an abdominal hysterectomy. Which statement indicates a need for further teaching?
    a. "I should report urinary incontinence or urgency."
    b. "I should report worsening pain."
    c. "Heavy menstrual-like bleeding is expected."
    d. "I should report a temperature over 100F."

▪ ▪ ▪   The Client with Menopausal Manifestations

14. Which of the following clinical symptoms is consistent with menopause?
    a. vaginal pH decreases
    b. vaginal lubrication increases
    c. menstrual cycles become erratic
    d. vaginal rugae increase in number

15. Name three health risks that increase after menopause.
    (a) _____
    (b) _____
    (c) _____

16. A client has been prescribed Estrace (oral estradiol). Which statement indicates an understanding of teaching regarding this medication?
    a. "I should have a mammogram after I start taking this medication."
    b. "I should have a mammogram before I start taking this medication."
    c. "This medication has no side effects."
    d. "I should take this medication only when I have menopausal symptoms."

17. List five self-care strategies for managing hot flashes.
    (a) _____
    (b) _____
    (c) _____
    (d) _____
    (e) _____

Read the following statements and determine if they are true or false. Correct any false statements.

_____ 18. Hot flashes are a result of vasomotor instability.

_____ 19. During menopause, estrogen levels decrease, follicle-stimulating hormone (FSH) levels fall, luteinizing hormone (LH) levels rise and then fall.

_____ 20. The primary purpose of hormone replacement therapy (HRT) is to manage symptoms of menopause.

_____ 21. A contraindication of hormone replacement therapy is a history of breast, ovarian, or cervical cancer.

22. List three long-term benefits of hormone replacement therapy.
    (a) _____
    (b) _____
    (c) _____

23. Which statement by a menopausal client on hormone replacement therapy indicates a need for further teaching?
    a. "Now I do not have to worry about my calcium intake."
    b. "I need 1000 mg of calcium a day."
    c. "I should do some type of weight-bearing exercise on a regular basis."
    d. "HRT can reduce my risks for fracture."

24. Which statement by a menopausal client indicates an understanding of teaching regarding altered sexuality patterns?
    a. "Vaginal lubrication can not be helped without HRT."
    b. "Most older adults stop having intercourse and find new ways to express intimacy."
    c. "Water-soluble gels can prevent vaginal irritation."
    d. "It is hard for women to maintain their interest in sex after menopause."

▪ ▪ ▪   The Client with Structural Disorders of the Female Reproductive System

25. Identify the three most common structural disorders of the female reproductive system.

(a) _____   (c) _____

(b) _____

26. The diagnosis of uterine displacement is usually made after:

a. pelvic ultrasonography.
b. laparoscopy exam.
c. physical exam.
d. pelvic x-ray exam.

27. List five teaching topics for the client with early stages of downward displacement of the uterus as it relates to stress incontinence.

(a) _____

(b) _____

(c) _____

(d) _____

(e) _____

Read the following statements and determine if they are true or false. Correct any false statements.

_____ 28. In procidentia, one would observe the uterus in the vagina.

_____ 29. Kegel exercises may assist a woman to strengthen her perineal muscles and minimize urine leakage.

Match the following descriptions (30–34) with the correct terms (a–f).

_____ 30. Herniation of the bladder into the vagina.

_____ 31. Flexing or bending of the uterine corpus in a backward manner toward the rectum.

_____ 32. A surgical procedure to shorten the pelvic muscles.

_____ 33. An opening between the urinary bladder and the vagina.

_____ 34. A device that provides temporary support for the uterus or bladder.

a. pessary
b. vescovaginal fistula
c. retroversion
d. retroflexion
e. cystocele
f. colporrhaphy

▪ ▪ ▪   The Client with Disorders of Female Reproductive Tissue

Read the statements below and determine if they are true or false. Correct any false statements.

_____ 35. Myomectomy is the treatment of choice for young women with fibroid tumors who wish to retain their reproductive capability.

_____ 36. Risk factors for the development of endometriosis include multiparity.

_____ 37. Endometriosis is an infectious process in the uterus.

_____ 38. The Papanicolaou smear is the primary screening tool for cervical cancer.

_____ 39. The recommended frequency of Papanicolaou screening is yearly until after the age of 65.

40. Risk factors for endometrial cancer suggest an increased risk with increased exposure to _____
_____.

41. Target areas of metastasis for endometrial cancer are (a) _____, (b) _____, and (c) _____.

42. A definitive diagnosis of endometrial cancer can be made after (a) _____ or (b) _____.

43. The treatment of choice for primary endometrial carcinoma is _____.

44. Which of the following diagnostic tests is useful in detecting ovarian cancer?
    a. "wet prep" with potassium hydroxide
    b. culture of vaginal secretions
    c. CA 125 antigen level
    d. complete blood count

45. A 78-year-old female tells the nurse at her senior center that she is experiencing abdominal bloating and constipation. The most appropriate response by the nurse is:
    a. "These symptoms may occur because your gastrointestinal tract slows down as you age."
    b. "Increase the amount of fiber and fluids in your diet."
    c. "You should see your physician for a pelvic examination."
    d. "Don't worry; many older women experience these symptoms."

46. Ovarian cancer is almost always asymptomatic. What percent of those diagnosed with this disease do not have local disease at the time of diagnosis? _____

47. The nurse is providing discharge teaching to a client who just underwent a vulvectomy. Which statement by the client indicates a need for further teaching?
    a. "I should wear support hose and elevate my legs regularly."
    b. "I should irrigate the vulvectomy wound as directed."
    c. "I should eat a diet high in protein, iron, and vitamin C."
    d. "I should use a 75-watt light bulb to provide dry heat to my perineum."

48. List at least four risk factors for cervial cancer.

49. Which statement by a client following a cervical biopsy indicates a need for further teaching?
    a. "I should expect minor bleeding."
    b. "I can not have intercourse for 14 days."
    c. "I should report heavy bleeding."
    d. "I should avoid tampons."

50. Ovarian cancer is often diagnosed when the prognosis is poor. What is the major reason for delayed diagnosis?

▪ ▪ ▪ The Client with Infections of the Female Reproductive System

Match the terms for different types of vaginal infections (a–d) with the correct statements listed in questions 51–54.

_____ 51. usually caused by a protozoan infection carried asymptomatically by the male partner

_____ 52. may be treated with topical estrogen cream and water-soluble lubricants

_____ 53. indicated by the presence of "clue cells" on microscopic examination of vaginal secretions

_____ 54. clinical manifestations include thick white patches that adhere to the cervix and vaginal walls

a. candidiasis
b. simple vaginitis
c. trichomoniasis
d. senile vaginitis

55. List three strategies that provide protection against vaginal infections.
    (a) _____
    (b) _____
    (c) _____

56. The client with repeated infections of the reproductive system should be assessed for:
    a. diabetes   b. endometriosis   c. dysmenorrhea   d. rectovaginal fistula

Read the statements below about pelvic inflammatory disease (PID) and determine if they are true or false. Correct any false statements.

_____ 57. PID has little or no effect on fertility.

_____ 58. PID is usually polymicrobial in origin.

_____ 59. PID is most common in postmenopausal women.

_____ 60. Typical treatment of PID involves anti-inflammatory drugs and analgesics.

61. Which of the following statements indicates that a client needs further teaching about toxic shock syndrome (TSS)?
    a. "I wash my hands before inserting my tampons."
    b. "I don't use my diaphragm during my menstrual period."
    c. "I always use the highest absorbency tampons to meet my menstrual needs."
    d. "Early symptoms of TSS can resemble the flu."

▪ ▪ ▪ The Client with Disorders of Sexual Expression

62. List two commonly held stereotypes held by society about female sexual function and aging.
    (a) _____
    (b) _____

63. When interviewing a client experiencing inhibited sexual desire, the nurse should:
    a. ensure that the interview can be conducted in private.
    b. involve the client's partner in all levels of the assessment.
    c. explain that loss of desire is a normal part of the aging process.
    d. defer any uncomfortable questions to the physician.

Read the following statements and determine if they are true or false. Correct any false statements.

_____ 64. Loss of sexual function is an expected change of aging.

_____ 65. The normal female sexual drive can persist until a woman is 80 or 90 years old.

▪ ▪ ▪ Critical Thinking Exercises

66. Develop a flow chart that would assist a female client in making decisions about the use of hormone replacement therapy.

67. A nurse is caring for a client in the immediate postoperative period following an abdominal hysterectomy. She has an indwelling Foley catheter. There is no observable urine output. What is the most appropriate action by the nurse? What is the probable cause for this problem?

▪ ▪ ▪ Additional Learning Experiences

- Identify community resources for women without health insurance to obtain health screenings such as Pap smears and mammograms.

- Visit the local pharmacy and familiarize yourself with the various feminine hygiene products that are available. Ask the pharmacist about over-the-counter medications to treat vaginal infections such as candidiasis.

- Attend a menopause support group and learn more about the experience from the women attending the session.

CHAPTER 48

Nursing Care of Clients with Breast Disorders

■ ■ ■ **Focused Study Tips**

- Discuss the risk factors and treatment options for breast cancer. Describe the emotional, psychologic, functional, and sexual significance of breast cancer and its treatments.

- Compare and contrast the meanings and implications of each stage of breast cancer.

- Describe the nursing care associated with the different types of tests performed to diagnose breast cancer.

- Review the client teaching required for the client receiving pharmacologic and radiation treatments for breast cancer.

- Explain the nursing care of the client with benign breast disease.

- Describe the appropriate technique for self-examination of the breasts.

■ ■ ■ **The Client with Breast Cancer**

Read the following statements and determine if they are true or false. Correct any false statements.

_____ 1. The mortality rate from breast cancer is higher in African American women than in European American women.

_____ 2. Family history has little or no impact on an individual's risk of developing breast cancer.

_____ 3. The majority of carcinomas of the breast occur in the lobular areas of the breast.

_____ 4. Breast cancer is usually painless.

_____ 5. Most types of breast cancer are detected during routine mammography.

6. Explain the difference between invasive and noninvasive carcinomas of the breast.

7. The two most significant risk factors for breast cancer are (a) _____ and (b) _____.

8. Paget's carcinoma of the breast involves infiltration of the _____.

9. Breast cancer can metastasize to other sites through the (a) _____ or (b) _____.

Match the terms used to classify invasive types of breast cancer (a–e) with the descriptions listed in questions 10–14.

_____ 10. slow growing and bulky; may have sharp edges and be confused with fibroadenoma

_____ 11. relatively uncommon; characterized by thickened, ill-defined areas of the breast

_____ 12. characterized by a stony hardness of the breast and metastasis to axillary lymph nodes

_____ 13. often called a "well-differentiated" cancer

_____ 14. usually well-circumscribed, small tumors; may be mistaken for a cyst

a. infiltrating ductal carcinoma
b. tubular carcinoma
c. medullary carcinoma
d. mucinous carcinoma
e. infiltrating lobular carcinoma

15. Describe the three characteristics that determine the staging of breast cancer.
    (a) _____
    (b) _____
    (c) _____

16. In which of the following stages of breast cancer would the findings include distant metastasis?
    a. stage I   b. stage II   c. stage III   d. stage IV

17. List the three recommended screenings for breast cancer.
    (a) _____
    (b) _____
    (c) _____

18. When implementing educational programs aimed at increasing compliance with breast cancer screening, it is important for the nurse to remember that:
    a. content should be culturally sensitive to the intended audience.
    b. the effectiveness of breast cancer screening in reducing breast cancer deaths has not been documented.
    c. breast self-exam should be performed monthly by all women over 40 years old.
    d. media campaigns about breast cancer screening have reached a wide and diverse audience.

19. List the four positions in which a female client should inspect her breasts when conducting breast self-exam.
    (a) _____
    (b) _____
    (c) _____
    (d) _____

20. When palpating the breasts during breast self-exam, the nurse should teach the client to:
    a. divide the breast into quadrants and palpate one quadrant at a time.
    b. avoid compressing the nipple and areolar regions.
    c. palpate all areas of the breast using concentric circles.
    d. palpate the breast from the nipple outward.

Match the following tests used to detect breast cancer (a–e) with their correct descriptions listed in questions 21–25.

_____ 21. A large piece of tissue from the breast lesion is surgically removed for histologic exam.

_____ 22. The client is injected with radioactive glucose molecules which are then absorbed by the cancer tissue.

_____ 23. This test produces a low-dose radiographic image of palpable breast lesions.

_____ 24. Faster, less painful, and more cost-efficient, this procedure removes a core of breast lesion tissue for histologic exam.

_____ 25. A fine needle is used to remove cells or fluid from a breast lesion.

a. diagnostic mammography
b. positive emission tomography (PET)
c. aspiration biopsy
d. incisional biopsy
e. stereotactic biopsy

26. The term "breast conservation treatment" refers to therapies that include (a) _____ _____ and (b) _____.

27. A 67-year-old client with breast cancer tells the nurse, "The doctor says she has good news about my hormone receptor assay." The nurse knows that this means the test results were:
   a. progesterone-receptor negative.
   b. estrogen-receptor negative.
   c. progesterone-receptor positive.
   d. estrogen-receptor positive.

28. Following a mastectomy, a client asks why she needs chemotherapy. The most appropriate response by the nurse is:
   a. "You will have to ask your doctor."
   b. "Breast cancer is a systemic disease."
   c. "Chemotherapy is part of the standard therapy."
   d. "Chemotherapy will eliminate the risks of metastasis."

29. A client is diagnosed with stage IV breast cancer with metastasis to her spine and hip. The radiologist schedules her for radiation therapy. The purpose of radiation therapy in this situation is to:
   a. control pain and prevent fractures.
   b. shrink the tumor prior to surgery.
   c. destroy cancer cells present in those areas.
   d. prepare the spine and hip for surgery.

30. To decrease the risk of a fibrous capsule forming around a breast reconstruction implant, it is important to teach the client to:
   a. discontinue the use of powders and lotions on the breast.
   b. wear a loose-fitting bra for the first 2 weeks.
   c. avoid abduction and external rotation exercises of the upper extremities.
   d. perform breast massage as instructed.

31. Which of the following statements indicates that the client taking tamoxifen (Nolvadex) needs further teaching?
    a. "While taking this drug, I will use a barrier form of contraception."
    b. "I will make an appointment for my annual endometrial biopsy."
    c. "Weight loss is a common side effect of this drug."
    d. "I will call my health provider if I have any leg pain."

32. While caring for the client who has just undergone a radical mastectomy, the nurse should:
    a. use the nonsurgical side when obtaining blood pressure readings.
    b. elevate the affected arm above the level of the shoulder to prevent lymphedema.
    c. assist the client to perform abduction exercises to prevent muscle atrophy.
    d. place the client surgical side down to facilitate drainage.

33. A client is being discharged following a modified radical mastectomy. Which statement by the client would indicate a need for further teaching?
    a. "I should wear gloves when I work in the garden."
    b. "I may experience feelings of numbness or tingling in my axillary area."
    c. "When my incision is healed, I can start carrying in the groceries."
    d. "I may experience feelings of loss, anxiety, or fear after discharge."

34. When giving advice regarding exercise to a client who just underwent a mastectomy and has a wound drain in place, the most appropriate statement by the nurse is:
    a. "Hold your arm still to prevent an increase in drainage."
    b. "Do not abduct the arm or raise the elbow above shoulder height."
    c. "Gradually increase your activity to tolerance."
    d. "You can do anything that does not cause pain or discomfort."

35. The nurse is caring for an 80-year-old woman with breast cancer. Based on research findings, the nurse plans care with an awareness that older women with breast cancer have:
    a. more emotional and physical distress than younger women.
    b. less emotional distress than younger women.
    c. needs equivalent to younger women for personal services and home care.
    d. higher pain thresholds and are less likely to complain of pain.

▪ ▪ ▪ **The Client with Gynecomastia or Male Breast Cancer**

Read the following statements and determine if they are true or false. Correct any false statements.

_____ 36. Lobular cancer is the most common type of breast cancer found in males.

_____ 37. Male breast cancer accounts for 1% of all breast cancers.

_____ 38. Most male breast cancer tumors are estrogen-receptor positive.

_____ 39. Males with breast cancer do well with adjunct tamoxifen (Nolvadex) therapy.

▪ ▪ ▪ The Client with Fibrocystic Breast Changes or Benign Disorders of the Breast

40. Fibrocystic breast changes are benign changes in the female breast that are thought to be due to
    (a) _____ and (b) _____.

41. Which of the following dietary modifications might be helpful for a woman with fibrocystic breast changes?
    a. increasing dietary fiber
    b. increasing amount of saturated fats
    c. eliminating food and drinks containing caffeine
    d. avoiding foods with high amounts of vitamin E

Match the types of benign breast disorders (a–e) with the correct descriptions listed in questions 42–46.

_____ 42. chronic or acute inflammation of the breast

_____ 43. an abnormal enlargement of the male breast

_____ 44. a wart-like growth on the peripheral mammary duct

_____ 45. an overgrowth of connective tissue that results in mobile, firm, nontender lumps

_____ 46. a palpable lumpiness found beneath the areola in perimenopausal women

a. fibroadenoma
b. intraductal papilloma
c. duct ectasia
d. mastitis
e. gynecomastia

▪ ▪ ▪ Critical Thinking Exercises

47. A nurse's good friend has just been diagnosed with breast cancer. She has no known risk factors for breast cancer. She is unsure how to decide on the various treatment options. How might the nurse support her in the decision-making process?

48. Develop a class for teenage women to learn about breast self-examination and their risks for breast cancer as well as prevention strategies.

▪ ▪ ▪ Additional Learning Experiences

▪ Attend a breast cancer support group and listen to the content of the discussion. If the group is willing, encourage participants to discuss ways that nurses can better assist women with breast cancer.

▪ Interview a woman who has experienced breast cancer and one or more therapies. Encourage her to verbalize about the diagnostic evaluation, the various treatments, and its physiologic and psychologic impact.

CHAPTER 49

Nursing Care of Clients with Sexually Transmitted Diseases

■ ■ ■ **Focused Study Tips**

- Compare the infecting organism, incubation period, and clinical presentation for each sexually transmitted disease.

- Describe client education related to safe sex, compliance with treatment regimens, and the evaluation and treatment of partners.

■ ■ ■ **Overview**

1. List three factors that explain the escalating incidence of STDs.
   (a) _____
   (b) _____
   (c) _____

2. Name the two population groups that the Centers for Disease Control has identified as having the highest incidence of sexually transmitted disease.
   (a) _____
   (b) _____

3. The spread of sexually transmitted disease can be controlled through:
   a. the early use of antibiotics.
   b. the use of latex condoms.
   c. the use of oral contraceptives.
   d. routine screening.

4. Two-thirds of STDs occur in people under age _____.

5. HIV/AIDS, the five classic STDs, and viral hepatitis must be reported to _____
   _____.

■ ■ ■ **The Client with STDs Producing Ulcers or Chancres**

6. List three modes of transmission of *Treponema pallidum*.
   (a) _____   (c) _____
   (b) _____

7. A 17-year-old client sees the school nurse because he suspects that he has been infected with the syphilis spirochete (*Treponema pallidum*). Which of the following clinical manifestations would the nurse expect the client to have?
   a. pelvic pain   b. dysuria   c. genital chancre   d. urethral discharge

8. The laboratory test that is specific for *T. pallidum* is:
   a. VDRL.
   b. FTA-ABS.
   c. RPR.
   d. urine culture and sensitivity.

9. The treatment of choice for primary syphilis is:
   a. amoxicillin.
   b. erythromycin.
   c. benzathine penicillin G.
   d. ceftriaxone.

10. Education is an important part of the nursing care for the client with an STD. List five points the nurse should include in discharge teaching for the client with syphillis.
    (a) _____
    (b) _____
    (c) _____
    (d) _____
    (e) _____

■ ■ ■ The Client with Genital Herpes

11. Prodromal symptoms of genital herpes include:
    a. vaginal or urethral discharge.
    b. headache, fever, and malaise.
    c. urinary frequency and urgency.
    d. burning, itching, and tingling at the site.

12. Which of the following findings would be most characteristic of genital herpes?
    a. macular lesion of the face and trunk
    b. genital chancres
    c. purulent discharge
    d. painful papules below the trunk

13. The client with genital herpes would be prescribed:
    a. antibiotics.
    b. antihistamines.
    c. anti-inflammatories.
    d. antivirals.

14. When teaching a client with genital herpes about perineal care, the nurse should instruct the client to use Burrow's solution or a solution of warm (a) _____, (b) _____, and (c) _____.

15. List the two complications that women of childbearing age with genital herpes may experience.
    (a) _____
    (b) _____

■ ■ ■ The Client with STDs Primarily Infecting Epithelial Surfaces

16. Clinical findings in a male client with gonorrhea would reveal:
    a. painful vesicles.
    b. milky, purulent discharge.
    c. maculopapular rash.
    d. hematuria.

17. To prevent the spread of gonorrhea, infected clients should be advised to:
    (a) _____
    (b) _____

Read the following statements and determine if they are true or false. Correct any false statements.

_____ 18. A positive culture is required before starting treatment for a woman with gonorrhea.

_____ 19. Clinical findings can guide the treatment of gonorrhea.

_____ 20. The treatment of choice for gonorrhea is oral doxycycline for 7 days.

_____ 21. Common symptoms of gonorrhea in women include dysuria, urinary frequency, or abnormal vaginal discharge.

■ ■ ■ The Client with a Chlamydial Infection

22. Which of the following statements is the most accurate about a chlamydia infection?
    a. Chlamydia is a virus.
    b. Chlamydia affects only women.
    c. Chlamydia causes no symptoms.
    d. The incubation period of chlamydia is 4–6 weeks.

23. List four possible complications of a chlamydia infection for a woman.
    (a) _____
    (b) _____
    (c) _____
    (d) _____

24. Which of the following facts is important for the female client with genital warts to know?
    a. She should have an annual Pap smear.
    b. Genital warts are always cancerous.
    c. She can never have children.
    d. The appearance of genital warts is always associated with HIV infection.

■ ■ ■ The Client with Genital Warts

Read the following statements and determine if they are true or false. Correct any false statements.

_____ 25. HPV is considered an acute, temporary problem.

_____ 26. The incubation period of HPV is approximately 7 days.

_____ 27. HPV is a reportable disease.

_____ 28. HPV is associated with a higher risk of vaginal, vulvar, penile, and anal cancers.

_____ 29. Most individuals know they have HPV as soon as it occurs.

_____ 30. An individual with HPV should have a VDRL and gonorrheal culture prior to treatment.

▪ ▪ ▪   Critical Thinking Exercises

31. Develop a community health program for young adults on the prevention and detection of sexually transmitted diseases.

32. The nurse is caring for a young adult who needs treatment for a sexually transmitted disease. The woman has limited financial resources and does not want to tell her parents that she has been sexually active. How might the nurse most effectively assist her?

▪ ▪ ▪   Additional Learning Experiences

- Identify community resources for individuals with sexually transmitted diseases.
- Contact the public health nurse in your community and learn more about the incidence of sexually transmitted diseases in your community.
- Contact the school nurses in your community and ask them about the resources they have to teach high school students about sexually transmitted diseases.

Answer Key

1. (a) adult, (b) human responses, (c–e) answers include: social, cultural, economic
2. Answers include: caregiver, educator, advocate, leader, manager, researcher
3. b. The role of nurse as a research-based scientist and educator may be relevant. The role of dependent practitioner has evolved in the last 40 years to one of independent and collaborative practitioner.
4. a. Interpersonal skills are crucial to teaching.
5. Answers may include: making referrals; identifying community and personal resources; arranging for necessary equipment and supplies for home care
6. (a) ethnocentrism, (b) prejudice
7. c. The primary focus of nursing care is the client.
8. d. The nurse acts as client advocate and supports the client's decisions.
9. (a) Quality assurance, (b) answers may include: hospital accreditation, licensure, and certification
10. a. Nursing research may be helpful for other reasons, but improving client care is the most important.
11. diagnosis   12. planning
13. assessment   14. evaluation
15. implementation
16. c   17. b   18. a   19. e   20. c   21. a
22. d   23. b   24. d   25. a   26. e   27. b
28. c
29. (a) Focused, (b) Initial
30. P = Problem, which is the NANDA diagnostic label; E = Etiology of the problem, which is indicated by the phrase "related to"; S = signs and symptoms, which are indicated by the phrase "as manifested by."
31. ethics   32. standard   33. dilemma
34. True. The nurse is morally obligated to provide care to the client with AIDS when all four of the criteria set by the ANA in 1986 are met.
35. c

36. The nurse must first establish that the client is competent.
37. True   38. True
39. False. The number of older adults has increased significantly in the 1990s.
40. True   41. d
42. b. Homelessness is defined, in part, as the condition experienced by an individual who lacks a fixed, regular, and adequate nighttime residence.
43. Answers include: ambulatory care, intensive care with rehabilitation
44. Answers may include: achieve realistic, expected client and family outcomes; promote professional and collaborative practice and care; ensure continuity of care; guarantee appropriate use of resources; reduce costs and length of stay; provide a framework for continuous improvement of care
45. Answers may include: program the administration rate of fluids; order supplies and services for clients; store and provide immediate access to the results of diagnostic tests; develop and implement client acuity classification systems used to predict staffing needs of nursing personnel; generate staffing schedules; provide continuing education programs; provide medication documentation records; document ongoing nursing assessments and care; develop nursing care plans
46. (a) health, (b) illness

■ ■ ■ Chapter 2

1. Answers include: physical, intellectual, spiritual
2. a   3. c   4. b   5. a   6. b
7. c   8. a   9. b   10. a   11. c
12. c   13. a   14. a   15. b
16. Answers include: health-related courses and seminars at colleges and universities, workplace programs, community programs
17. male

18. Answers may include: nails grow more slowly and may become thick and brittle, systolic blood pressure rises and cardiac output decreases, large and small intestines have some atrophy with decreased peristalsis (see page 34 of main text for additional answers)
19. Answers include: falls, fires, motor vehicle accidents
20. b. Diet should be low in fat; dental and vision exam should be done annually; exercise should be in moderation.
21. d   22. d   23. a   24. d
25. c   26. c   27. d   28. d
29. a. The definition of family changes as society changes.
30. Answers include: high cholesterol diet, overweight, hypertension, smoking, alcohol abuse, physical inactivity, negative health habits, exposure to environment, depression
31. c
32. Answers may include: behavior problems, speech and vision problems, learning disabilities, physical abuse, obesity, underweight
33. wellness
34. health
35. Answers may include: genetic makeup, cognitive ability, educational level, ethnicity, cultural background, age, gender, developmental level (refer to text for examples)
36. (a) preventive, (b) community
37. b   38. c   39. c   40. a   41. b   42. a
43. *Healthy People 2000*
44. (a) nursing, (b) medicine
45. acute illness
46. c   47. a   48. d   49. b   50. e
51. d. The client must adjust to changes in the course of the disease.
52. d
53. rehabilitation
54. Answers may include: implementing an individualized teaching plan with emphasis on home care, developing an exercise plan with the client, teaching the client how to prevent complications such as injury and skin breakdown, teaching the client about the disease process, providing care as necessary, promoting independence
55. c
56. Answers may include: functional level and self-care abilities, educational needs, psychosocial needs, the home environment,

client and family goals, concerns of the client and family, stage of grief and loss, educational levels, learning style, availability of resources
57. Answers include: preventing complications, providing care as necessary and appropriate, implementing individualized teaching plans, providing information about the disease process or disability and about health promotion and health maintenance activities

■ ■ ■ **Chapter 3**

1. a. individual   b. family
2. (a) promoting (b) maintaining (c) restoring (d) maximizing the level of independence
3. DRGs   4. c   5. a
6. c. Legal and reimbursement agencies require a physician-approved treatment plan prior to initiation of home health care.
7. b
8. referral source
9. Answers include: licensing, certification, accreditation
10. a. Medicare   b. out-of-pocket funds
11. a   12. d
13. Items (b) and (c) are the only reimbursable services. Items (a) and (d) are health maintenance visits, and items (e) and (f) are emotional and economic problems—none of which are reimbursable.
14. c
15. Answers may include: nursing process, interdisciplinary collaboration, quality assurance, professional development, research
16. National Association for Home Care Bill of Rights
17. a
18. False. It is a nursing intervention to initiate a client referral.
19. Answers include: establish trust and rapport, set mutual goals and boundaries, promote learning, assess home environment, prioritize
20. (a) draw up, (b) store, (c) inject
21. Answers may include: talking the client through learning tasks, encouraging the client to listen to their own bodies and to ask questions, urging the client to write down questions or concerns and bring them up at the next visit or doctor's appointment

22. Answers may include: signs of abusive behavior, electrical hazards, absence of smoke detectors, slippery throw rugs, supply of expired medications, inappropriate clothing, chipping paint
23. health teaching
24. Answers may include: effective hand washing, the use of gloves when appropriate, proper disposal of wastes and soiled dressings, proper handling of linens, and the practice of universal precautions
25. (a) personal friend, (b) financial advisor, (c) psychologist
26. (b) Within the home setting, ignoring an unsafe environment is considered nursing negligence. Documentation should address the information the nurse has covered, the client's and family's response to the teaching, and assessment of their ongoing practice of safety precautions.
27. (a) Experts suggest that the greatest level of success is achieved when the client feels ownership of the plan. It is essential to set mutually acceptable goals.
28. cooperative working agreement between the nurse and client
29. (a) Formative, (b) summative
30. Answers may include: increased client comfort, lower financial costs
31. c   32. c
33. Answers may include: acute, chronic, hospice

▪ ▪ ▪ Chapter 4

1. b. Pain can be experienced only by the person affected and has a very personal meaning. Pain is not always an indicator of tissue damage. Therapies such as nutritional counseling, biofeedback, and massage are examples of ways other than pharmacologically that effective pain relief can be achieved.
2. b   3. f   4. c   5. e
6. d   7. a   8. c
9. d. The most clearly defined chemical inhibitory mechanism is fueled by endorphins.
10. d
11. pattern theory
12. specificity theory

13. gate-control theory
14. c   15. b   16. a
17. b. The other statements are incorrect. Acute pain is localized, has an identifiable course, and lasts for less than six months.
18. c. Recurrent acute pain is characterized by relatively well-defined episodes of pain interspersed with pain-free episodes.
19. d. Psychogenic pain is pain that is experienced in the absence of any diagnosed physiologic cause or event.
20. lower back pain.
21. c   22. a   23. b   24. d
25. phantom pain
26. False. There is complete mental awareness that the limb is gone. The client does experience pain in the missing body part, which is thought to be due to stimulation of the severed nerves at the site of the amputation. Treatment is complex and often unsuccessful.
27. Answers may include: age, sociocultural influences, emotional status, past experiences, the meaning associated with the pain, the knowledge level of the client, the source of pain
28. (a) threshold, (b) tolerance
29. The client could receive a more serious injury.
30. (a) serotonin, (b) pain sensations
31. b. Answers (a), (c), and (d) are myths.
32. a
33. tolerance
34. drug abuse
35. physical drug dependence
36. c. NSAIDs may increase the hypoglycemic effect.
37. a. Administer oral hypoglycemic agents with meals, milk, or a full glass of water to decrease gastric irritation.
38. Answers may include: guaiac all stools, since NSAIDs may cause gastrointestinal bleeding; share with Ms. Avery the importance of avoiding alcohol; advise Ms. Avery to take the medication with food to decrease gastric irritation.
39. True   40. True
41. True. Naloxone should be immediately available, as morphine sulfate can cause respiratory depression.
42. True
43. equianalgesic dosage chart

44. c   45. e   46. a   47. b   48. d

49. d. With PCAs there is a potential for infection and cost for disposable supplies. PCAs may or may not save nursing time.

50. Answers include: develop a more hopeful attitude that pain relief is possible, allow local procedures to be performed without causing discomfort, exercise and move the affected part.

51. c. A TENS unit consists of a low-voltage transmitter connected by wires to electrodes that are placed by the client as directed by the physical therapist. The client experiences a gentle tapping or vibrating sensation over the electrodes.

52. a. Relaxation helps the client avoid the anxiety that often accompanies and complicates pain.

53. assist the client to achieve optimal control of the pain

54. pain behaviors

55. b. The most reliable indicator of the presence and degree of pain is the client's own statement about the pain.

56. Answers include: relaxation, distraction, cutaneous stimulation

57. The use of the imaginative power of the mind to create a scene or sensory experience that relaxes the muscles and moves the attention of the mind away from the pain experience.

58. Answers may include: the redirection of the client's attention away from the pain and onto something that the client finds more pleasant, listening to music, any rhythmic activity to music (such as singing and tapping), viewing a comedy, reading a joke book

59. Answers may include: touch, massage, heat, cold, therapeutic touch, vibration

60. a. Noninvasive methods of pain management are useful when used in conjunction with pain medications. The use of narcotics to treat severe pain is unlikely to cause addiction.

61. b. Both these techniques may initiate gate closure. Heat is best for localized pain.

62. c. These complaints are consistent with a chronic pain experience.

63. d. Grimacing and guarding are observed in acute pain. The other findings are consistent with chronic pain.

■ ■ ■ **Chapter 5**

1. (a) homeostasis, (b–e) answers include: volume, composition, distribution, pH

2. (a) 60, (b–c) answers include: intracellular, extracellular

3. body fat

4. (a) an elderly client, (b) an obese client, (c) a female client

5. c   6. c   7. b   8. a   9. b

10. c   11. a   12. d   13. e   14. f

15. a   16. b   17. c   18. b   19. a

20. a   21. c   22. a   23. c   24. a

25. b   26. c   27. a

28. (a) low, (b) high, (c) high

29. b   30. b   31. b   32. c

33. Monitor intake and output for the last 24 hours; assess weight, skin turgor, and oral mucous membranes; and assess vital signs, especially for tachycardia

34. (a) low, (b) low/borderline, (c) normal, (d) normal, (e) normal

35. An increase in pulse of more than 15 bpm and a decrease in BP of 15 mm Hg with position change equals orthostatic hypotension and is an indicator of hypovolemia.

36. side rails up, assist to bathroom

37. IV site must be patent; ensure correct solution and correct rate; assess for fluid overload

38. Discharge teaching would include: drink clear liquids to DAT and force fluids; administration instructions for the prescription compazine; provide client with a stool container and instructions regarding how to collect the stool for the lab

39. In the older client, fluids would be given slowly; lab results could be different because the older client is more susceptible to fluid loss and inefficient kidneys; vital signs may not return to within normal limits as quickly; the older client may need to be admitted.

40. c   41. a   42. d   43. b

44. place client in high Fowler's, turn IV to keep vein open rate, administer oxygen, have someone stay with client, notify physician

45. (a) diuretic to excrete extra fluid, (b) determine the amount of extra fluid in the lungs, (c) determine amount of urine output and assess level of fluid balance, (d) increased BP and bounding pulses indicate hypervolemia,

(e) to avoid excess fluid intake, (f) determine status after receiving Lasix (furosemide), (g) increase indicates fluid retention

46. Take the diuretic in the morning; monitor for sudden weight gain or loss; eat bananas or drink orange juice when taking Lasix (furosemide); never double doses; continue taking Lasix even when feeling well; report dizziness, trouble breathing, and swelling of hands and feet; elevate lower extremities

47. Answers include: potassium, phosphorus

48. Answers include: sodium, chloride

49. (a) 136, (b) 148

50. Answers include: kidneys, gastrointestinal tract, skin

51. c   52. a

53. (a) anorexia, nausea, vomiting, abdominal cramping, diarrhea; (b) headache, depression, dulled sensorium, personality changes, irritability, lethargy, hyperreflexia, muscle twitching, tremors, convulsions, coma

54. c   55. a   56. d

57. Answers may include: obtain baseline neurologic data as well as ongoing assessments, maintain a quiet environment, institute safety precautions, monitor and maintain fluid replacement, provide orientation

58. True   59. True

60. False. Salt substitutes may contain high levels of potassium and should be used sparingly.

61. True

62. False. The preference for salt will eventually diminish.

63. (a) 3.5, (b) 5.0   64. b

65. (a) hypokalemia/many drugs such as penicillin promote potassium loss; (b) hypokalemia/there is insufficient dietary potassium intake with continued renal excretion, and laxative abuse is possible; (c) hyperkalemia/the client is taking a potassium-sparing diuretic; (d) hypokalemia/diarrhea is a potassium-rich solution; (e) hyperkalemia/acidosis moves potassium out of the serum

66. b

67. b. Reporting the potassium level and collaborating about the medication are the only appropriate nursing actions.

68. a

69. Do not give the medication as ordered, and inform the physician of the findings.

70. 37.5 drops in one minute

71. check the IV for infiltration; inform the client that the IV medication may be irritating to the vein; discuss with the physician the possibility of slowing the infusion rate

72. c

73. Take medication as prescribed, dilute or dissolve in fruit or vegetable juice; chill

74. generalized muscle weakness, leg cramps, nausea or vomiting, paresthesias, irregular weak pulse, decreased BP

75. (a) cardiac, (b) EKG

76. b

77. Aldactone (spironolactone) is a potassium-sparing diuretic; the potassium supplement increased the client's serum potassium; most salt substitutes contain potassium.

78. Kayexalate (sodium polystyrene sulfonate) exchanges sodium or calcium for potassium in the gastrointestinal tract and promotes bowel removal of the potassium-containing resin.

79. bananas, lowfat yogurt, tuna, broccoli, orange juice, turkey, beef

80. b

81. (a) 8.8, (b) 10

82. c   83. b   84. d   85. a   86. b

87. (a) deep bone pain, flank pain indicative of renal calculi; (b) anorexia, nausea, abdominal pain; (c) vomiting and constipation, (d) behavioral changes: irritability, depression, confusion

88. (a–b) answers include: sodium phosphate, potassium phosphate, (c–d) answers include: 0.45% normal saline, normal saline, (e–g) answers include: diuretics, intravenous plicamycin, cortisone

89. b

90. (a) 2.5, (b) 4.5

91. phosphorus levels drop during alcohol withdrawal

92. c   93. a   94. c

95. The cellular release of phosphorus occurs following cellular destruction.

96. b

97. (a) 1.3, (b) 2.1

98. a   99. b   100. d   101. d   102. b

103. c   104. c   105. a   106. b

107. (a) 7.35   (b) 7.45

108. (a) 35   (b) 45

109. a   110. b   111. c   112. b   113. a

114. (a) high, (b) excess, (c) low

115. (a) low, (b) deficit, (c) high
116. hypotension, tachycardia, confusion, decreasing levels of consciousness, hyper-reflexia, tetany, dysrhythmias, seizures, and respiratory failure
117. protect the client from injury: side rails up, padded side rails, bed in low position, room close to nursing station, frequent checks
118. (a) greater than, (b) less than
119. hyperventilation associated with anxiety
120. Answers include: administering prescribed sedation or tranquilizers; administering oxygen as needed; maintaining safety, providing support, reassurance and assisting with definitive therapy; instructing client to breathe into a paper bag to rebreathe carbon dioxide; monitoring laboratory and diagnostic tests; providing support and reassurance; assisting with definitive therapy
121. b. Oxygen should be administered with extreme caution to the client with chronic respiratory acidosis.
122. a 123. a 124. b 125. a 126. b

■ ■ ■ **Chapter 6**

1. a systemic imbalance between oxygen supply and demand
2. c   3. b
4. Answers include: heart rate, respiratory rate, systemic vascular resistance
5. a. An increase in cardiac output raises the BP and allows for more efficient delivery of oxygen to the tissues. It does not affect the serum potassium level, respiratory rate, or heart rate.
6. b. There are shock states that are not due to blood loss and not all shock results in death.
7. a sustained drop in MAP (mean arterial pressure)
8. b. The client may have no symptoms in the initial stages. The other symptoms listed are found in the compensatory, progressive and irreversible stages of shock.
9. d. The other answers can be eliminated because peripheral pulses are decreased in the progressive stage of shock and heart sounds are generally not used as an indicator of shock. The respiratory rate changes

(increase) are due to a beta two response in the compensatory stage of shock. The level of consciousness changes in the progressive or irreversible stage of shock.
10. b. By definition, HR (heart rate) × SV (stroke volume) = CO (cardiac output). When a decrease in CO (such as in blood loss, which decreases the stroke volume) is sensed, the body attempts to compensate and balance this formula by increasing the HR.
11. d
12. b. Water and sodium retention are a renal response for regulating fluid volume. The other answers refer to systems other than renal.
13. Answers include: sodium potassium pump fails, cells absorb water and are damaged, cells switch from aerobic to anaerobic metabolism
14. a. In the progressive stage of shock, the sodium-potassium pump fails; there is cellular anoxia leading to acidosis; and plasma proteins diffuse out of the vascular space, decreasing renal blood flow, which results in oliguria.
15. e. An MI is the most common cause of cardiogenic shock.
16. e. Histamine release and vasodilation in response to an antigen may cause anaphylactic shock.
17. d or a. Major burns have tremendous fluid losses initially and may present with hypovolemic shock. Septic shock may occur later in the hospitalization due to infected wounds.
18. b. A cervical spine injury can cause neurogenic shock as a result of an imbalance between parasympathetic and sympathetic responses. These responses can cause severe vasodilation.
19. a. A bowel obstruction can cause the pooling of several liters of fluid in the abdomen, and the client may present with hypovolemia.
20. a. Due to blood loss and therefore loss of circulating volume.
21. b. Insulin reactions cause hypoglycemia, which decreases glucose to the medulla.
22. d. Immunocompromised clients (such as those receiving chemotherapy drugs, the client with leukemia, and others) do not

have the immune response to destroy pathogens.

23. e. Histamine release and vasodilation in response to an antigen may cause anaphylactic shock.

24. a. An arterial bleed will cause rapid loss of blood and decreased circulating volume.

25. d. Urinary retention is not an issue since Mr. Conor has a Foley catheter. His low urine output would rule out fluid volume excess. Septic shock is the most likely problem; the findings are not consistent with hypovolemic shock.

26. Answers include: age, postprocedure (cystoscopy), or indwelling Foley catheter.

27. c. Answers (b) and (d) generally refer to hypovolemic shock, which is not Mr. Conor's problem. The nurse does need to measure and record urine output, but monitoring cardiovascular function is a first priority.

28. a. Decreased cerebral perfusion may cause a change in mental status, but there is no evidence to support this. A low urine output or fatigue should not alter mental status.

29. d. This solution is not appropriate because it is a hypotonic solution and will cause water to enter the cells. The goal in shock is to increase volume in the vascular system so that isotonic solutions such as lactated Ringer's or NS will stay in the intravascular system and raise blood pressure. Albumin is also a volume expander.

30. c. Answers (a), (b), and (d) are interventions for some types of shock but may be inappropriate for other types. Oxygen therapy increases the amount of available oxygen to the client.

31. a. Hemoglobin and hematocrit (H&H) are values related to the total amount of fluid in plasma. Therefore, a decreased H&H may indicate fluid volume overload, and an increased H&H may indicate fluid volume deficit.

32. c. Antibiotics would treat the underlying cause of septic shock.

33. b. Assessing the client's vital signs will give an indication of his cardiovascular status. Auscultating breath sounds is appropriate, but not for the first action. Trendelenberg is not a current intervention in shock, but rather, ele-

vating the legs 20 degrees. Administration of pain medications is inappropriate without knowledge of the client's BP.

34. b. An isotonic solution would raise his blood pressure because it stays in the intravascular space. Option (c) is incorrect because a hypertonic solution would draw fluid out of the cell. Option (a) is incorrect because although the physician should be notified, the RN needs to intervene with the client in shock immediately.

35. d. 20–30 mL urine output indicates an adequate renal blood flow. Less than this may indicate renal ischemia.

36. c. This is the accepted first aid intervention for obvious bleeding. Options (a) and (d) may be ineffective in controlling the bleeding and (b) a tourniquet may cause tissue necrosis.

37. b. This is the correct position to increase flow to essential organs in blood loss. It may also help to prevent loss of consciousness (LOC). Answer (a) is incorrect because the client may have a LOC and aspirate. She may also need to go to the operating room when she arrives at a hospital. Pillows under the knees reduce the venous return.

38. Answers include: relieve the client's pain, provide supplemental oxygen, administer vasodilating medications.

39. a. The client needs to be very closely monitored, and vital signs should be frequently assessed. Options (b), (c), and (d) are all true relating to the administration of the drug. Infiltration of the drug can cause tissue necrosis.

40. d   41. b   42. c   43. a   44. c

45. Answers may include: speak slowly and calmly, using short sentences; allow visitors as appropriate; listen carefully to the client; use touch to provide support; assess the cause of anxiety; provide periods of rest; administer prescribed medications; provide interventions to increase comfort and reduce restlessness; support client and client's family; provide information to client and family (see pp. 180–181 of main text for more specific interventions)

46. e   47. d   48. b   49. b
50. a   51. c   52. d   53. e
54. c   55. b   56. d   57. a

▪ ▪ ▪ **Chapter 7**

1. a
2. a. In palliative surgery, disease symptoms are alleviated but not cured.
3. d. The purpose of reconstructive surgery is to rebuild tissue or organs that have been damaged.
4. c. An emergency surgical procedure must be performed immediately and includes such cases as obstetric emergencies, bowel obstructions, life-threatening trauma, and ruptured aneurysms.
5. c. The purpose of diagnostic surgery is to determine or confirm a diagnosis.
6. a. If the client has a low H & H and significant blood loss during surgery is anticipated, the surgeon may order a type and cross-match of the client's blood for a possible transfusion.
7. a. An EKG is prescribed routinely for clients who are undergoing general anesthesia and who are 40 years of age or have cardiovascular disease.
8. d
9. b. During this phase the client is positioned, the skin is prepared, and surgery is performed.
10. c. Atropine sulfate, an anticholinergic drug, reduces oral and respiratory secretions to decrease risk of aspiration.
11. c. The client should be npo after midnight for morning general anesthesia. Mouth care will diminish the discomfort the npo status along with the medication may cause.
12. b. famotidine (Pepcid), along with cimetidine (Tagamet) and ranitidine (Zantac), are H_2-receptor antagonists that are given preoperatively to increase gastric pH and decrease gastric volume.
13. d   14. c   15. e   16. a   17. b
18. Answers include: bed rest, maintaining hydration, application of pressure to infusion site
19. a. Pain is more easily treated soon after its onset than it is after it is established. Therefore, postoperative analgesics should be administered initially at regular intervals to maintain a therapeutic blood level.
20. (a) uncommon, (b) rarely

21. c. It is the responsibility of the surgeon who will be performing the procedure to obtain the client's informed consent.
22. (a) patency of airway
    (b) naloxone hydrochloride (Narcan)
    (c) flumazenil (Romazicon)
23. d. If the client has questions or concerns that were not discussed or made clear, or if the nurse questions the client's understanding, the surgeon is responsible for supplying further information.
24. a
25. c. Surgery is a significant and stressful event in the life of the client and family. Regardless of the nature of the surgery, anxiety will be present.
26. c. Most teaching takes place prior to surgery because pain and effects of anesthesia can diminish the client's ability to learn.
27. Answers include: loosen, mobilize, remove
28. thrombophlebitis
29. a. The nurse should verify that the informed consent has been signed prior to administering preoperative medications. The risks and benefits should be explained prior to the day of surgery.
30. c. Dentures and contact lenses should be removed preoperatively. A hearing aid may be left in place if the client cannot hear without it.
31. a. The circulating nurse is a highly experienced registered nurse who coordinates and manages a wide range of activities before, during, and after surgery.
32. b
33. Answers include: injury to the client; sensory and motor dysfunction, resulting in nerve damage; pressure on the peripheral blood vessels decreasing venous return
34. c   35. b   36. a
37. Answers include: keeping the height of the client's bed in the lowest position, raising the side rails of the bed, placing the client's call bell within reach
38. d. Clients at risk for developing DVT include those who are over age 40 and who have varicose veins.
39. a
40. b. The nurse must ensure that the affected area is not rubbed or massaged.

41. b. Conversations during surgery should be maintained on a professional level. Psychologic trauma can result from intraoperative awareness.

42. Answers include: hypotension, hypothermia, hypoxemia

43. c. Nursing care includes encouraging the client to turn, cough, and perform deep-breathing exercises at least every 2 hours.

44. Answers include: applying a pressure dressing to the area, applying mechanical pressure with a gloved hand, preparing the client and the client's family for possible emergency surgery

45. 2

46. a. Nursing care includes encouraging early ambulation in postoperative clients within prescribed limits.

47. False. Nursing care of the client with urinary retention includes increasing the daily oral fluid intake to 2500 to 3000 mL if the client's condition permits.

48. b. Healing by primary intention takes place when the wound is uncomplicated and clean and has sustained little tissue loss. Edges of the incision are well approximated, with sutures or staples.

49. (a) sanguineous, (b) serous, (c) purulent

50. d

51. c. When dehiscence occurs, the wound should be covered immediately with a sterile dressing moistened with normal saline.

52. Answers include: proper wound care, signs and symptoms of wound infection, how to monitor temperature, proper activity level, how to control pain

53. Answers may include: minimizing noise in the environment; providing adequate room light; staying within the client's field of vision when speaking; speak low, not loud; encourage client to wear hearing aid to operating room; provide comfort measures

54. Answers may include: applying warm blankets over the client upon arrival in the OR, covering as much of the client's body surface as possible during skin preparation and throughout the surgery, using a heating lamp to provide warmth to the client's extremities during surgery, administering warmed intravenous fluids and irrigants

55. d. This is directly related to the shortened stay in the hospital.

56. c. There is less time for the nurse to assess, evaluate, and teach the client and family.

57. stable vital signs, pain must be controlled or alleviated, client demonstrates understanding of postoperative instructions.

58. d. The use of suggestive voiding techniques, such as running water, may stimulate voiding. The client should not be discharged prior to voiding. An order to catheterize the client should be obtained prior to insertion. The surgeon should only be called after suggestive voiding techniques are attempted.

59. b. This decrease in blood pressure and increase in pulse may be consistent with signs of shock. Increasing the frequency of assessment and assessing the wound are the only appropriate interventions.

60. a. Activity is generally restricted to walking for at least 7 to 14 days following laparoscopic surgery.

▪ ▪ ▪ **Chapter 8**

1. Answers include: defending and protecting the body from infection, removing and destroying damaged or dead cells, identifying and destroying malignant cells

2. a. Leukocytes are responsible for phagocytosis and chemotaxis.

3. c. Marginated cells are lymphocytes that adhere to vascular epithelial cells along the vessel walls, in other tissue spaces, or in the lymph system.

4. b. An elevated white blood cell count (leukocytosis) is seen in most infections.

5. b. The WBC differential identifies the portion of the total represented by each type of leukocyte.

6. e   7. b   8. c   9. a   10. a   11. d

12. b   13. f   14. a   15. b   16. e   17. a

18. g   19. d   20. a   21. d   22. b   23. d

24. Answers include: filter foreign antigens from lymph, support proliferation of lymphocytes and macrophages

25. c. White pulp is lymphoid tissue that serves as a site for lymphocyte proliferation and immune surveillance and B cells predominate the white pulp.

26. d. The spleen is not essential to life, and the liver and bone marrow can assume its functions.

27. a

28. (a) vasoconstrict, (b) vasodilate, (c) histamine, (d) kinins, (e) redness, (f) heat, (g) serosanguineous, (h) phagocytosis, (i) reconstruction, (j) resolution, (k) repair

29. b. Immunocompetent individuals have immune systems that are able to identify antigens and effectively destroy or remove them.

30. d. Immune defenses are decreased in the older adult.

31. b. Confusion is one of the most frequent atypical signs of infections in older adults. The WBC would most likely elevate only slightly and fever and chills will most likely be absent.

32. c. Limiting fluid may increase the chances of infection. The other interventions will limit the risks of infection.

33. c

34. b. IgE plays an important role in allergic and other hypersensitivity reactions.

35. d. T-lymphocytes are initiators of a cell-mediated immune response.

36. decrease

37. b. Lymphadenopathy describes swollen and tender lymph glands.

38. Answers include: erythema, hyperemia, swelling, pain, loss of function

39. Answers include: temperature over 38C or under 36C, pulse >90/min, R >20/min, WBC >12,000 mm^3 or >10% bands

40. b. Pus forms from dead neutrophils, necrotic tissue, and digested bacteria.

41. d. An elevated ESR is indicative of an inflammatory response.

42. c. Chronic diseases such as diabetes impair healing and diabetes is a common cause of poor healing. The other clients may be at risk, but the client with DM is at greatest risk of impaired healing.

43. c. Stopping the medication may result in adrenal crisis. Prior to stopping corticosteroids the dose must be gradually tapered.

44. a. Aspirin is an anti-inflammatory; acetaminophen is not.

45. a. Aspirin should be taken with food or milk.

46. Answers include: sufficient kilocalories, adequate protein, adequate carbohydrates, vitamin A, B-complex vitamins, vitamin C, vitamin K, zinc

47. c. Normal saline will result in the least amount of drying and tissue damage. The other solutions may result in tissue damage or drying.

48. b. The use of boiling water may result in tissue injury and burns and there should be protection between the compress and the skin. The other statements are true.

49. b. Option (a) describes artificially acquired immunity. Options (c) and (d) describe passive immunity.

50. c. Artificially acquired immunity occurs as the result of immunizations or vaccines.

51. c. Measles vaccine provides active artificial immunity.

52. c. Protein electrophoresis breaks down globulin into its specific components.

53. b. Adults born before 1956 are generally considered to be immune to measles.

54. a. Most younger adults who received primary immunizations for tetanus and a client with a contaminated wound should receive a booster if immunization history is unclear.

55. d. Hepatitis B vaccine is used cautiously in individuals with active infection. All the other individuals are at risk for hepatitis B and should receive the vaccine.

56. d. Anergy occurs when there is no reactivity to injected known antigens.

57. c. Selected vaccines such as gamma globulins stimulate an intermediate immune response.

58. b. Tetanus antitoxins are usually made from horse serum. Invasive dyes are usually made of iodine which is also contained in shellfish. Egg allergies should be assessed when administering MMR and influenza. Beef and pork are not associated with immunizations and vaccines.

59. b. Live virus vaccines should not be administered to immunocompromised individuals or to clients who are in close contact with an immunocompromised individual. In this situation, immunizations may not be required for school. There is no solid research to date that confirms an association between polio vaccine and HIV infection.

60. d. The most serious complication of an immunization immediately after administration is anaphylaxis, and airway distress could be fatal. Redness may occur at the injection site, but usually not immediately. The client should be observed for at least 20 to 30 minutes. Irritability and restlessness may occur following an immunization, but generally not immediately unless associated with airway distress and hypoxia.

61. (a) Viruses, (b) Parasites, (c) Bacteria, (d) Mycoplasma

62. (a) prodromal, (b) incubation, (c) carrier

63. c. Early signs of septic shock include restlessness, hypotension, and tachycardia. Early in septic shock the urine output would be normal. Symptoms would not include hypertension, bradycardia, or decreased urine output.

64. d. Foley catheters are associated with urinary tract infections. Removing a Foley catheter as soon as possible reduces the risk. The other interventions may reduce the risks of infections, but the highest risk is presence of a Foley catheter.

65. c. The most common change one would expect is a change in mental status. Signs of infection are less dramatic in the older adult. The older adult usually has subtle signs of infection and not usually fever, chills, shivering, or restlessness.

66. a. There are more often immature neutrophils in circulation, causing a "shift to the left," when infection occurs.

67. c. For IV medications, the peak is 30 minutes after administration and the trough is a few minutes before the next scheduled dose. Options a and d are incorrect because it would take at least 30 minutes to administer the medication.

68. b. Bacteriostatic drugs inhibit the growth of the microorganisms, but do not necessarily kill them.

69. Answers include: history of sensitivity, the age and childbearing status of the client, renal function, hepatic function, site of infection, other host factors such as chronic diseases and other medications

70. b. Resistance that kills all of the pathogens, making it vital for patients to take all the prescribed doses.

71. (a) local erythema and rash at the injection site; (b) fever, chills, skin rashes, and hives; (c) acute respiratory distress and anaphylaxis

72. b. The nurse should contact the physician to make certain he or she is aware of the penicillin allergy and possibility of a cross-sensitivity to a cephalosporin. Some clients experience a cross-sensitivity reaction to cephalosporins if allergic to penicillin. The nurse should not refuse to give a medication without conferring with the physician. Administering Benadryl (diphenhydramine) in this situation is generally not recommended.

73. b. Gentamicin is nephrotoxic and the nurse should monitor the BUN and creatinine as indicators of renal function. The other tests do not specifically measure renal function.

74. a. The client should report an upset stomach and not stop the medication without consulting the physician. The other statements are true.

75. c. If blood is not present in sweat, universal precautions are not required. All the other situations place the nurse at risk of body fluid contamination.

76. d. Hand washing is the most important step in preventing infection.

77. c. Anaphylaxis is an immediate hypersensitivity reaction. All the other situations are not immediate reactions.

78. b. A wheal and erythema are the findings with a positive skin test. You would not expect to find crusting or cyanosis. No observable change would indicate a negative skin test.

79. b. Identifying allergens by a careful nursing assessment is critical to minimizing exposure. The other interventions are important but not the most important.

80. d. A concentration of 1:100,000 is used in a more severe anaphylactic reaction, and is indicated in this situation. A concentration of 1:1000 is used for mild reactions. Cromolyn sodium and oral diphenhydramine hydrochloride are not appropriate in this situation.

81. c. The most important assessment is patency of the airway. The rate and quality of respirations should be assessed after airway. Blood pressure and pulse should be assessed following airway and breathing. Neurovital signs are not of the highest priority in anaphylaxis.

82. c. The priority and most appropriate action is to stop the blood, but the IV should be maintained with normal saline. A patent IV will allow an access to administer IV medications if needed. The other interventions would not be appropriate.

83. c. It is during the first 15 minutes that a blood transfusion reaction is most likely to occur. The other statements are not correct.

84. b. Alcohol should not be used when taking prescription antihistamines. The other statements are correct.

85. c   86. a

87. b

88. b. Acute tissue rejection occurs 4 days to 3 months after a transplant. It is the most common and most treatable form of rejection. An immediate reaction occurs 2 to 3 days after transplant and organ failure usually follows. Reactions from 4 months to years after transplant are chronic tissue rejections and there is gradual deterioration of the transplanted organ. Reactions during the first 100 days after transplant may include immediate and acute tissue rejections.

89. b. Following a transplant, the client should not be exposed to minor infections. A mask may not completely protect the client. There is no way to be certain that the visitor is getting over an infection. Stating that the client might die creates unnecessary fear.

90. a. An itchy maculopapular rash is typical of graft-versus-host disease.

91. many of these drugs alter the normal response to infection such as temperature

92. Answers include: signs and symptoms of infection, importance of medication regime, side effects of immunosuppressive drug therapy, (d) the importance of avoiding infection, the importance of wearing a medical alert bracelet, the importance of follow-up visits

93. c. AIDS is the leading cause of death in men ages 35–44.

94. a. Sexual contact is thought to be the primary mode of transmission. Breast milk, saliva, and needlestick injuries may result in transmission of HIV.

95. d. HIV transmission is associated with behaviors such as sexual practices and IV drug use. Heterosexuals are at risk for HIV.

Behaviors such as unprotected sex and sharing needles results in HIV transmission. Being a homosexual or a prisoner does not place an individual at risk.

96. b. ELISA tests have the highest sensitivity when performed at least 12 weeks after infection. The test may be negative early in infection. ELISA is the most appropriate test and it tests for antibodies. The effectiveness of AZT in preventing infection has not been established.

97. c. Helper T cells are infected by the HIV virus.

98. a. Opportunistic infections occur when the CD4 cell count drops lower than 200/µl.

99. a. Tuberculosis is the most common opportunistic infection. The other infections may occur but not at the rate of TB. Lymphoma is a cancer, not an infection.

100. a. Kaposi's sarcoma is the most common cancer. Lymphomas and cervical cancers may occur with AIDS, but not usually oat cell cancer.

101. b. Natural skin condoms allow HIV to pass through. Latex condoms should be used instead. Water-soluble lubricants should be used because they are compatible with latex condoms. Oil-based lubricants will break down latex products.

102. c. The Western blot test is confirmatory for a positive ELISA. The other tests are not indicated.

103. a. The antivirals act on different parts of the viral replication cycle and diminish resistance. The other answers are incorrect. The antivirals are readily available once they are approved by the FDA. These medications would not be used if ineffective. Toxic effects may occur despite this schedule.

104. c. Most clients with HIV-wasting syndrome have diarrhea, not constipation. Weight loss, fever, and fatigue are common symptoms of HIV-wasting syndrome.

■ ■ ■ **Chapter 9**

1. 42

2. b. Cancer occurs when abnormal cells become tumor cells.

3. address the client's response to the diagnosis

4. two 5. lung cancer

6. (a) women (b) African Americans

7. (a) prostate, (b) breast, (c) lung, (d) colorectal

8. d. Cancer is described as a disease of aging, with 66% of cancer deaths occurring after age 65.

9. interphase 10. interphase 11. mitosis

12. (a) G_1 (growth 1); (b) S (synthesis); (c) G_2 (growth 2)

13. identical genetic material

14. b 15. d 16. b 17. a 18. c

19. b. The impairment of the immune system applies to all present theories about the etiology of cancer.

20. d. Some cancers such as cervical cancer may have a viral etiology. Option (a) is incorrect as in this instance a viral etiology is of high probability. Option (b) is incorrect because not all cancers have a viral etiology. Option (c) is incorrect because the nurse can respond to this client's question.

21. d. Breast and colon cancers and melanomas have been demonstrated to have a familial association.

22. d. An English teacher should have the lowest theoretical risk for an occupational exposure. Miners, construction workers, and health care workers are exposed to possible carcinogens.

23. Answers include: stress, diet, occupation, infection, tobacco use, alcohol use, use of recreational drugs, obesity, sun exposure

24. Answers may include: older clients often mistake cancer symptoms for the normal aging process; chronic conditions often seen in older adults may mask cancer symptoms; there are greater side effects from cancer chemotherapy in older clients; older adults do not participate in screenings or seek treatment for cancer

25. d. The other characteristics relate to malignant neoplasms.

26. a, d, e

27. Answers include: embolism in the blood or lymph, spread by way of body cavities, iatrogenesis

28. impairment or alteration of the immune system

29. b. Relieving and/or managing stress may improve the immune system's function. Chemotherapy may be essential to treatment.

Depression may weaken the immune system, but antidepressants may not be indicated. Herbal remedies have not been proven to strengthen the immune system.

30. d. Aggressive therapy may kill the cancer cells. Metastasis is not consistent with a death sentence. If cancer is in the lymph system it may have spread to other organs. Chemotherapy and radiation may result in a cure.

31. f 32. e 33. d 34. c

35. a 36. b 37. h 38. g

39. c. Lung cancers may cause ectopic secretions of insulin, which would decrease blood sugar.

40. (a) acute, (b) chronic

41. d

42. (a) prostatic, (b) cervical, (c) bone

43. (a) grading, (b) staging, (c) classification

44. d. Papilloma is a benign tumor. It is not related to cancer, malignancy, or metastatic lesions

45. b

46. c. An MRI uses radio frequency signals, not sound waves. Radioactive substances and dyes are generally not used for this procedure.

47. b

48. (a) germ cell tumors, testicular cancers; (b) leukemia or metastatic liver; (c) breast, thyroid, lung; (d) colon, lung, breast, ovary, stomach, pancreas; (e) liver

49. c. Responding by listening and giving support is the most appropriate response by the nurse. The other responses minimize her experience and do not convey warmth, caring, and respect.

50. a. Chemotherapy is not a local treatment, it is a systemic treatment. The other statements are true.

51. d. This is the only statement that relates to the cell-kill hypothesis.

52. (a) plant alkaloids, (b) alkylating agents, (c) antimetabolites, (d) miscellaneous agents, (e) cytotoxic antibiotics, (f) hormone, (g) hormone antagonist

53. a. The Hickman is the only example of a tunneled catheter. Mediports and Port-a-Caths are surgically implanted ports and a PICC is a peripherally inserted catheter.

54. c. Fluids should be encouraged during chemotherapy. The other interventions are appropriate.

55. b. Cardiac toxicity can occur when a client is taking Adriamycin. It is not prevalent with the other listed medications.

56. c. Wearing gloves, a mask, and a gown are the appropriate safety measures. Chemotherapeutic agents are not given through peripheral veins.

57. b. The client should avoid her school-aged grandchildren while she is immuno-compromised. She may not have adequate protection against childhood illnesses. The other steps are appropriate.

58. b. The nurse should arrange for the client to confer with the surgeon and oncologist so that she fully understands treatment options. The nurse should never try to persuade the client to accept any option. The other answers are not appropriate in this situation.

59. b. Brachytherapy involves placing radioactive material directly in the tumor site.

60. d. Body fluids are disposed in a specially marked container. An abdominal apron is not required. The client with internal radiation should not have a roommate. Any dislodged implants should be moved with long-handled forceps.

61. c. The client should protect the skin during and after the treatment period. Heat or ice should not be applied to the site. Clients receiving external radiation can have intimate physical contact. Washing the skin with soap and hot water can dry the skin and wash off treatment marks.

62 Answers include: immunotherapy such as biologic response modifiers (BRMs); photo-dynamic therapy and/or bone marrow trans-plantation

63. d. Fluids should be encouraged, not limited. The other steps are appropriate, as confusion is a side effect, the medication is given sub-cutaneously, and flulike symptoms can occur.

64. True   65. False   66. True
67. True   68. False
69. b, c, d, f
70. c
71. b. This is an indicator of poor nutrition. The other findings do not support a diagnosis of poor nutrition.

72. b. These symptoms are consistent with anxi-ety. The other problems may be contributing to anxiety, but are not directly related to the symptoms described.

73. d. Hair often grows back in after chemo-therapy, but the color and texture may be different. The other statements are correct.

74. c. The immunosuppressed client with cancer may not have a fever when infection is pres-ent. The nurse should expect that the pulse rate and respiratory rate would increase with an infection. An elevated blood pressure may indicate uncontrolled pain.

75. b. When the temperature is 101.5F or higher, the friend should call. The other situations would require a call for help.

76. b. A positive PPD (5 mm or greater of indura-tion and redness) indicates immunocompe-tence which is consistent with improved nutrition. The other findings are consistent with malnutrition.

77. c. Dry foods are best tolerated by the nause-ated client. The other interventions may increase nausea.

78. b. Clients with leukemia should not floss, as it might result in sepsis. The other interven-tions are appropriate.

79. b. If the client refuses to acknowledge the change in body image, allow the client to engage in denial as it is a protective mecha-nism. The other interventions are not appro-priate as they are not empathetic and do not convey respect for the client's experience.

80. b. Mr. Rodriguez should be included in the funeral planning if he wishes as it will pro-vide him with a sense of control. Keeping the information from Mr. Rodriguez may be upsetting to him. Stating that treatment might be still effective is inappropriate. Wait-ing until death may add stress at an extremely stressful time.

81. d. Warm spiced foods may be irritating to the oral mucosa. The other interventions would be appropriate.

82. d. The ACS recommends a high-fiber, low-fat diet, not a high-fat diet. The ACS recom-mends minimal use of salt-cured foods and using foods high in vitamins, not supple-ments.

83. d. Facial and arm edema are early signs and symptoms of superior vena cava syndrome. The other problems do not cause facial and arm swelling.

84. b. Changes in neurologic function may be related to spinal cord compression. Spinal cord compression is an emergency as it can lead to irreversible paraplegia.

85. (a) manifested by fever, vascular dehydration, peripheral edema, hypotension, tachycardia, hot flushed skin

    (b) manifested by hypotension, rapid thready pulse, respiratory distress, cyanosis, subnormal temperature, cold clammy skin, decreased urinary output, altered mentation

▪ ▪ ▪ **Chapter 10**

1. c   2. a   3. b

4. Answers include: The greater the momentum of the moving object, the greater the force that will be transferred to the object that is struck; the amount of damage that will result from the transfer of the energy varies at different parts of the body; as a force is applied to a body, there is a reciprocal force applied to another body.

5. Answers include: mechanical, gravitational, thermal, electrical, physical, chemical

6. (a) penetrating, (b) thermal, (c) penetrating, (d) inhalation, (e) penetrating, (f) blunt, (g) thermal

7. (a) Assessment: no evidence of breathing, violent respiratory effort, deep intercostal/substernal retracting; Interventions: open airway, clear airway, use airway adjuncts, intubation, cricothyrotomy

    (b) Assessment: tracheal shift, decreased/absent chest expansion, distended neck veins; Interventions: needle thoracostomy, oxygen

    (c) Assessment: decreased LOC, delayed capillary refill, restlessness, increased pulse rate; Interventions: determine cause and location, control bleeding, initiate volume replacement

8. c

9. Answers include: insert a Foley catheter into the bladder, insert a nasogastric tube, determine allergies to drugs or solutions

10. d   11. d   12. c   13. c
14. c   15. a   16. d   17. b

18. This injury may cause significant blood loss and/or provide clues to the presence of other serious injuries, such as ruptured bladder.

19. Answers may include: safe transport to the hospital, primary and secondary assessments, accurate documentation, facilitation of diagnostic tests, continuous assessment of vital signs and neurologic status, provision of pain medication

20. Answers may include: long-term disability, loss of income, high cost of trauma care, anger, guilt, anxiety

21. Answers include: loss of consciousness, altered mental status, weakness or paralysis

22. Answers include: (a) ensure the cervical spine is immobilized, (b) assess the airway, (c) assess breathing, (d) assess circulation, (e) perform a brief neurologic assessment, (f) assess the integumentary system, (g) perform a brief health history interview

23. (a) head to toe assessment; thorough evaluation of the client's anterior body and a brief assessment of the posterior body, (b) completion of the primary assessment, (c) life-threatening injuries have been stabilized, (d–f) pre-hospital care providers, trauma nurse, the medical-surgical nurse

24. (a) to prevent tetanus, an exotoxin produced by *Clostridium tetani,* which is usually introduced through an open wound in a client whose status is outdated or unknown; (b) to prevent additional injury to the extremity, circulation could be compromised or obstructed after splinting; (c) to prevent cerebral spinal fluid leak; (d) to keep family/friends informed and to help with decision making and crisis intervention

25. discontinue the transfusion, keep the vein open, send unused blood and bag to the laboratory, recheck blood bank information, report and record, intervene as directed by the physician, continuously observe the client for further distress

26. assess for: anger/fear, flashbacks, psychic numbing, calm, shock, terror, disbelief

27. be available if client wishes to talk, teach relaxation techniques, allow family/friends to be present, establish short-term realistic goals; refer for counseling

28. (a) optimize organ perfusion and minimize the development of infection, (b–d) Answers include: systolic BP of 90 mm Hg, oxygen saturation at 90%, an hourly urine output of 30 mL.

29. a. Brain death occurs when cerebral functioning ceases. Clinical signs of brain death include: known cause of injury, irreversible condition, apnea with $PaCO_2$ greater than 60 mm Hg, no spontaneous movement, no gag or corneal reflex, no occulocephalic or oculovestibular reflex, normothermic, acceptable levels of central nervous system depressants and neuromuscular blocking agents, absence of toxic or metabolic disorders.

30. penetration of tissues, with damage to heart and lungs, intestines, and vascular system; fractured bones

31. death in the ED within a short time after admission; a sudden, violent unexpected death

32. place clothing in a breathable bag; wrap hands in paper bags; leave all tubing and apparatus in the body cavities; do not clean the body

33. document the presence of entrance/exit wound(s); information from witnesses about the incident should be documented as quotes

34. all articles found on the client will be signed for and turned over to the authorized receiving person

35. assess airway for secretions, obstructions, and foreign debris; monitor oxygen saturation; assess LOC; assess for signs and symptoms of airway obstruction; observe for increasing facial and neck edema

36. *Risk for Ineffective Breathing Pattern, Risk for Fluid Volume Deficit, Risk for Altered Family Processes, Fear, Risk for Injury, Pain*

37. use strict aseptic technique; monitor wounds for redness, odor, heat, swelling and drainage; wash wounds with normal saline or antimicrobial solution as ordered; cover with DSD

38. The nurse should provide a wound care demonstration and written instructions, head injury sheet, a tetanus immunization card and information regarding follow-up care.

39. Mr. Adams needs education about safety precautions and minimizing risk factors related to road conditions, unsafe vehicles, lack of restraining devices, presence of guns or knives, and high crime areas.

40. Key interventions include assessing the client's emotional responses, encouraging client to express his feelings, teaching relaxation techniques, and referring client and family for counseling.

■ ■ ■ Chapter 11

1. (a) mourning, (b) loss, (c) grief
2. Freud   3. Carter   4. Engel
5. Kübler-Ross   6. Cody   7. Lindemann
8. (a) protest, (b) despair, (c) detachment
9. Answers include: the psychic pain of the broken bond, living without the assets and guidance of the lost person or resource, reduced cognitive and problem-solving effectiveness
10. d. Viewing death as a spiritual reunion with deceased loved ones does not occur until the adult reaches this stage in life.
11. c. As middle-aged adults grow older, they begin to accept their own mortality and experience waves of death anxiety.
12. b. Before children are 6 years old, they view death as similar to sleep. Between 6 to 10 years of age, children begin to accept the finality of death.
13. d. Adults ages 22 to 45 typically think of death only when confronted with it. Adults ages 46 and older tend to experience death anxiety. Children ages 11 to 12 may think about the afterlife. Adolescents ages 13 to 21 often view death as distant and may see themselves as invulnerable to death.
14. Answers may include: guilt about things other than actions taken or not taken, morbid preoccupation with worthlessness, marked psychomotor retardation, prolonged and marked functional impairment, hallucinatory experiences, thoughts of death
15. c. Her suicidal ideation, her guilt regarding the care she provided her husband, and her marked functional impairments are evidence of a major depression. The only appropriate intervention listed is referral for evaluation of her depression.
16. The nurse's conscious or unconscious reactions to loss may influence the outcome of interventions.
17. b. Expressions of loss are often evidenced in physical symptoms. These are not symptoms of phantom or referred pain or normal bereavement.

18. Spiritual beliefs and practices greatly influence people's reaction to loss. Assessment helps identify spiritual support systems.

19. b. Focusing on the meaning of the loss is much more important than establishing the phase of the grief process. Both the client and her husband will be experiencing grief and both need to be assessed and supported by the nurse.

20. b   21. a   22. c   23. e   24. d
25. c   26. d   27. b   28. a   29. e

30. Answers include: perceived inability to share the loss, lack of social recognition of the loss, ambivalent relationship prior to the loss, traumatic circumstances of the loss

31. Ceremonies are part of the work of mourning and grieving a loss.

32. d. These are symptoms of dysfunctional grieving. The family is not necessarily dysfunctional. Their symptoms are not those of a normal stress response or denial.

33. anticipatory grieving

34. dysfunctional grieving

35. c. Crying helps provide relief from feelings of acute pain and stress. Encouraging him to stop crying, telling him to be strong, or leaving him alone are not supportive interventions.

36. c. There is not enough assessment data to support the diagnosis of depression. There is no evidence to support the belief that his condition is chronic or that he cannot be responsible for treatment goals. The best answer is c, as there are nursing interventions that are appropriate to address his needs.

37. c. Encouraging the client to talk about the loss will help the client process the loss. Asking direct questions or discouraging the client's anger may block communication.

38. c. This is the most reflective response, allowing the client to express thoughts and feelings. The other responses block communication.

39. c. The client is angry. This anger should be acknowledged and he should be encouraged to verbalize regarding his loss. Being alone will not help him process his anger. His behavior is part of the grief process, but the best response is to assist the client in processing his feeling. Telling him that his behavior is unacceptable is a judgmental response.

40. c. This response acknowledges her loss and feelings regarding her change in body image. The other responses minimize her loss.

41. life review

42. framing memories

43. b. According to Kübler-Ross, fear of dying alone is the greatest fear. The other responses may be fears, but they are not the greatest fears.

44. d. This response focuses the client on her own feelings of loss. The other responses do not provide an opportunity to further assess the family's responses to this loss.

45. b. This is the only factual statement. The other statements provide false hope.

46. c. Although the other factors may contribute to dysfunctional grieving, the client's prior methods of coping with loss will provide a basis for predicting whether or not an individual may develop dysfunctional grieving.

47. a. The other responses are correct, but the primary reason for not using antianxiety drugs is so not to interfere with the normal grieving processes.

48. d. This response acknowledges the client's loss and offers the client an opportunity to reflect on the loss. The other responses block communication.

49. d. Recalling positive and negative memories is evidence that she has resolved her loss. The other signs and symptoms are evidence that she has dysfunctional grieving.

50. b. When one stays busy with work or activities, it may indicate that they are postponing the work of mourning.

51. (a) family cohesiveness/social support, (b) community-based support groups

52. d. Hearing may be the last sense to be lost. If the client is near death, the family may want to communicate their presence and concern and remain at the bedside.

53. acknowledge the loss

54. Answers may include: accept the reality of the loss, regain a sense of self-esteem, begin to put the loss into perspective, griever breaks ties with lost object or person

55. the ending of another life for reasons of mercy

56. In voluntary euthanasia, consent is given by a competent adult client, health care providers, and the client's family. Involuntary euthanasia is performed without consent.

57. a   58. c

59. d. There is no legal basis for a "slow code." A client's decisions regarding end-of-life interventions should be made in advance and clarified through advanced directives.

60. b. The client should be encouraged to make decisions when he is ready. There never should be any coercion to sign the document. All the other interventions are appropriate.

61. A living will and a durable power of attorney for health care are both legal documents. A living will expresses a person's wishes regarding life-sustaining treatment in the event of terminal illness or permanent unconsciousness, whereas a durable power of attorney for health care empowers another competent adult to make decisions on the person's behalf in the event of incapacitation.

62. b. The client with dysfunctional grieving should be encouraged to verbalize her feelings and thoughts and should not be told what to do or feel. All the other interventions are appropriate.

63. Clients who present a brave, stoic front have a history of frequent/multiple losses, are socially isolated, and have a history of dealing ineffectively with loss.

64. a. Talking about the loss and past is evidence of dysfunctional grieving. All other responses are evidence of grief resolution.

Chapter 12

1. (a) move, (b) absorption, (c) blood, (d) lymph

2. c. Absorption of acids is not a function of the GI tract. It secretes enzymes and mucus and moves wastes.

3. (a) pharynx, (b) esophagus, (c) stomach, (d) small intestine, (e) large intestine, (f) rectum

4. to moisten food, dissolve food chemicals, and provide enzymes

5. alternating waves of contraction and relaxation of involuntary muscle

6. c   7. d   8. a.

9. b. The small intestine begins at the pyloric sphincter and ends at the ileocecal junction.

10. b. The liver has many functions, but its digestive function is to produce bile.

11. f   12. h   13. a   14. e

15. g   16. d   17. c   18. b

19. plant foods

20. (a) 4, (b) 125, (c) 175

21. b. Potatoes, milk, and whole grains are high in complex carbohydrates The other menu selections do not include as many foods that are high in complex carbohydrates.

22. (a) complete, (b) incomplete

23. 0.8

24. c. All the other selections include either animal or plant fat.

25. b. All the other selections include foods that are high in cholesterol.

26. (a) 30, (b) 10, (c) 250

27. g   28. a   29. c   30. e

31. h   32. f   33. d   34. b

35. (a) onset, (b) characteristics and course, (c) severity, (d) precipitating factors, (e) relieving factors, (f) associated symptoms

36. c

37. a. Pale conjunctiva are a sign of anemia, which can be related to malnutrition. The other findings are normal.

38. 117.6%   39. 104.4%

40. 6.82 inches

41. f   42. d   43. e   44. g   45. h

46. a   47. b   48. j   49. i   50. c

51. (a) percussion, (b) palpation

52. c   53. d

54. c. One could not examine the abdomen if the client were in the prone position. A reclining position or one with the head elevated would make it difficult to accurately assess the location of internal organs.

55. d. There is no evidence that older adults have decreased nutritional requirements.

56. subjective findings: 63 years old, retired, widow, not sexually active, would like a boyfriend, recently relocated to Florida, dark brown and hard bowel movement 4 days ago, complaints of tenderness right lower quadrant objective findings: adbomen soft and non-distended, quiet bowel sounds in all four quadrants
abnormal findings and possible etiologies: No bowel movement in 4 days, possibly from constipation or diverticulitis; quiet bowel sounds, possibly from constipation; right lower quadrant tenderness, possibly related to appendicitis, constipation, or diverticulitis

57. auscultation
58. presses the fingers into the abdomen slowly and then releases the pressure quickly.
59. raise her head and shoulders.
60. a mass in the abdomen may become more prominent with this maneuver.
61. hyperactive, high-pitched, tinkling, rushing, or growling bowel sounds
62. It may indicate diarrhea or the onset of a bowel obstruction.

■ ■ ■ **Chapter 13**

1. (a) obesity, (b) overweight, (c) morbid obesity
2. Answers may include: arteriosclerosis; arthritis; atherosclerosis; cancers of the breast, uterus, prostate, and colon; cardiac enlargement; cholecystitis and cholelithiasis; chronic renal failure; congestive heart failure; diabetes mellitus; hiatal hernia; hypertension; impaired pulmonary function; low back pain; muscle strains and sprains; postoperative complications; stress incontinence; thrombophlebitis; varicosities
3. Answers include: client's height and weight, standard height and weight tables
4. composition
5. females
6. (a) to assess for diabetes mellitus; (b) assess for elevated cholesterol levels that may be from a diet high in saturated fats; (c) to confirm that high-density lipoproteins are reduced, while low-density lipoproteins are elevated; (d) to rule out myocardial infarction or heart enlargement, which are associated with morbid obesity
7. Answers may include: abundant and readily accessible food, fast-food restaurants, advertising, vending machines
8. aerobic exercise for 30 minutes per day, 3 to 5 times per week
9. c
10. Answers may include: lipectomy, liposuction, jejuneleal bypass, gastric bypass, and gastroplasty.
11. Answers include: *Altered Nutrition: More than Body Requirements, Self-Esteem Disturbance, Powerlessness, Activity Intolerance, Ineffective Management of Theraputic Regimen*

12. Answers may include: acute respiratory failure, aging, AIDS, alcoholism, burns, COPD, eating disorders, GI disorders, neurologic disorders, renal disease, short bowel syndrome, surgery, trauma
13. c   14. a   15. e
16. b   17. d   18. c
19. (a) Physiologic data: changes in taste and smell, a higher incidence of gastrointestinal disease, poor oral health, loss of teeth or ill-fitting dentures, anorexia caused by medications used to treat chronic conditions, and functional limitations that impair the ability to shop and cook

    (b) Psychologic issues: older clients live on fixed incomes, many at the poverty level; may not be able to afford well-balanced meals; loss of appetite as seen in depression; social isolation and loneliness
20. Clients with kwashiorkor have inadequate protein intake; their weight can be normal; and their serum protein, hemoglobin, and hematocrit are decreased. Clients with marasmus have an inadequate intake of calories.
21. d   22. c   23. c   24. b
25. b. Only after x-ray documentation that the tip of the catheter is placed correctly (for example in the subclavian vein) can TPN be initiated. The nurse never adds medications to the TPN solution. The other choices are important but not essential before starting the TPN.
26. Answers may include: pneumothorax, infection, hyperglycemia, hypoglycemia, circulatory overload, air embolism, hyperosmolar nonketotic dehydration
27. b
28. (a) oral hygiene and a pleasant environment make food more appetizing; small, frequent meals are generally more appealing and less overwhelming; (b) dry mucous membranes, somnolence and an increased specific gravity may indicate dehydration; dehydration may result in electrolyte disturbances; (c) hand washing is the best strategy to prevent the spread of pathogens; sterile technique is required for procedures such as inserting central lines and changing dressings
29. a   30. b, c   31. f
32. a, d   33. a, d, e, f
34. Answers include: infection, mechanical trauma, irritants

35. Answers include: pain, malodorous breath, blood-tinged saliva
36. b   37. d   38. c
39. b   40. a   41. c
42. (a) maintain adequate hydration, (b) assess for airway patency so client is receiving oxygen, (c) place in Fowler's position, (d) assess client's knowledge and provide teaching, (e) turn, cough, and deep breathe the client q2–4h
43. inform the client that an emergency call system will be in place and that staff will respond promptly
44. Answers may include: obesity, smoking, drinking alcohol and caffeine, eating peppermint and chocolate, fatty meals, increased gastric volume
45. d
46. (a) neutralize gastric acid, thus diminishing the pain of GERD; (b) inhibit the secretion of gastric acid by inhibiting histamine action; (c) inhibits the hydrogen-potassium pump, thereby reducing gastric secretions
47. d. EGD is a test where the esophagus and duodenum are visualized. In order to pass the instrument (endoscope), the throat must be anesthetized.
48. (a) dysphagia, chest pain, nocturnal cough, regurgitation, weight loss; (b) small frequent feedings of soft, warm foods and fluids; avoiding hot, spicy foods and alcohol; (c) lower esophageal sphincter pressures
49. d   50. a   51. c
52. b. A high-calorie diet would promote weight gain. Weight loss is associated with esophageal cancer.

■ ■ ■ **Chapter 14**

1. b   2. d   3. d
4. pernicious anemia
5. b. An NG tube is not necessary for a gastroscopy.
6. c. The gag and swallow reflex must be present before eating to prevent aspiration.
7. mixing alcohol with aspirin
8. Nursing reponsibilities include: check allergies, give deep IM Z track, be alert for side effects, teach not to drive or operate machinery while taking medicine, take 30 to 60 minutes before eating.
9. (a) clear liquids; (b) broth, tea, gelatin; (c) heavier or full liquids; (d) cream soups, puddings, milk
10. a. Carafate (sucralfate) coats the ulcer and protects it from acid and pepsin.
11. c
12. (a–c) answers include: nausea, vomiting, abdominal distress, (d) inadequate, (e-f) answers include: fluid, electrolyte
13. a   14. c
15. b. Recent findings indicate that in up to 90% of people with PUD, helicobacter pylori may be responsible.
16. *Helicobacter pylori*
17. c   18. a   19. b   20. d
21. Answers include: diaphoretic skin; tachycardic pulse; rapid, shallow respirations
22. (a) pain, (b) mental confusion (and other nonspecific symptoms)
23. b
24. Curling's ulcers
25. Cushing's ulcers
26. d
27. a. Steatorrhea results from impaired fat digestion and absorption.
28. a. Antacids interfere with the absorption of some drugs.
29. Answers include: alternate magnesium-based antacids with aluminum-based antacids, continue taking an antacid for 6 to 8 weeks for mucosal healing, report continued constipation
30. (a) to determine the extent of the bleeding, (b) to evacuate blood and clots
31. 14–16
32. normal saline
33. room
34. severe vasoconstriction
35. aspirate gastric contents and test pH of aspirate
36. b. Fluid imbalances are related to the antidiuretic properties of vasopressin.
37. d. The client remains npo until bleeding is controlled.
38. c   39. b   40. 5 to 30
41. Answers may include: nausea, vomiting, epigastric pain with cramping, borborygmi, diarrhea
42. Answers may include: tachycardia, orthostatic hypotension, dizziness, flushing, diaphoresis

43. c
44. d. A truncal vagotomy eliminates all vagal input to liver, pancreas, and other viscera.
45. c. The nurse assesses patency if the tube becomes clogged.
46. Answers include: metabolic alkalosis, hypokalemia, imbalances of sodium
47. c. This delays gastric emptying.
48. d. The supine position delays gastric emptying.
49. sterile water may result in water intoxication
50. d. Digestion and absorption of blood in the GI tract may result in elevated BUN.
51. Answers may include: male gender, low socioeconomic status, urban residence, familial disposition, diet high in nitrates, type A blood group
52. b   53. c   54. d   55. a
56. b. The client should receive irrigations of water after each feeding to maintain patency. The other interventions are appropriate.
57. c. Self-care, independence, and self-image must be encouraged. Gastrostomy tubes do not become easily displaced, clean technique can be used once healing has occurred, and mouth care should be given on a regular basis.
58. Remove old dressing wearing nonsterile gloves; inspect the skin surrounding the insertion site; cleanse the site with antiseptic swabs; redress the wound using a folded 4 × 4 pad
59. The physician would order a complete blood count, an upper GI x-ray study with barium swallow, and perhaps, an ultrasound or gastroscopy with biopsy.
60. The blood count would indicate anemia from chronic blood loss. The upper GI x-ray study would assist in the identification of a lesion. An ultrasound might demonstrate a mass lesion, a gastroscopy would assist in visualization of any mass, and a biopsy would provide a definitive diagnosis.

▪ ▪ ▪ **Chapter 15**

1. c
2. Answers include: stasis of bile in the gallbladder, increased bile concentration
3. female
4. c   5. a   6. d   7. b

8. c. The pain occurs in the right upper quadrant of the abdomen in the area of the gallbladder and common bile duct.
9. a. Murphy's sign is pain on inspiration.
10. b. Clients with cholelithiasis have intolerance to fat-containing foods.
11. c. An HIDA, ultrasound, and cholecystogram are more specific tests to visualize gallstones.
12. d. Gallstones may recur when dissolvers are used. These drugs can cause diarrhea, but this is not considered a major disadvantage.
13. c. A laparoscopic procedure results in minor incisions that do not require an abdominal dressing.
14. a. Following a laparascopic cholecystectomy, a client is generally held overnight to observe for complications such as bleeding.
15. b. A T-tube is required following a common bile duct exploration.
16. c. A T-tube maintains the patency of the common bile duct in the period immediately following surgery.
17. c
18. d. Stools should be of normal color before removing the T-tube. The other symptoms are indications of complications.
19. a. The nurse should tell the client that there may be colicky pain, hematuria, and nausea postprocedure.
20. d. Morphine sulfate may cause spasms in the sphincter of Oddi.
21. d. Upper abdominal surgery will increase the client's risk for respiratory problems. The client should be encouraged to cough and deep breathe.
22. a. Fever and chills are not normal after surgery and may indicate an infection such as a subphrenic abscess. The client should see her surgeon as soon as possible. There is nothing in the question that indicates that she needs more fluids.
23. b   24. e   25. d
26. c   27. a   28. b
29. a. During the preicteric phase, a primary symptom would be nausea leading to anorexia.
30. d. Diffuse abdominal pain is a common symptom of hepatitis.
31. c   32. c
33. d. The other tests relate to liver function, but are not the most appropriate for determining liver dysfunction.

34. Answers include: hepatotoxic drugs, hepatitis B, hepatitis C

35. b. All health care workers should receive hepatitis B protection. Hepatitis B vaccine has just been added to infant's protection. Gloves or immune globulin may not fully protect an individual.

36. c.

37. d. HBIG and HBV are the recommended treatments for a hepatitis B exposure without prior protection.

38. private

39. b. Following hepatitis, individuals are hungrier in the morning and tend to have less appetite later in the day.

40. Answers include: detoxify substances, produce essential proteins, regulate glucose and bilirubin metabolism, serve as a blood volume regulator

41. d. An elevated blood pressure would not be observed in portal hypertension. The other symptoms would occur.

42. b. Thrombocytopenia does not cause fluid volume excess. Portal hypertension, hypoalbuminemia, and hyperaldosteronism do contribute to fluid volume excess.

43. b. Smoked ham is high in sodium. The client with cirrhosis of the liver should avoid salt in the diet. All the other foods listed contain little or no sodium.

44. Answers may include: confusion, altered mentation, altered motor function, changes in handwriting, speeech and development of asterixis, changes in personality, agitation, restlessness, inability to concentrate, altered sleep patterns, impaired judgment, forgetfulness

45. a   46. c

47. d. Hypoalbuminemia results in anasarca.

48. (a) diuretic, (b) aldosterone

49. c. Neomycin can interfere with the absorption of digoxin.

50. A sodium of 127 mEq/L indicates an overload of body water and hemodilution. Sodium below 125 mEq/L is an ominous sign and should be reported to the physician. The nurse should monitor the client for fluid volume overload and signs of hyponatremia.

51. A potassium of 3.6 mEq/L is low, but within normal limits. It should be monitored carefully. There is no urgent need to notify the physician. The nurse should monitor for hypokalemia and assess whether the client is on potassium-wasting diuretics or if the client is malnourished.

52. A GGT of 230 U/L is consistent with the diagnosis of cirrhosis. The physician would expect to see an elevated level with this diagnosis. There is no urgent need to report this finding. The client should be monitored for signs of decreasing hepatic function.

53. A glucose of 250 mg/dL is consistent with liver disease. This result should be reported to the physician so that appropriate therapy can be initiated. The nurse should monitor the client for signs and symptoms of hyperglycemia.

54. A serum albumin of 3.0 mg/dL is consistent with the diagnosis of cirrhosis. This low level may further contribute to edema. The physician should be notified of this laboratory finding and of the serum sodium level.

55. A prothrombin time of 24 seconds is markedly prolonged. The physician should be notified of this result as soon as possible. The nurse should protect the client from injury and monitor the client for signs and symptoms of bleeding.

56. d. This is the only correct response, the others are false.

57. d. The indications for a parencentesis are shortness of breath and labored respirations.

58. b. The client would experience some pain or discomfort, not severe pain.

59. a. Riopan is a low-sodium antacid and most appropriate for the client with cirrhosis.

60. Answers may include: monitor vital signs and for evidence of bleeding, avoid injections and other invasive procedures, apply pressure to venipunctures for at least 5 minutes, prevent constipation, institute bleeding precautions

61. Answers include: careful assessment of the nasal area for tissue damage, keep the head of the bed elevated to prevent aspirations, maintain suction and monitor drainage, release balloon pressures per protocol

62. b. Although antihistamines may be prescribed, they must be taken cautiously, as hepatic dysfunction may increase the risk for adverse drug reactions.

63. b. Evidence to date suggests that primary liver cancer is the result of chronic infections and environmental toxins.
64. Answers may include: malaise, anorexia, lethargy, weight loss, fever of undermined origin, fullness in epigastric area
65. c. Liver trauma places the client at high risk for bleeding—not ascites, hepatitis, or cirrhosis.
66. a. Repair of bleeding would necessitate a high abdominal or thoracic incision placing the client at risk for respiratory problems. Bleeding would not be expected. The client would be held npo until there is a return of bowel sounds. Ambulation is not appropriate immediately following surgery.
67. The onset of pyrogenic abscesses is sudden, and the onset of amebic abscesses is insidious.
68. Answers include: Flagyl (metronidazole), Diquinol (iodiquinol)
69. Answers include: avoiding contaminated food and water, washing hands thoroughly
70. a   71. a   72. b
73. Turner's sign
74. Cullen's sign
75. c   76. d
77. d. Pancreatic enzymes should be taken regularly, not just with symptoms.
78. c. A urine output of less than 20–30 mL/hr may suggest dehydration or impending renal failure and should be reported.
79. c. This position will increase comfort and may decrease the metabolic rate and rate of gastrointestinal secretion. The HOB should be elevated to prevent aspiration. The other positions may not promote comfort.
80. b. The diet should be low in fat, high in carbohydrate, and low in protein. The other diets would increase the secretion of pancreatic enzymes.
81. Answers include: frequency, color, odor, consistency
82. His major risk factors for pancreatic cancer include smoking, history pancreatitis, and a high fat diet (cheddar cheese).
83. The nurse should assess his vital signs, weight, perform an abdominal assessment, collect a urine specimen, and assess his skin for color or pruritus.
84. The nurse should acknowledge Mrs. Salvitori's distress over the diagnosis. The nurse should assess Mrs. Salvitori's knowledge about pancreatic cancer and her husband's specific situation. She should be provided with accurate information about her husband's condition and expected treatment. His prognosis will determine the level and type of support she will need at this point in time. An early diagnosis of pancreatic cancer may be treated effectively with surgery. Radiation and chemotherapy may also be used. Unfortunately, 85% of clients with pancreatic cancer are not diagnosed in time to receive treatments that will cure their cancer.
85. d. Irrigation of a Salem tube following a Whipple's procedure should only be done with a physician's order and only with minimal pressure. Forceful irrigations and repositioning of the tube may disrupt the suture line. Drainage would be expected following this type of surgery.
86. hemorrhage, hypovolemic shock, and hepatorenal failure
87. Monitor vital signs on a regular basis; monitor laboratory results; monitor intake and output (including all intravenous fluids, drainage tubes, and wound drainage); assess skin color, temperature, moisture, and turgor.

▪ ▪ ▪ **Chapter 16**

1. Answers include: skin, glands, hair, nails
2. f   3. c   4. a   5. e
6. g   7. b   8. d   9. a
10. b   11. d   12. c   13. a
14. (a) dead cells, (b) matrix, (c) lunula
15. (a) onset; (b) characteristics, course; (c) severity; (d) precipitating, relieving; (e) associated symptoms
16. Skin problems may be manifestations of other disorders, such as cardiovascular disease, endocrine or hepatic disease, or hematologic diseases.
17. Answers include: ruler, flashlight, rubber gloves
18. vitiligo. Vitiligo is an abnormal loss of melanin typically found over the face, hands, or groin; thought to be an autoimmune disorder.
19. anemia
20. keloid. Keloid is more commonly found in clients of African ancestry.

21. d
22. vascular
23. d   24. b   25. e   26. g   27. f
28. a   29. h   30. c   31. d
32. nutritional deficiencies
33. liver spots
34. c   35. g   36. b   37. d
38. f   39. a   40. e   41. d
42. c   43. e   44. a   45. b

▪ ▪ ▪ Chapter 17

1. c. Objective data observed in pruritus includes skin excoriation, erythema, wheals, changes in pigmentation, and infections. The other findings are not necessarily related to pruritus.

2. b. Pruritus may be the direct result of a drug reaction. Whenever possible, the physician would recommend stopping all unnecessary medication. Rubbing the skin with a dry towel and taking hot baths can only add to itching and drying. Eliminating citrus fruits will help only if they are the causative agent.

3. d. Hydrocortisone is the only anti-inflammatory listed. Vaseline and Lubriderm may help dryness, but will not affect the immune response. Xylocaine is an anesthetic and will relieve itching.

4. b. Creams with alcohol will cause skin drying and increase itching. All the other statements are actions that should be taken.

5. a. A therapeutic bath should not be too hot or too cold.

6. d

7. b. Limiting baths will limit drying. Hot water and deodorant soap are drying. Fluids and bath oils should increase moisture.

8. c. The use of extra soap will dry skin. The client should take less frequent baths, but use less soap. All of the other responses will decrease dryness.

9. f   10. a   11. c
12. e   13. b   14. a
12. b   13. d   14. c

15. d. This response acknowledges Hannah's feelings of self-esteem and body image. The other responses minimize her experience.

16. c. Topical lotions should be applied in a thin layer. Using a thick layer may reduce the medication's effectiveness.

17. c. Any client with skin lesions is at high risk for infection, as the body is the first line of defense.

18. a. The skin is the first line of defense, and keeping it clean helps minimize the risks of infection. Squeezing lesions and leaving draining lesions uncovered will only add to the spread of infection. If antibiotics are prescribed, they should be taken for the entire course prescribed. Taking antibiotics until the lesions disappear may result in resistance or a secondary infection.

19. d. The objective findings are consistent with a furuncle. Cellulitis is a localized infection of the dermis and subcutaneous tissue. Impetigo begins as vesicles or pustules, whereas erysipelas appears as firm, red spots that enlarge to form a circumscribed, bright red, raised, hot lesion.

20. b. Furuncles often appear in systemic diseases such as diabetes.

21. c. Systemic antibiotics are the primary treatment. The other measures may be used in combination with a systemic antibiotic, but they are not the primary intervention.

22. c. Careful and thorough hand washing is one of the most effective measures to prevent the spread of infection. Antibiotic soaps may not help if careful hand washing is not practiced. The other measures are not among the most effective or feasible.

23. b   24. c

25. c. Fungal infections are contagious. The other steps should be taken to reduce the risks of exposure to others.

26. d. Pregnancy, diabetes, and immunosuppression place individuals at higher risk for candidiasis infection. A 22-year-old following an appendectomy is generally not at high risk.

27. d. All family members and sexual partners must be treated for the parasite. Universal or body fluid precautions are not indicated. Ensuring that there are no eggs on the client's head does not mean that other members of the family have not been exposed or have the parasite.

28. c
29. The mother should be instructed to use a lin-dane-containing shampoo and apply it to Anissa's dry hair and massage it into the hair. A small amount of water can be added to help produce a lather. The head should be scrubbed for 4 minutes and then rinsed. The treatment may need to be repeated in 7 days. The hair should be combed with a fine tooth comb to remove the dead nits. Linens and clothing should be washed with hot soapy water or they should be dry cleaned. Ironing of clothes kills lice eggs. Personal care items, such as combs and brushes, should be boiled. All family members and their sexual partners should be treated. The use of combs, brushes, and hats of others should be avoided. Lice can infest anyone.
30. *Anxiety, Risk for Infection, Knowledge Deficit,* and *Impaired Skin Integrity*
31. The nurse should reassure the mother that this infestation is not related to poor hygiene or dirty living conditions. The mother should be instructed on how to prevent the spread of the infestation and on how to check her daughter for any recurrent infestations.
32. a. Contact isolation should be practiced unless the client is immunocompromised and requires strict isolation.
33. c. The most appropriate treatment is acyclovir (Zovirax), which is an antiviral. Topical steroids, antibiotics, and salicylic acid are not indicated.
34. c. The fact that the lesions have spread over the entire trunk, face, and thorax is indicative of disseminated herpes zoster.
35. c. Warm compresses are likely to make the skin itch more.
36. a
37. c. Dietary and environmental factors that cause the dermatitis must be identified and changes made. Medications do not necessarily prevent recurrence or cure the problems. Oral steroids should always be tapered prior to stopping them completely.
38. b 39. d 40. a 41. c
42. b. Isotretinoin (Accutane) is absolutely con-traindicated in pregnant women.
43. a. The cause of acne is multifactorial and poor hygiene may make acne worse, but it is not the cause.

44. When a client receives plasmapheresis, the plasma that contains autoantibodies is selec-tively removed. The antibody-free plasma is then reinfused into the client.
45. Answers include: skin care, oral care, diet, pain management, prevention of infection, medications
46. sepsis
47. allergic
48. Answers may include: fluid and electrolyte imbalances, blindness, urethral slough, sec-ondary infections, lacrimal duct occlusion, scarring and contractures, loss of nails, esophageal strictures, glomerulonephritis, dis-orientation, coma
49. b. The client is at high risk for infection, and reverse precautions will minimize risks within the environment.
50. d. If the client can ingest fluids, then cool or room temperature liquids would be best toler-ated, as they are nonirritating and easily swal-lowed. Warm fluid and foods would be irritating.
51. d. It is important the client monitor the lesions for any changes as these may indicate malignant changes. Seborrheic keratoses are not cancer, not a result of the sun, and are common in adults.
52. limit exposure to sun and use sunscreens.
53. carefully monitoring skin for any changes and seeking regular professional examinations.
54. c. Any lesion that does not heal within a 2-week period should be evaluated by a physician.
55. b
56. a. All of the answers are causes of non-melanoma skin cancer; however, ultraviolet radiation is most commonly implicated.
57. b. Fair skin individuals of Irish, Scandinavian, or English ancestry are more likely to develop nonmelanoma skin cancers.
58. d
59. punch   60. incisional
61. excisional   62. shaved
63. Answers may include: (a) minimize exposure to the sun between the hours of 10 AM and 3 PM; (b) wear a wide-brimmed hat, sun-glasses, long-sleeved shirt, and long pants; (c) use a sunscreen with an SPF of 15 or more on sunny days; (d) use sunscreen when you

are on or near sand, snow, concrete, or water; (e) avoid tanning booths

64. A: asymmetry, B: border irregularity, C: color variation, D: diameter greater than 6 mm

65. d

66. Answers include: teaching techniques for avoiding sun exposure, teaching skin self-examination, showing pictures of skin cancers

67. c

68. c. Using a pull sheet would minimize shearing forces. Keeping the HOB up, giving a massage, and using a donut-type device would only increase pressure.

69. a   70. d

71. Answers may include: black eschar, yellow slough

72. Due to slow wound healing in the elderly, the nurse should assess the client's mobility after his recent hip replacement. The nurse should also assess the caregiving capabilities of his elderly sister, as well as the client's nutrition, his finances, and the size and cleanliness of his wound.

73. b. When outdoors and treating superficial frostbite, one should apply firm pressure with a warm hand. Continued skiing might result in more severe frostbite. Hot compresses could result in tissue injury. Covering the nose with a scarf would do nothing to treat the already present frostbite.

74. c. In the hospital, severe frostbite is treated with rapid rewarming in circulating warm water.

75. excision   76. curettage

77. sclerotherapy   78. electrosurgery

79. cryosurgery   80. chemical destruction

81. c. A full-thickness skin graft contains both epidermis and dermis. They are not used on infected sites or areas with a poor blood supply.

82. c. The donor site should be protected from injury. Palpating the graft site is not indicated; positioning the client on the graft site may restrict blood flow; and if a dressing is present, it would not be changed every 2 hours.

83. d   84. c   85. a   86. b   87. e

88. b   89. d   90. e   91. d

92. A list of "at risk for" and actual nursing diagnoses includes *Ineffective Individual Coping, Risk for Self-Care Deficit, Body Image Disturbance, Self-Esteem Disturbances, Knowledge Deficit, Social Isolation,* and *Impaired Skin Integrity*.

93. a. Alopecia areata is characterized by patchy areas of hair loss on the scalp and other parts of the body. It is usually self-limiting and reverses without treatment, though it may reoccur.
    b. In contrast to alopecia areata, alopecia totalis involves all the scalp hair and is irreversible.

94. For her alopecia and exfoliative dermatitis, it would be important to assist Ms. Parker in identifying strategies to help her manage stress. These might include counseling, progressive muscle relaxation, stress management exercises or classes, physical exercise. Ms. Parker also may need help learning how to manage her condition. It would be important to ascertain that she has received an appropriate evaluation for her hair and skin problems and is receiving any appropriate medical therapies. She also may need assistance learning self-care routines, grooming her hair, or obtaining and styling a wig. For her birthmark, it would be important to assess her feelings regarding her appearance and strategies she has used to either cope with its appearance or change its appearance (makeup or other therapies). She may not be aware of medical interventions that might change the appearance of the birthmark. If she is not interested in exploring this option, she may be interested in working with a cosmetologist to cover the birthmark. Ms. Parker may also need to explore strategies to increase her self-esteem.

95. Outcome statements include: 1) The client will state an increased ability to cope with the stress of changing jobs. 2) The client will verbalize the need to start a stress reduction program prior to starting her new job. 3) The client will begin a stress reduction program prior to starting her new job. 4) The client will verbalize an understanding of her self-

care routines related to her hair and skin problems prior to starting her new job. 5) The client will choose and initiate interventions to assist her with her grooming and appearance prior to starting her new job.

▪ ▪ ▪ ▪ Chapter 18

1. b　2. a　3. d　4. a　5. c
6. Answers include: children, older adults
7. True
8. False. This is a minor burn injury.
9. True
10. True
11. d. Older adults are at higher risk for burns of all degrees of severity.
12. prevention
13. Answers include: massive infection, fluid and electrolyte imbalances, hypothermia
14. Burn shock
15. Answers include: fluid replacement, maintenance
16. Inhalation injury　17. Curling's ulcer
18. (a) ebb, (b) flow
19. c. The blood pressure rises as carbon dioxide increases and urinary output improves.
20. b. The compromise in the humoral and cell-mediated immune systems constitutes a state of acquired immunodeficiency, which places the burn client at risk for infection.
21. b　22. a　23. c　24. c　25. a　26. b
27. c. "Stop, drop, and roll" is done to extinguish the flame and limit the extent of the burn.
28. d. Use blankets to maintain body core temperatures at 99.6–101F.
29. Answers include: extent of the burn (percentage of body surface area involved), depth of the burn (layers of tissue affected)
30. a　31. c　32. b　33. c
34. Answers include: rule of nines, Lund and Browder method
35. c. lactated Ringer's most closely approximates the body's extracellular fluid composition.
36. a　37. c　38. b　39. d　40. f　41. e
42. Answers include: carry out hydrotherapy, apply skin grafts, calculate fluid replacement, maintain laminar flow environments, assess the extent and depth of the burn injury

43. Answers may include: physician, physical therapist, social worker, nutritionist, and burn technician
44. (a) indicates the presence of infection in sputum, blood, urine, and wound tissue; (b) indicates the client's nutritional status and the adequacy of renal perfusion; (c) decreased secondary to hemolysis; (d) elevated in the presence of infection and depleted in immuno-deficient states; (e) transiently elevated after major burn injury
45. Serial ABGs indicate the presence of hypoxia and acid-base disturbances, and indicate client responses to changes in oxygen therapies.
46. c. The intramuscular route of administration should be avoided until the client is hemo-dynamically stable and adequate tissue perfusion is restored.
47. Answers include: silver nitrate, silver sulfadiazine, mafenide acetate
48. d. To prevent Curling's ulcer, hyperacidity must be controlled. To control gastric acid secretion during the acute phase, histamine H_2 blockers can be administered intravenously.
49. Curling's ulcer, bowel obstruction, feeding intolerance, pancreatitis, and septic ileus.
50. (a) enzymatic, (b) surgical, (c) mechanical
51. a　52. b　53. d　54. b　55. c　56. a
57. True　58. True
59. False. The nurse should enhance mobility.
60. True
61. b. Powerlessness derives from the belief that one is unable to influence the outcome of a situation.
62. b　63. a　64. c
65. Answers include: sunburn, scald burn
66. b. Range-of-motion exercises are not a priority in this situation. Mild analgesics and implementation of alternative pain management therapies may be sufficient for minor burns. Liquid intake should be increased.
67. b. Swelling and erythema may be signs of impaired wound healing and/or infection. The other indicators demonstrate improvement.
68. d. Assessment of the airway is a priority, as inhalation burns may have occurred. The other assessments are important but not the highest priority.

69. d. Range-of-motion exercises should be performed to all joints every 2 hours as ordered. Antideformity positioning would be used and the client should be repositioned every hour. Lying still will lead to the development of contractures.

70. a. Psychological counseling is indicated. Antidepressants may be ordered if the episodes are severe or associated with suicidal ideation.

71. The purpose of hydrotherapy is to promote mechanical debridement, while the purpose of silver sulfadiazine is to eliminate infection of the surface of the burn wound.

72. The client and family need to understand the purpose of his treatment as well as how frequently they will be performed. The client and family need to understand how these interventions will contribute to eventual healing and preparation for skin grafting.

73. The nurse should first determine if and how the client's pain has been anticipated and managed before hydrotherapy treatments. He should be pre-medicated and if this has not occurred, perhaps offering medication will change his decision about not going for hydrotherapy. If this is not effective, the physician should be notified. Hydrotherapy is an important component of the client's care. Perhaps the physician can change the prescription for pain medication or increase the dose. It is important to develop a plan with the client that will ensure that he will cooperate with the plan of care.

74. The client's pain should be assessed on a regular basis and he should receive pain medication on a regular basis and prior to any painful treatments. All procedures should be explained and the client should understand any anticipated discomfort. Nonpharmacologic pain-relief measures may enhance pain relief. He should be encouraged to verbalize about his discomfort and his pain experience.

75. His white blood count and temperature should be monitored on a regular basis. He should maintain a high calorie and nutrient intake. Although the whirlpool is not a sterile environment, wound care should otherwise be performed using aseptic technique. His wounds should be monitored for evidence of infection.

■ ■ ■ **Chapter 19**

1. serves as an essential regulator of the body's internal environment and assists the body in adapting to constant alterations in internal and external environment

2. growth, reproduction, metabolism, fluid and electrolyte balance, and sex differentiation

3. e   4. c   5. a   6. b   7. d   8. d

9. g   10. f   11. d   12. h   13. f   14. b

15. c   16. f   17. e   18. d   19. e

20. (a) renin, (b) aldosterone

21. (a) stress, (b) depress

22. (a–b) endocrine, exocrine; (c–d) hormones, digestive enzymes

23. (a) Hormones, (b) endocrine, (c) target

24. b   25. d   26. c   27. a   28. b

29. manifestations of dysfunction are often non-specific and may affect all body tissues and organs.

30. a   31. client's family

32. the ability to recognize a familiar object using only the sense of touch

33. protruding eyes

34. excessive facial, chest, or abdominal hair

35. The nurse inflates a blood pressure cuff above the antecubital space to occlude the blood supply to the arm. Decreased calcium levels cause the client's hand and fingers to contract.

36. Using a finger, the nurse taps in front of the client's ear at the angle of the jaw. Decreased calcium levels cause the client's lateral facial muscles to contract.

37. d   38. e   39. g

40. e   41. e, h   42. i

43. h   44. c, g, h   45. d

46. a   47. a, b   48. c

49. inspect skin color; palpate skin; assess texture and condition of nails and hair; inspect facial symmetry and form; inspect position of eyes; palpate thyroid gland; assess deep tendon reflexes; assess for Trousseau's sign; assess for Chvostek's sign

50. c   51. a

52. subjective data: family history of obesity; feeling "dragged out"; prolonged stress and worry; chronic fatigue
objective data: weight 245 lb.; height 6' 1"; dry, rough, yellowish skin; dry, thick, brittle nails
possible etiologies: thyroid dysfunction; prolonged stress

53. Have you ever experienced any endocrine problems? If so, describe the problem and how it was treated. Do you drink alcohol? If so, what kind and how much? How do you care for your health in general? Have you experienced a recent weight gain or loss? If so, how many pounds over what period of time? Describe a typical 24-hour dietary intake. Have you experienced headaches, memory loss, changes in sensation, or depression? Have you experienced any pain or stiffness in your muscles and joints? Has anyone in your family had a condition similar to the one you are experiencing? What have you been doing to cope with your condition?

54. Mr. Thomas needs to learn the effects, dose, frequency, route, and side effects of his medication. He also needs to know the signs and symptoms that indicate whether his condition is improving or worsening. He also needs to know about the schedule of follow-up visits and laboratory tests. He needs to know that his condition will require lifetime monitoring and treatment.

55. A plan to manage his stress includes eating a well-balanced diet, exercising on a regular basis, modifying stressors, learning relaxation exercises, and getting adequate sleep.

▪ ▪ ▪ Chapter 20

1. Answers include: increased metabolic rate, cardiac output, peripheral blood flow, oxygen consumption, body temperature
2. thyrotoxicosis
3. Answers include: Graves' disease, toxic nodular goiter
4. multisystem autoimmune disorder
5. small, discrete, independently functioning nodules in the thyroid gland tissue that secrete TH
6. Thyroid crisis (thyroid storm)—an extreme state of hyperthyroidism. Manifestations may include hyperthermia, tachycardia, systolic hypertension, GI symptoms, agitation, restlesssness, and tremors.
7. goiter
8. thyroiditis   9. exophthalmos
10. subjective: increased appetite, agitation, restlessness, irritability, complaints of emotional

lability, palpitations, nausea, nervousness objective: weight loss, hypermotile bowels and diarrhea, heat intolerance and increased sweating, fine hair, smooth, warm skin, exophthalmos

11. c. All the other answers are clinical manifestations of hypothyroidism.
12. c. With hyperthyroidism there is an increase in the client's metabolism. The client would have an increased appetite.
13. a   14. a   15. a, b
16. b   17. b   18. a   19. b
20. d. Following a total thyroidectomy, a client would require lifetime therapy with thyroid medication and routine follow-up care. Weight loss or palpitations may indicate that the client is taking too much thyroid replacement. Propylthiouracil (PTU), which suppresses thyroid function, is not required following a total thyroidectomy.
21. (a) hypothyroid, (b) thyroid hormone replacement
22. c. It is common to administer iodine preparations prior to surgery to decrease the vascularity of the gland.
23. Answers include: administering antithyroid medications and iodine preparations, teaching the client how to support the neck, answering the client's questions and allowing the client to verbalize concerns
24. b. Assessment of a patent airway is of the highest priority. Other priority interventions include assessing breathing pattern and respiratory rate and blood pressure and pulse. The nurse should not expect to observe hypokalemia.
25. assess the client's ability to speak aloud, and note the quality and tone of the voice
26. c. Hypocalcemia may occur secondary to incidental removal of the parathyroid glands during a thyroidectomy.
27. tingling of toes, fingers, and lips; muscular twitches, positive Chvostek's and Trousseau's signs, and decreased calcium levels
28. Answers include: tracheostomy set, suction equipment, calcium gluconate or calcium carbonate
29. b. To protect the eye from injury and maintain visual acuity, the nurse uses artificial tears.
30. c. The client with hyperthyroidism needs a cool environment and adequate rest and

relaxation in order to conserve energy and maintain oxygen requirements.

31. Answers include: weigh and record the client's weight daily; teach the client to eat a diet high in carbohydrates and protein, with frequent between-meal snacks; monitor the client's serum albumin, transferrin, and total lymphocyte counts

32. increased serum thyroid antibodies, Graves' disease

33. serum TSH and T4

34. c. Because hypothyroidism is often characterized by a decrease in metabolic functioning, it is often confused with normal aging rather than identified as a pathologic process.

35. d. Primary hypothyroidism may be caused by the loss of thyroid tissue following treatment for hyperthyroidism with surgery or radiation or antithyroid medications. Secondary hypothyroidism is the result of pituitary TSH deficiency or peripheral resistance to thyroid hormone.

36. b

37. nonpitting edema in the connective tissues throughout the body, a puffy face, and an enlarged tongue

38. subjective: dyspnea, muscle stiffness, fatigue, decreased appetite
objective: fluid retention, edema, weight gain, constipation, dry skin, elevated serum cholesterol and triglyceride levels

39. Answers include: congenital defects; treatment of hyperthyroidism (surgery, radiation, antithyroid medications); thyroiditis or endemic iodine deficiency; pituitary TSH deficiency or peripheral resistance to thyroid hormones; iodine deficiency or Hashimoto's thyroiditis

40. Myxedema coma—a serious complication of extreme or prolonged hypothyroidism. It is characterized by severe metabolic disorders, hyponatremia, hypoglycemia, lactic acidosis, hypothermia, cardiovascular collapse, and coma.

41. (a) Hashimoto's thyroiditis, (b) females

42. a. Clients with hypothyroidism develop lipid abnormalities, including elevated serum cholesterol and triglyceride levels, which places clients at high risk for atherosclerosis.

43. d. Clients with hypothyroidism commonly experience edema, not dehydration. Expected clinical manifestations of hypothyroidism include slowed heart rate, weight gain, and dry skin.

44. elevated

45. a. Teaching for a client taking thyroid replacement hormones includes how to avoid excessive intake of foods that inhibit thyroid hormone utilization, such as spinach, cabbage, carrots, and peaches.

46. a. Answers (c) and (d) can be excluded because they are not electrolytes. A client who has not taken thyroid replacement hormone for long periods of time is at risk for developing myxedema coma. This is characterized by hyponatremia.

47. Answers include: decreased thyroid hormone, decreased T4, decreased T3

48. a. Frequent changes in position will help prevent tissue injury. Clients with hypothyroidism should avoid frequent bathing and alcohol-based lotions, which will further dry skin. Sheepskins and foam cushions may relieve pressure.

49. b. With the increase in PTH, there is an increased release of calcium and phosphorus by bones that results in subsequent fractures.

50. c. Although all of the laboratory data are important, excretion of phosphorus by the kidneys may lead to hypophosphatemia.

51. d. In hyperparathyroidism, large doses of Lasix (furosemide) are administered in an effort to lower calcium levels. Calcium levels are normally elevated, and thus calcium would not be administered. There is no indication for digoxin.

52. b. Clients with hyperparathyroidism are at risk for pathologic fractures, placing them at risk for injury.

53. b

54. d. The incidental removal of the parathyroid glands during thyroid surgery often results in hypoparathyroidism. Radiation, congenital defects, or cancer may result in hypoparathyroidism, but are not common causes.

55. (a) tetany, (b) death, (c) Chvostek's, (d) Trousseau's

56. a. In hypoparathyroidism, paresthesias, diarrhea, dry skin, and hyperactive reflexes are common clinical manifestations.

57. (a) vitamin D, (b) calcium

58. Altered glucose metabolism may lead to dia-

betes mellitus. Because of the hyperglycemia, the nurse could also see polyuria, polydipsia, and glycosuria.

59. Altered protein metabolism may lead to muscle weakness and wasting. There may also be poor wound healing.

60. Altered fat metabolism may lead to fat being deposited in the abdominal region (truncal obesity). The client may also develop a buffalo hump over the upper back and a "moon" face.

61. long-term administration of steroids

62. a. The other symptoms are associated with hypofunction of the adrenal gland.

63. c. Individuals at highest risk for Cushing's syndrome are those taking steroid preparations.

64. a

65. d. Excessive cortisol secretion in Cushing's syndrome results in sodium and water reabsorption.

66. the morning sample

67. elevated

68. a. Following a bilateral adrenalectomy, the client will require lifelong therapy with steroids.

69. body image disturbance

70. a private room. A client with Cushing's syndrome is at increased risk for infection and should be placed in a private room. There are no indications for protective isolation.

71. d   72. c   73. a, e, g

74. f   75. b

76. long-term, high-dose steroid therapy

77. a. In Addison's crisis the nurse would see decreased sodium, decreased blood glucose, increased potassium, and decreased cortisol level.

78. Place the client on cardiac monitoring because of the electrolyte abnormalities associated with Addison's disease. Administration of potassium may be appropriate, but only after cardiac monitoring is instituted.

79. c. This serum sodium level is very low, which increases the client's risk for seizures.

80. d. Weight gain may indicate fluid retention. Cortisol replacements should be taken with milk or food. The client should be instructed to eat a diet high in potassium, low in sodium, and high in protein. Individuals on cortisol replacement therapy should not abruptly stop therapy.

81. c. Fluid volume deficit occurs due to the loss of water and sodium. Potassium levels and the hematocrit will increase due to hemoconcentration.

82. b. The client with Addison's disease should sit and stand slowly to avoid orthostatic hypotension and dizziness. Generally a high fluid and salt intake is encouraged and potassium intake is limited.

83. d. These symptoms are associated with sympathetic stimulation.

84. c. This is the only appropriate answer. These tumors are most often benign.

85. benign adenoma

86. Answers may include: pituitary tumors, surgical removal of the pituitary, infarctions, infection, trauma, radiation

87. a   88. a   89. b   90. a

91. b   92. b   93. a   94. a

95. a, b, d, g

96. b. An increase in urine specific gravity would indicate that urine is less dilute and more concentrated.

97. vasopressin

98. d. In SIADH, hypertonic fluids are administered to correct fluid and electrolyte problems.

99. a. Oral fluids should be encouraged and not restricted. All other interventions are appropriate.

100. c. Fluids should be restricted to less than 800 cc/day. All other interventions are appropriate.

▪ ▪ ▪ Chapter 21

1. (a) chronic disorders, (b) pancreas

2. d

3. educator

4. (a) 8–16, (b) 4, (c) 7

5. (a) 200, (b) 4, (c) 6

6. c

7. (a) diabetes mellitus, (b–d) atherosclerosis, coronary artery disease, CVA (stroke)

8. Answers include: carbohydrates, fats, proteins

9. (a) glucagon, (b) decrease glucose oxidation and increase blood glucose levels

10. (a) insulin, (b) facilitating movement of glucose across the cell membrane, (c) the excessive breakdown of glycogen in the liver and the muscle

11. (a) somatostatin, (b) production of glucagon and insulin
12. e   13. a   14. b   15. d   16. c
17. (a) blood glucose, (b) increases, (c) 30, (d) 60, (e) 2, (f) 3
18. True   19. False   20. False
21. Answers include: epinephrine, growth hormone, thyroxine, glucocorticoids
22. c   23. a   24. a   25. b
26. b   27. a   28. b   29. a
30. True   31. False   32. True
33. Answers include: genetic predisposition, viral or toxic chemical agents, autoimmune attack
34. Answers include: polydipsia, polyuria, polyphagia
35. Answers include: weight loss, malaise, fatigue
36. (a) hyperglycemia acts as an osmotic diuretic, (b) glucose level exceeds renal threshold for glucose and is excreted in the urine, (c) increased urine output leads to dehydration and thirst, (d) glucose cannot enter cells without insulin, thus stimulating hunger
37. False   38. False   39. False
40. Answers may include: untreated IDDM, physical or emotional stress, infection, illness, missed insulin doses
41. Answers include: severe dehydration and acidosis
42. Answers include: lowering blood sugar, correcting fluid and electrolyte problems, returning pH to normal
43. d. Plasma bicarbonate would be less than 10 mEq/L. All other findings would be present.
44. fruity breath odor
45. Answers may include: heredity, obesity, increasing age, belonging to a high-risk ethnic group
46. Answers include: decrease insulin resistance, improve insulin release
47. c. The blood sugar may exceed 300 mg/dL, Type II diabetics may require insulin, and ketosis does not occur because whatever insulin is present prevents the breakdown of fat.
48. c. All other symptoms would be present, but polyphagia is rarely present in Type II diabetes.
49. True   50. False
51. True   52. True
53. b   54. c   55. e   56. a   57. d

58. a. The nurse would assess for hunger and nausea. The client would be hypotensive and anxious, with a rapid pulse, difficulty concentrating, and have moist skin.
59. True   60. False   61. True
62. False   63. True   64. False
65. True   66. True
67. subjective feeling of a change in sensation
68. isolated peripheral neuropathies affecting a single nerve
69. changes in sensation
70. d. The only symptoms of peripheral vascular insufficiency is intermittent claudication. The other symptoms are not consistent with arterial problems.
71. I   72. I   73. I   74. I   75. I
76. D   77. I   78. D   79. I
80. b. The diabetic should never go barefoot; pain at rest is a sign of severe arterial insufficiency; cracks, fissures, and calluses contribute to ulcerations and infections. An important outcome of foot care is the early detection of painless ulceration.
81. Answers may include: (a) increase fiber, limit fat and salt; (b) stop smoking; (c) engage in moderate exercise
82. Answers may include: chronic nature of the problem, dietary restrictions, income, physical limitations, cultural background, and visual/hearing deficit
83. False   84. True   85. True
86. c. An elevated glycosylated hemoglobin indicates poor diabetic control and would not be directly affected by diet intake the evening before. The client may require more insulin. This test does not reflect iron balances.
87. b. Aspirin should have no effect on the need for urine testing. All the other conditions would indicate a need for urine or blood testing.
88. d. The testing schedule for SGBM depends on the client's particular situation. Times any diabetic should test include hypoglycemia, hyperglycemia, and during illness.
89. b. Most strips are read by comparing the color against a chart.
90. d. Insulin needs remain constant or increase during illness and should be taken as ordered. The other statements are true.

91.

Insulin Type	Insulin Preparation	Onset of Action	Peak of Action	Duration of Action
rapid-acting	regular	½–1 hour	2–4 hours	4–6 hours
intermediate-acting	NPH	1–2 hours	8–12 hours	16–24 hours
long-acting	Protamine zinc	4–8 hours	16–18 hours	>36 hours

92. regular insulin
93. True   94. False   95. False
96. True   97. True
98. 90 degrees
99. a. Regular (clear) insulin is drawn first, and then intermediate-acting (cloudy) insulin is drawn up next.
100. Answers include: obtain a fingerstick BS, administer glucose
101. c. Blurry vision occurs related to the fluid changes. Seeing an ophthalmologist can be deferred for 8 weeks unless there are other indications for a visit. Blindness is a complication that can be minimized by good control, and these symptoms are not an allergic reaction.
102. The nurse should advise the client to take his regular dose of insulin and monitor his blood glucose level while he is ill.
103 (a) hypertrophy of subcutaneous tissue; (b) atrophy of subcutaneous tissue; (c–d) reusing injection sites; using cold insulin; (e) altered insulin absorption
104. D 105. D 106. I 107. I
108. I 109. D 110. D 111. I
112. (a) provide food plan teaching so that client maintains desirable weight; (b) teach client calories needed to attain and maintain reasonable weight; (c) individualized, with complex carbohydrates making up 90–95% of daily carbohydrates; (d) should be 10–20% of total daily kcal intake; (e) should be less than 10% of daily calories and cholesterol should not exceed 300 mg daily; (f) 20–35 g of fiber daily; (g) should be the same as for general population—no more than 2400–3000 mg per day; (h) no more than 2 alcoholic drinks at one time—use as a fat exchange; (i) use non-nutritive sweeteners—be careful of nutritive sweeteners
113. b. One tortilla is equal to one bread exchange or ½ cup rice.

114. d. Fluids are needed during illness to prevent dehydration. During illness, blood glucose would increase, blood sugar should be tested more frequently, and the client should take his/her regular dose of insulin.
115. a
116. b. High-impact aerobic exercise is not indicated for the client with DM. The client with DM can usually participate in low-impact aerobic exercise. All the other statements are true.
117. a, b, c, d, e
118. After initially treating hypoglycemia with 15 g of carbohydrates, wait 15 minutes and then, if still symptomatic, treat again with 15 g of carbohydrate.
119. c. The fastest way to increase the blood glucose is to administer IV glucose. The patient is unconscious and cannot take food or fluids. Glucagon would be appropriate in the outpatient setting, but does not elevate blood sugar as quickly as IV glucose.
120. b. Soaking feet in hot water may result in tissue injury. It is generally advised that the client wash the feet with warm water, but avoid soaking. All the other statements are true.
121. c. The potassium level will initially be normal, but will fall when insulin and fluids are given. During rehydration, the body loses potassium from increased urine output, acidosis, catabolic state, and vomiting or diarrhea.
122. b. The highest priority is to monitor for dysrhythmias, which may occur as the result of potassium loss.
123. electrolyte imbalances
124. d. An ingrown toenail should be evaluated and treated as soon as possible. The other interventions may cause trauma or delay appropriate treatment.

125. Answers include: have dental exams every 4–6 months; brush and floss teeth twice a day; report symptoms of dental/periodontal disease; if dental surgery is required, monitor blood glucose and need for adjustments of insulin

126. *Candida albicans* vaginitis

127.

Hypoglycemia Signs and Symptoms	Hyperglycemia Signs and Symptoms
hunger	thirst
nausea	warm, dry skin
anxiety	dry mucous
pale, cool skin	membranes
sweating	soft eyeballs
shakiness	weakness
irritability	malaise
rapid pulse	rapid, weak pulse
hypotension	hypotension
headache	nausea and vomiting
difficulty thinking	ketone breath odor
inability to	lethargy
concentrate	coma
change in emotional	abdominal pain
behavior	Kussmaul's
slurred speech	respirations
blurred vision	
decreasing levels of	
consciousness	
seizures	
coma	

128. c. This is the most appropriate response. The nurse does not have enough information to advise the client. The other answers are incorrect and do not elicit further information regarding the client's concern.

129. Answers may include: information regarding illness and signs and symptoms of hypo/hyperglycemia, diet planning, medications and medication administration, self-monitoring of blood glucose, relationship of blood glucose to exercise, healthy lifestyle

130. Five areas include: (a) difficulty in implementing diet, (b) exercise may not be part of activities of daily living and must be individualized, (c) the older adult may experience feelings of dependence and low self-worth, (d) money for care may not be available on a fixed income, and (e) visual deficits may make self-care difficult

131. Interventions include: assessing the client's priorities and providing teaching based on those needs, assisting the client with meal planning that is reflective of likes and dislikes, using language that the client understands, using positive reinforcement and setting goals that assist the client in adjusting to the disease, repeating and reinforcing information as many times as is necessary, using a variety of teaching materials, developing an exercise program that incorporates exercise in daily activities, and validating the person's knowledge and skills

■ ■ ■ **Chapter 22**

1. Answers include: duodenum, jejunum, ileum
2. All three structures increase surface area of the small intestine to enhance absorption of food.
3. Answers include: ascending colon, transverse colon, descending colon
4. anus
5. a 6. bowel sounds
7. a. Clients may feel embarrassed and hesitant to provide information about bowel elimination patterns. Choices (b), (c), and (d) do not acknowledge this. The nurse should not assume to know how the client is feeling or what the client is experiencing.
8. False
9. d. Begin the interview by inquiring about any medical conditions that may influence the client's bowel elimination pattern, such as a stroke or spinal cord impairment, inflammatory gastrointestinal diseases, or allergies. The other choices would come later in the interview.
10. a 11. d 12. e 13. c 14. b
15. b. Current use of anticholinergic drugs, antihistamines, tranquilizers, or narcotics may cause constipation.
16. Retention of flatus (gas) or stool may cause generalized abdominal distention.
17. Decreased bowel sounds suggest changes in colon motility and may be a sign of obstruction. Bowel sounds may be absent in later stages of a bowel obstruction or after surgery of the abdominal organs.

18. gurgling or clicking sounds that last from 5 to 30 seconds

19. d

20. d. The colon does not atrophy until after the age of 90 years.

21. Answers include: color, odor, consistency

22. a   23. melena

24. b. Greasy, frothy, yellow stools, called steatorrhea, may appear with fat malabsorption.

25. within. Blood on the stool results from bleeding from the sigmoid colon, anus, or rectum.

26. Answers include: rectal exam, anal exam, the client's stool

27. Answers include: inspection of the abdomen, auscultation of bowel sounds

28. (a) left lateral, (b) Sims'

29. b. The nurse should explain that this is a normal feeling. Choices (a) and (c) do not acknowledge the client's statement. Choice (d) is incorrect because it is unnecessary to interrupt the exam. This prolongs the procedure for the client.

30. Answers include: diarrhea, onset of bowel obstruction

31. Answers include: lack of bulk in diet, decreased fluid intake, decreased activity, laxative abuse

32. an involuntary release of feces from the rectum.

33. Answers include: lead a more active lifestyle, improve fluid and dietary intake

34. (a) anal fisures, (b) hemorrhoids, (c) prolapsed rectum

35. True   36. True

37. False. The finger must be rotated in both directions.

38. True

39. False. The nurse should lubricate the gloved index finger to enhance client comfort during the exam. Testing the feces for occult blood is not affected by the lubricant.

40. Subjective assessment data includes complaints regarding the presence or absence of pain and nausea, time as well as the date of last bowel movement and description of usual bowel pattern, personal and family history of gastrointestinal problems, and dietary history. Assessment questions should also address current medication routines, history of surgery, and usual bowel elimination patterns.

41. Objective assessment data includes auscultation of bowel sounds, and inspection, palpation, and percussion of abdomen. Respiratory and cardiac assessments should also be completed. Any bowel movements should be assessed for the presence of blood and described in terms of color, amount, odor, and consistency. If abnormal distention is present, measuring and recording abdominal girth may be indicated.

42. Assessment findings would include absence of nausea and vomiting and abdominal pain. Abdominal distention would be lessening while bowel sounds would return to normal. The nurse would expect that the client would start passing flatus per rectum and return to usual bowel elimination pattern. The client's abdomen would be soft and nontender when palpated.

▪ ▪ ▪ **Chapter 23**

1. direct: food intake and bacterial population
   indirect: psychologic stress and voluntary postponement of defecation

2. An increase in the frequency, volume, and fluid content of the stool.

3. Answers may include: water and electrolytes are lost; the client can become dehydrated; vascular collapse and hypovolemic shock may occur; potassium and magnesium are lost; the client may develop metabolic acidosis due to the loss of bicarbonate in the stool

4. Answers may include: stool specimen, stool culture, serum electrolytes, serum osmolality, arterial blood gases

5. a. A scope is inserted and advanced through the sigmoid colon.
   b. to report these symptoms to the physician as soon as possible.

6. c. The client should avoid food in the first 24 hours of acute diarrhea to provide bowel rest. Clear liquids should be encouraged if tolerated, milk should be avoided.

7. b. As a general rule, avoid taking aspirin while taking bismuth subsalicylate. Bismuth subsalicylate tablets should be chewed, not swallowed, for maximal effectiveness. The darkening of the tongue and stool that may be caused by this medication is harmless. This medication should not be taken for more than 24 hours.

8. Answers include: (a) Record intake and output, weigh the client daily, assess skin turgor. These assessments help monitor fluid volume status. (b) Monitor and record vital signs, including orthostatic blood pressures (BPs); if the BP drops more than 10 mm Hg when the client moves from a lying to a sitting position, or from a sitting to a standing position, orthostatic hypotension, an indicator of fluid volume deficit, may be present. It is typically accompanied by an increase in pulse rate. (c) Remind the client to seek assistance when getting up; the client with orthostatic hypotension may become dizzy or light-headed on rising.

9. Answers include: (a) Provide good skin care; poorly hydrated skin is at increased risk for breakdown. (b) Assist the client with cleaning the perianal area using warm water and soft cloths; this will help prevent tissue irritation and trauma. (c) Apply protective ointment to the perianal area. Protective ointment or creams help prevent breakdown of affected tissue.

10. (a) constipation, (b) presbycolon, (c) prevention

11. Answers may include: decreased activity, inadequate fluid intake, use of antacids containing aluminum or calcium salts, impaired health status, medications, low-fiber diet, large bowel diseases, pregnancy, chronic laxative use (see Table 23-2 of main text for other possible answers)

12. c. The client should avoid heavy lifting and straining for at least 7 days. He should avoid a high fiber diet for 1 to 2 days. Returning to activity too soon may result in bleeding from the site where polyps were removed.

13. c. Fluids are important to maintain bowel motility and soft stools. The client should eat less refined foods; increase the amount of fiber in the diet; and eat raw fruits and vegetables, which are good sources of dietary fiber.

14. b. The others are irritants.

15. c. The drug should be taken in the morning or with meals. To reduce the risk of impaction, the drug should not be taken at bedtime.

16. d. Grape juice is a gas-forming food.

17. True

18. b. A low-residue diet may be encouraged to reduce the frequency of defecation.

19. Glycerine suppositories help to stimulate evacuation.

20. Putting the client in the normal defecation position at a consistent time each day stimulates the defecation reflex.

21. Toilet tissue is more irritating to the skin and less effective in removing fecal material.

22. Applying skin cream will help protect the skin from irritating substances in the feces.

23. False. It is usually located in the *right* iliac region, at McBurney's point.

24. c. Antibiotic therapy with a third-generation cephalosporin effective against many gram-negative bacteria is initiated prior to surgery.

25. prevent complications

26. d. An increased pulse rate and rapid, shallow breathing can indicate perforation of the appendix. The temperature may be elevated and the blood pressure may fall if sepsis is present.

27. d. An elevated white blood count between 10,000/mm^3 and 20,000/mm^3 may be indicative of appendicitis.

28. b. Hematuria and pyuria may indicate a urologic cause for these symptoms. Microscopic hematuria and pyuria might be observed in acute appendicitis. These are not normal findings in any adolescent or adult and not consistent with a contaminated urine.

29. Answers may include: diminished or absent bowel sounds, diffuse or localized abdominal pain, boardlike abdominal rigidity, abdominal distention, abdominal tenderness with rebound, anorexia, nausea, vomiting, fever, malaise, tachycardia, tachypnea, restlessness, confusion, disorientation, oliguria

30. a. An older, chronically ill client may not experience the classic signs of peritonitis such as diffuse abdominal pain. They are more likely to experience confusion and restlessness, decreased urinary output, and vague abdominal complaints.

31. False   32. True   33. True   34. False
35. False   36. True   37. False

38. a. His skin turgor would be assessed every 4 to 8 hours. It is unnecessary to assess his skin turgor more frequently. All other interventions are appropriate.

39. (a) bacterial infections, (b) viral infections, (c) parasitic infections, (d) toxins
40. (a) production of endotoxins, (b) invasion and ulceration of the mucosa
41. e   42. f   43. d   44. a
45. b   46. g   47. c   48. b
49. Botulism
50. c. *Fluid Volume Deficit* is a priority nursing diagnosis, as is *Diarrhea.*
51. b   52. c   53. a
54. c   55. a   56. b
57. c. There are no medications that safely or effectively prevent protozoal infections of the bowel. All other reponses are correct.
58. b   59. a
60. d. Hand washing will help prevent the spread of a helminthic disorder. All the other responses are correct statements.
61. b   62. c
63. c. The other choices refer to Crohn's disease.
64. b. One should not take aspirin, vitamin C, or any other over-the-counter medication containing aspirin or vitamin C without con-sulting with the primary care provider.
65. d. During an acute exacerbation of ulcerative colitis, the client is usually kept npo. TPN is administered to maintain the client's nutri-tional status.
66. b   67. c   68. a
69. d. This behavior is not appropriate or indicated.
70. False   71. True   72. False
73. False   74. False
75. d. The physician should be contacted and the instructions clarified. Harsh bowel prepara-tions in any amount may exacerbate the disease.
76. A high-calorie, high-protein, low-fat diet with restricted milk and milk products (if client is lactose intolerant) is prescribed.
77. The client's likes and dislikes and usual dietary habits should be assessed. The client should be provided with food lists that describe high-calorie, high-protein, lowfat foods. Milk and milk products should be limited. The client should use nutritional supplements as pre-scribed. The family should be included in all diet and nutrition teaching. The client should understand the reasons for the importance of ensuring adequate nutrition.
78. d. The other choices are local manifestations of malabsorption.

79. (a) sprue, (b) lactose intolerance, (c) short bowel syndrome
80. Celiac disease
81. Tropical sprue
82. (a) wheat, (b) rye, (c) barley, (d) oats
83. d   84. a   85. c
86. e   87. d   88. b
89. The client and his family should be taught to monitor the frequency and character of the clients' stools. The client should monitor weight on a regular basis and report weight loss. The client should be taught to keep perianal area dry and clean. The client should increase oral fluid intake and ingest a gluten-free, lactose-reduced diet. The client should be provided with opportunities to explore how diarrhea affects one's lifestyle.
90. d
91. lower abdominal cramping, pain, and diar-rhea following milk ingestion.
92. (a) education, (b) support
93. significant portions of the small intestine are resected
94. Nursing care includes alleviating symptoms and providing frequent, small, high-calorie, high-protein feedings, multivitamin and mineral supplements, and adequate fluids. The client may need support managing diar-rhea and skin care in the perianal area. The client and family will need extensive educa-tion regarding the condition and ongoing care.
95. b   96. b   97. c   98. a   99. c
100. a. Regular follow-up is crucial to detect any future problems. The other responses are incorrect. Depending on the type of polyp, follow-up is usually at 1 year and 3 years with colonoscopy.
101. bleeding   102. b
103. b. The distal bowel carries no fecal contents and does not need irrigation.
104. a   105. c   106. b
107. c. The bag should be emptied when it is no more than one-third full so it does not affect the seal and cause leakage. A drainable bag should be applied so the skin is not irritated by frequent appliance changes.
108. c. In an abdominal perineal resection, the rectum and anus are removed and the colostomy is permanent.

109. a. These are the expected findings of a healthy stoma. The other findings are evidence of an unhealthy stoma and should be reported.
110. strangulated hernia
111. a. The risk of strangulation with any hernia makes this a high-priority nursing diagnosis.
112. An indirect hernia results from the improper closure of the tract that develops as the testes descend into the scrotum before birth. A direct hernia is an acquired defect that results from weakness of the posterior inguinal wall.
113. (a) obesity (b) pregnancy
114. Have the client pull into a sitting position from a lying position and assess for a bulge at the incisional site.
115. The client should be taught how to splint the incision and how to care for the incision. The client should be taught to avoid lifting for 2 to 6 weeks after surgery and to avoid driving for at least 2 weeks. The client should be taught about the dose, frequency, route, and side effects of any medications that are prescribed. The client should be encouraged to eat a well-balanced diet and to drink adequate amounts of fluid.
116. (a) paralytic ileus, (b) mechanical obstruction
117. (a) adhesions, (b) surgery, (c) inflammatory processess
118. Manifestation of a small bowel obstruction includes cramping or colicky abdominal pain that may be intermittent. Vomiting is common.
119. The most common manifestations of a large bowel obstruction are constipation and abdominal pain. Vomiting is a late sign. The abdomen is distended with high-pitched bowel sounds.
120. Complications include hypovolemia and hypovolemic shock with organ failure, strangulation, death, fluid and electrolyte disturbances, dehydration, renal insufficiency, and respiratory distress.
121. b
122. a. A high-fiber diet increases stool bulk, decreases intraluminal pressures, and may reduce spasm.

123. c. This diet selection has the highest amounts of fiber. Raw apples must be peeled, white bread or bagels are not wholegrains. Bananas are not a high-fiber fruit.
124. Symptoms include pain, constipation or an increased frequency of defecation. Nausea, vomiting, and a low-grade fever may be observed. A distended abdomen, tenderness, and a palpable mass may also be noted.
125. The care for uncomplicated diverticulosis is changes in diet. The care for acute diverticulitis is bowel rest and broad-spectrum antibiotic therapy. Surgery may be required.
126. c. Drink at least 2000 mL of fluid per day.
127. hemorrhoids
128. a 129. b 130. c
131. False. These clients should maintain a high-fiber diet and liberal fluid intake to increase stool bulk and softness, thus decreasing discomfort with defecation.

■ ■ ■ **Chapter 24**

1. Answers include: to regulate body fluids, to filter metabolic wastes from the bloodstream, to reabsorb needed substances and water into bloodstream, to eliminate metabolic wastes and water as urine
2. c
3. Answers may include: regulate acid-base balance; excrete metabolic waste products; balance solute and water transport; conserve nutrients; form urine; and secrete hormones to help regulate blood pressure, erythrocyte production, and calcium metabolism
4. (a) The cortex contains glomeruli that bring blood to and carry waste products from the functioning units of the kidneys (nephrons); (b) the medulla contains collecting tubules that channel urine into the innermost region, the renal pelvis; (c) the renal pelvis contains branches that collect urine and empty it into the pelvis for movement through the ureter and storage in the bladder.
5. a   6. g   7. c   8. f   9. d
10. e   11. h   12. a   13. b
14. A passive, nonselective process in which fluid and solutes are forced through a membrane by hydrostatic pressure; influencing factors

include total surface area available for filtration, permeability of the filtration membrane, and net filtration pressure.

15. c   16. (a) 1.5, (b) 8

17. c. An elevated white blood count in the urine is indicative of an infection. It is not a normal finding, or consistent with mucous. Any uninfected urine specimen should not have such an elevated white blood count.

18. b. An increased specific gravity is consistent with dehydration and fluids should be encouraged, not restricted. This is not a normal finding and the nurse should not increase the IV rate without an order.

19. Answers may include: negative to trace of protein, negative glucose, pale to deep yellow or clear color, negative ketones, pH between 4.5–8.0, specific gravity between 1.001–1.030

20. tubular reabsorption

21. d

22. (a) erythropoietin, (b) natriuretic hormone

23. Erythropoietin stimulates bone marrow to produce red blood cells in response to tissue hypoxia. The stimulus for production from kidneys is decreased oxygen delivery to kidney cells. Natriuretic hormone is released from the right atria of the heart in response to increased volume. Its presence inhibits ADH secretion, causing large amounts of dilute urine to be produced.

24. e   25. b   26. f   27. c   28. d

29. a   30. b   31. c   32. c

33. uremic frost 34. a.   35. b

36. (a) stress incontinence, (b) prostate enlargement

37. a

38. nocturia, frequency, urgency

39. complaints of frequency, urgency, dysuria, report of fluid restriction

40. urine is positive for white blood cells and bacteria, tenderness in the suprapubic area, kidneys nontender to palpation and percussion

41. Questions should be asked about her usual urine elimination pattern, history of urinary infections or disorders and their treatment, age, general health, current medication therapy, likelihood of pregnancy, history of renal colic, personal hygiene habits, history of incontinence, time and amount of last voiding, lifestyle, and health habits.

▪ ▪ ▪ Chapter 25

1. c   2. acidic   3. d

4. (a) they prevent the flushing action of voiding, (b) they act as a conduit for ascension of bacteria into the urinary tract

5. d

6. Answers may include: nocturia, incontinence, confusion, behavior changes, lethargy, anorexia, "not feeling well," hyperthermia or hypothermia, classic symptoms

7. b

8. (a) a Gram's stain allows for rapid identification of the probable pathogen and timely therapy, (b) urine culture and sensitivity allows for definitive identification of the infecting organism and the prescription of the proper antibiotic

9. b

10. c. Cranberry juice contributes to urine acidity.

11. d. Sulfa drugs, such as Bactrim (sulfamethoxazole), may turn the urine orange.

12. (a) sulfonamides are poorly absorbed in urine and may crystallize if the urine output falls, (b) clients receiving oral hypoglycemic agents are at increased risk for hypoglycemia, (c) sulfonamides potentiate the effects of oral anticoagulants

13. a. A small percentage of clients on Macrodantin (nitrofurantoin) may develop interstitial pneumonitis.

14. Answers include: for increased compliance; to lower the rate of side effects; for reduced cost

15. c. Kidney pain is often referred to flank pain.

16. Lab tests would show: urinalysis with a bacteria count of greater than 100,000; a urine culture that identifies the infective organism; and an elevated WBC with increased neutrophils.

17. b. Choice (a) is a true statement; however, it is not a therapeutic response. Choice (c) would give the client false hopes that the pain will be obliterated. A sitz bath would provide only some relief.

18. b

19. c. Drinking cranberry juice or orange juice will keep the urine pH lower than 5 and inhibit bacterial growth.

20. b. Increased fluids help prevent urostasis and the formation of stones.

21. c. Anticholinergics reduce vasospasm of the ureters.

22. a. Stones are analyzed to determine their constituents and thus help in establishing a medical plan to prevent stone formation.
23. c
24. (a) lithotripsy, (b) hemorrhage and shock, (c) red, (d) cloudy
25. b
26. Answers include: nausea, vomiting, pallor, cool and clammy skin
27. (a) chills, fever, frequency, urgency, dysuria; (b) gross or microscopic hematuria; (c) impaired urine outflow, urinary stasis; vague abdominal, back, or flank pain with slow development; severe pain in flank or genital region with acute development
28. (a) to maintain patency and promote healing of ureters; (b) careful labeling facilitates close monitoring of output from all sources; (c) the stent can precipitate calculus formation and urinary tract infection, and fluids will help prevent these complications
29. a. This is the only method that ensures an accurate 24-hour collection.
30. Answers include: presence of carcinogens in the urine; inflammation or infection of the bladder mucosa
31. d   32. c
33. Answers include: removal or destruction of the cancerous tissue, prevention of further invasion of metastasis, maintenance of renal and urinary function
34. d. Remaining perfectly still is not necessary during the treatment. The other statements are true.
35. c   36. a   37. d   38. b
39. f   40. e   41. d   42. d
43. a. A dark purple stoma may indicate a decreased blood supply and should be reported immediately.
44. Answers may include: Use therapeutic communication techniques, actively listening and responding to the client's and family's concerns. Recognize and accept behaviors that indicate the use of coping mechanisms, encouraging use of adaptive mechanisms. Encourage the client to look at, touch, and care for the stoma and appliance as soon as possible. Discuss client and family concerns about returning to usual activities, perceived changes in relationships with family and friends, and resumption of sexual relations.

Initiate referral to a support group or provide for contact with someone who has successfully adjusted to a urinary diversion.
45. The cystectomy client will need to learn about external appliances and skin care, while the client with a Koch's pouch will need to learn about clean intermittent self-catheterization.
46. b. Detrusor muscle tone is lost in a chronic overfill condition.
47. Answers may include: BPH; surgery, especially abdominal or pelvic; medications; voluntary urinary retention; mechanical obstructions
48. (a) prevents overdistention and retention, (b) promotes detrusor muscle contraction and bladder emptying, (c) enables urine to flow by gravity
49. (a) 400; (b) trauma; (c–d) central, peripheral; (e) neurogenic; (f) neuropathies; (g) diabetes mellitus
50. (a) increase sphincter tone.
    Example: NeoSynephrine (phenylephrine HCI)
    (b) stimulate contraction of the detrusor muscle in flaccid neurogenic bladder.
    Example: Urecholine (bethanechol)
    (c) relax the detrusor muscle and contract the internal sphincter.
    Example: Ditropan (oxybutynin chloride)
    (d) increase the tone of detrusor muscle.
    Example: Mestinon (pyridostigmine)
    (e) decrease internal sphincter tone.
    Example: Dibenzyline (phenoxybenzamine)
51. b. Autonomic dysreflexia may occur.
52. Answers include: the ability of the bladder to expand and contract, the ability of the sphincters to maintain a urethral pressure higher than that in the bladder
53. c   54. a   55. b   56. e   57. d
58. (a) enlarged prostate; (b) weak abdominal and pelvic muscle tone, cystocele or urethrocele, atrophic vaginitis
59. c
60. Answers include: use of analgesia, deep breathing, movement after surgery, avoid straining, and Valsalva maneuver
61. Answers include: bright red urine, excessive vaginal drainage, incisional bleeding
62. self-care, recognizing signs of possible complications
63. Voiding and stopping the flow of urine midstream are the steps of a Kegel's exercise.

64. Limit intake of caffeine, alcohol, citrus juices, and artificial sweeteners. Fluids should be limited to 1.5–2 liters per day.

■ ■ ■ **Chapter 26**

1. (a) 20 million, (b) 1, (c) 1000
2. b   3. (a) 1:10, (b)1:15   4. higher
5. Answers include: arteriosclerosis, a smaller renal vascular bed, decreased cardiac output
6. half
7. creatinine clearance
8. Answers include: cardiac drugs, antibiotics, histamine H_2 antagonist, antidiabetic agents
9. b   10. d   11. c   12. a
13. c. There is an increased incidence of incompetent cardiac valves in clients with polycystic kidney disease. Hypertension is also a clinical manifestation seen with polycystic kidney disease.
14. (a) 30 and 40
15. Answers include: hematuria, flank pain, proteinuria, polyuria, nocturia
16. have no associated systemic disease
17. d. Fluids should be encouraged to promote elimination of the dye. The client should be npo before, not after, the procedure; the nurse should not expect pain; and conductive gel is used for an ultrasound, not a CT scan.
18. a. Fluids should be encouraged, not restricted.
19. Vesicoureteral reflux is the backflow of urine from the bladders to the ureters.
20. preserve kidney function
21. c. Recurrent hydronephrosis may result in these symptoms and may occur if the tube is blocked. The nurse should assess the client further before medicating for pain. A nephrostomy tube is usually not irrigated, unless there is a specific order. These symptoms are not consistent with anxiety.
22. b
23. infection of the pharynx or skin with Group A beta-hemolytic streptococcus
24. c
25. Answers include: massive proteinuria, hypoalbuminemia, hyperlipidemia, edema
26. a. The entire procedure takes about 10 minutes and is uncomfortable but not painful.

27. b
28. d. Strep throat is caused by Group A beta-hemolytic streptococcus and is a precipitating factor in acute glomerulonephritis. She should be evaluated as soon as possible.
29. Answers may include: hematuria, proteinuria, salt and water retention, edema, hypertension, azotemia, fatigue, anorexia, nausea and vomiting, and headache
30. b. Bleeding can co-occur with Goodpasture's syndrome. The priority for the nurse is to assess for bleeding and monitor respiratory status.
31. b. The erythrocyte sedimentation rate is elevated in inflammatory conditions.
32. (a) kidneys, (b) ureters, (c) bladder
33. Void and discard her urine at 10:00 AM. All voided urine specimens should be collected in a container for a 24-hour period. The last specimen should be collected at 10:00 AM the next morning and placed in the 24-hour urine container. The client should keep the urine container on ice during the collection period.
34. (a) 5–20, (b) 0.5–1.1, (c) 0.5–1.2
35. b. When taking this medication, the client should protect against pregnancy. The other statements are true.
36. c. Maintaining the ordered fluid restriction is critical to preventing further edema. Oral or IV fluids should not be encouraged, nor should food high in sodium, as these actions will result in worsening edema.
37. b. Balancing activity and rest should minimize fatigue. Fatigue may only worsen in time and eating high-calorie foods will not necessarily increase energy. Telling him that he has to accept fatigue does not provide support or understanding.
38. c. Clients with renal disease have a depressed immune function and are at much higher risk for infection.
39. c. This statement encourages verbalization and provides support and understanding. The client should be assisted to address these issues with her family.
40. d. The kidneys depend on adequate blood flow.
41. c. Renal artery stenosis can cause secondary hypertension.
42. (a) 120, (b) 150–170

43. a. An elevated blood pressure in an individual under age 30 with an epigastric bruit may have renal artery stenosis and should be evaluated as soon as possible. The other responses would not be appropriate.

44. b. Hematuria is a common symptom of renal cell carcinoma. The other symptoms are not consistent with renal cell carcinoma.

45. Answers may include: fever, fatigue, weight loss, anemia

46. a. A nephrectomy requires a large incision and results in severe pain. The other interventions may be appropriate, but are not of the highest priority.

47. b. Bleeding is not expected and may indicate hemorrhage. It is not appropriate to start a continuous bladder irrigation or simply monitor the bleeding.

48. a. A fluid intake between 2000 to 2500 mL will prevent dehydration and help dilute any nephrotoxic substances.

49. c. Gymnastics should be avoided due to the chance of falls leading to kidney trauma.

50. postrenal   51. intrarenal
52. intrarenal   53. postrenal
54. prerenal   55. prerenal

56. c. In ARF, the specific gravity is fixed at 1.010.

57. a. Fluids should be increased to 2 to 3 L.

58. Answers include: BUN, creatinine, serum electrolytes

59. b. Older men are prone to prostatic disease, which can lead to a postrenal obstruction. The other situations do not place individuals at high risk for postrenal failure.

60. c   61. a

62. Diuresis indicates that the nephrons have recovered sufficiently to eliminate urine. However, they still are unable to eliminate waste production; hence, the continued rise in the BUN and creatinine.

63. c. Dopamine increases renal blood flow; it does not have any of the other actions.

64. a. With several loose stools, potassium will be lost, which is the desired outcome of taking Kayexalate.

65. d. The aluminum binds with phosphate and is excreted in the feces.

66. b

67. b. In PD, the peritoneum is the dialyzing membrane. In HD and PD, fluid and nephro-

toxins are removed. They can both be used in acute renal failure.

68. a. Hyporeflexia would not be observed. Hyperreflexia, paresthesias, and tetany would be observed.

69. c. All oral fluids have to be measured during acute renal failure.

70. d. Fluid and dietary recommendations must be followed as prescribed. She may be on a diet that controls the intake of protein.

71. c. Native Americans (and African Americans) have 3 to 4 times the incidence of end-stage renal disease when compared to European Americans

72. b. Edema is also seen, but is not the most common clinical manifestation.

73. b. Maintaining safety is critical for the client with progressive uremia. With progressive uremia, the client will have weakness, lethargy, and confusion. The other actions are inappropriate.

74. c. PD offers the control of treatment to the client. The other statements are false.

75. a. The client would be npo prior to surgery. The other actions should be taken.

76. Answers include: clotting, aneurysms, infection

77. b. The hematocrit drops in ARF as a result of reduced erythropoietin levels.

78. b. A diminished urine output following vascular surgery may indicate impending renal failure.

79. c. Lasix (furosemide) should be taken in the morning so as not to interrupt sleep patterns. If two or more doses are ordered, the last dose should be taken with the evening meal.

80. a

81. d. Clients on hemodialysis may void very infrequently.

82. b. Tenderness at the graft site is consistent with rejection of a kidney.

83. Answers may include: monitoring urine output every 30 to 60 minutes, maintaining adequate fluid replacement, monitoring electrolytes and urinary function, maintaining a closed urinary drainage system.

84. (a) addressing concerns, (b) reducing anxiety

85. (a) bacterial and viral infections, (b) tumors, (c) congenital anomalies, (d) bone problems, peptic ulcer disease, and cataract formation

▪ ▪ ▪ Chapter 27

1. d   2. c   3. f   4. e   5. h
6. g   7. j   8. a   9. d   10. b
11. c   12. i   13. a
14. (a) sympathetic, (b) parasympathetic
15. ejection fraction
16. stroke volume
17. c   18. b
19. From sinoatrial node, across atria, via internal pathways to atrioventricular nodes; then through bundle of His, down interventricular septum, through right and left bundle branches, and out to Purkinje fibers in ventricular walls
20. Depolarization   21. c
22. cardiac output   23. chief complaint
24. c
25. Answers include: apical impluse, retraction, lift, heave
26. b   27. i   28. g   29. c
30. h   31. k   32. a   33. j
34. e   35. f   36. d
37. Age and male gender may increase the risk of cardiac problems. Recurrent episodes of tachycardia and repeated episodes of abnormal cardiac findings increase the likelihood of finding an ongoing, abnormal cardiac condition. Lightheadedness, vertigo, and transient numbness of the left arm are symptoms that suggest occlusive disorders (an imbalance between supply and demand of oxygenated blood to the tissues). A history of smoking supports the risk for carotid artery and/or coronary artery occlusive disease. Symptoms of increasing fatigue and orthopnea would raise the suspicion of some cardiac failure, as in congestive heart failure (CHF). A positive family history increases client's risk of heart disease. He doesn't eat red meat, which shows that he has some knowledge of cholesterol, but he may have a knowledge deficit regarding other foods that are high in cholesterol. His alcohol intake needs to be further explored. Hypertension and tachycardia suggest that the heart is working hard to meet body needs. Bigeminy, atrial, and ventricular gallops are irregular heart rhythm and abnormal heart sounds which support the diagnosis of atrial dysfunction and myocardial failure.

38. apical impulse   39. d
40. (a) locate the major auscultatory areas on the precordium, (b) choose a sequence of listening, and (c) listen first to the client in the sitting or supine position, then with the client lying on the left side, and with the client sitting up and leaning forward. Listen in each area and position using the bell and diaphragm and the effect of respirations on each heart sound.
41. f   42. d   43. a   44. c
45. g   46. i   47. h
48. (a) thickening and hardening in the valves, (b) decrease in cardiac reserve, (c) fibrosis of the conduction system
49. True   50. False
51. False   52. False

▪ ▪ ▪ Chapter 28

1. (a) SA node, (b) 60–100, (c) AV node, (d) ventricles, (e) atrial kick, (f) bundle of His, (g) right and left bundle branches, (h) Purkinje fibers, (i) AV node, (j) Purkinje fibers, (k) slower
2. i   3. a   4. f   5. j   6. c
7. e   8. d   9. g   10. h   11. b
12. b   13. e   14. d   15. c   16. f
17. heart block
18. >100 per minute
19. c. Answers a, b, and d result in tachycardia.
20. (a) rapid heart rate, (b) inadequate ventricular filling.
21. atrial flutter
22. a. A 24-year-old, 6 hours following elective surgery, has no risks that would require monitoring. All the other clients would require monitoring.
23. d. Lidocaine is the drug of choice. Answers (a) and (b) would slow the rate, but not quickly enough in an emergency situation. Answer (c) is contraindicated because it will increase the rate.
24. b. The nurse must first assess the client to ascertain that the flat line is due to cardiac dysrhythmia rather than a mechanical problem.
25. c. Everyone must be "all clear" to avoid electrical injuries.

26. c. Initially, movement of the affected shoulder and arm should be restricted. Gentle ROM can start 24 hours after implantation. This activity restriction allows the leads to become anchored and minimizes the risks of dislodging.

27. b. This description is an AICD (automatic implantable cardioverter-defibrillator).

28. Answers may include: removing damaged electrical equipment from the client's room; wearing rubber or plastic gloves when handling equipment, testing the pacemaker battery prior to use; using ground equipment; insulating pacemaker terminals and wires with nonconductive, moisture-proof materials

29. a. The latest protocols for performing CPR recommend calling for help after assessing responsiveness.

30. defibrillation

31. d. If the client is alert and talking, thus tolerating the rhythm, the nurse has time to more adequately assess the situation.

32. CAD is the accumulation of atherosclerotic plaque in the coronary arteries that obstructs flow to the myocardium.

33. d

34. c. One can stop smoking, but one cannot modify one's gender, age, or race.

35. (a) 30%, (b) abdominal

36. LDL (low-density lipoprotein), HDL (high-density lipoprotein)

37. c. Smoking is the number one risk factor for heart disease. Providing this information may help the client understand the importance of quitting smoking.

38. (a) cigarette smoking—offer smoking cessation strategies, (b) obesity—provide information about weight-loss programs, provide diet teaching, (c) physical inactivity—provide education about the importance of regular physical activity, (d) personality type—provide information about stress reduction or modification, (e) women only: use of oral contraceptives—teach women on birth control pills about the importance of not smoking and the importance of modifying lifestyle risk factors that might contribute to CAD

39. c. This is the only correct answer. He should reduce his fat and cholesterol intake. Accepting it as normal or borderline high and not implementing a diet change would be inappropriate. Usually the cholesterol is interpreted along with the lipids.

40. c. The other diet selections include foods high in cholesterol (eggs, low-fat cream cheese) or foods potentially too high in fat (home fries, bran muffin). This diet choice is also high in fiber.

41. c. Muscle aches (myalgias) are potentially serious side effects of the cholesterol-synthesis inhibitors, such as lovastatin.

42. (a) supply, (b) demand

43. b. Angina can result from emotional stress or other factors such as excessive environmental temperatures. It is usually located substernally with radiation to the neck or left arm, and usually lasts no more than 10–15 minutes.

44. (a) downward sloping, (b) flattened, (c) inverted

45. d. ST depressions are positive findings during an exercise ECG.

46. (a) nitroglycerin, (b) sublingual

47. a. Taking the nitroglycerin every 5 minutes for three doses is the customary maximum dosage.

48. remove the patch or ointment at night and reapply it in the morning

49. Answers include headache, nausea, dizziness, hypotension

50. b. Atropine is an anticholinergic that decreases vagal tone and increases heart rate. Bradycardia is an unexpected complication of sheath removal. Oxygen and bedrest may also be appropriate, but are not priority interventions. An ammonia inhaler will not produce a quick enough response.

51. d. Recurrent chest pain may indicate ischemia and possible myocardial infarction. Chest pain is not an expected response and should be treated aggressively.

52. c. Following open heart surgery it is important to differentiate incisional and anginal pain. Then the nurse can implement appropriate interventions.

53. b. Assisting her to sit up and deep breathe will assist her to improve respiratory function by increasing lung expansion and helping her to mobilize secretions. Suctioning would only be appropriate if she is unable to deep breathe and expectorate secretions. A nurse does not

reintubate clients. A face mask might be helpful if the rate of oxygen flow is increased, but it is not the priority intervention.

54. c. The client will be npo after midnight the evening before the procedure; he should notify the catherization team if he experiences shortness of breath or chest pain during the procedure so that nitrate therapy or channel blockers are administered; he will be awake during the procedure, although a mild sedative will be administered.

55. Answers may include: frequently assess vital signs to detect any signs of retroperitoneal bleeding; assess for increased BP or heart rate, which might induce angina; frequently check catheterization site for bleeding or hematoma; check peripheral pulses and monitor color, sensation, and mobility (CSM) of lower extremities; maintain the client on complete bed rest

56. inferior (II, III, and AVF)

57. Answers may include: serum electrolytes, BUN, creatinine, CBC, PTT, cardiac enzymes

58. True

59. a. Choices (b), (c), and (d) may predispose a client to a myocardial infarction, but they are not the pathology that actually causes the infarction.

60. clot or thrombus

61. (a) left ventricle, (b) LAD

62. The pain of a myocardial infarction lasts longer (>15–20 minutes); is not always associated with activity or stress; is unrelieved by nitroglycerin; and is often accompanied by tachycardia, cold and clammy skin, nausea and vomiting.

63. dysrhythmias

64. b. The left ventricle is the largest muscle, or workhorse, of the heart and bears the major responsibility for cardiac output.

65. c   66. a   67. a

68. the inability of the heart to function as an effective pump

69. a. Chronic heart failure in African Americans is most frequently related to long-term, uncontrolled hypertension.

70. Answers include: Frank-Starling mechanism, neuroendocrine response, ventricular response

71. b. Marked dyspnea and rhonchi throughout the lungs are late manifestations of left-sided failure, and dependent edema may indicate

that right-sided failure has also occurred.

72. left-sided heart failure

73. b. The pulse may be full, bounding, or weak, but not thready. A thready pulse is a manifestation of shock.

74. d. Canned soups and meats, even those labeled as "low salt" or "lower salt," often have a high content of sodium.

75. left ventricular function and/or overall cardiac functioning

76. d. These symptoms are most consistent with pulmonary edema. The other conditions are possible, but not the most probable.

77. d. He should contact his physician as this weight gain is excessive. The other actions are inappropriate without first consulting with the physician.

78. c. He should contact his health care provider as these symptoms are consistent with digoxin toxicity. The other interventions are not appropriate without consulting with his health care provider.

79. Balancing activity, meals, and rest; when to stop activity; avoiding straining; beginning a graded exercise program; following a low-salt diet; signs and symptoms to report; and medication, dose, frequency, route, and side effects.

80. Left-sided heart failure: Causes include left ventricular muscle damage or overloading. Symptoms include dyspnea, shortness of breath, crackles, orthopnea, dry and hacking cough, tachycardia, palpitations, pallor, decreased urine output, activity intolerance, fatigue, weakness.
Right-sided heart failure: Causes include pulmonary hypertension or right ventricular infarction. Symptoms include elevated central venous pressure, jugular venous distention, peripheral edema, liver enlargement and tenderness, ascites, nausea, anorexia, abdominal distention, nocturia, hepatojugular reflux, and fatigue.

81. b. The other options are appropriate interventions, but are not goals.

82. (a) morphine sulfate, (b) intravenous

83. a. Pulmonary edema is a medical emergency. Delaying treatment could result in hypoxia, organ failure, or death. Calling the physician is the only correct option.

84. False   85. True   86. False

87. True   88. False

89. b. As blood backs up from the stenosed mitral value, fluid accumulates in the lungs.

90. d. Disturbance in the blood flow can result in stagnation of blood and clot formation. This can lead to an embolic stroke (CVA).

91. c. In aortic stenosis, the pulse pressure decreases to less than 30 mm Hg.

92. Clients with valvular disorders (or a history of cardiac surgery) need to have prophylactic antibiotics prior to any dental work or invasive procedures to prevent the occurrence of endocarditis.

93. PTCA

94. b. Option (a) is not correct because the systolic pressure will decrease; (c) and (d) are not correct because the weight and pulmonary and wedge pressures will increase.

95. b   96. c   97. a

98. Answers may include: helping the client to adjust to a gradual decrease in activity tolerance, teaching the client to maintain a fluid restriction of 1500 mL/day, teaching the client to recognize manifestation of organ rejection

99. Primary cardiomyopathies are idiopathic and their cause is unknown. Secondary cardiomyopathies occur as a result of other disease processes.

100. The prognosis for an individual diagnosed with dilated cardiomyopathy is grim; most clients get progressively worse and die within 2 years of the onset of symptoms.

101. (a) cardiomegaly (enlargement of the heart), (b) pulmonary congestion, (c) edema

102. A teaching plan for a client with cardiomyopathy should focus on self-care measures such as activity restrictions, dietary changes, and pharmacologic measures to reduce symptoms and/or prevent complications. The client and family need to understand the disease process and treatment options, as well as teaching specifics to ongoing care, treatments, and diagnostic evaluation.

103. a

104. d. Group A streptococcus is a precipitating cause of rheumatic fever.

105. c. Damaged valves are especially vulnerable to infectious organisms.

106. b

107. abrupt-onset chest pain, aggravated by respiratory movements and position changes

108. upright, leaning forward

109. c. Cor pulmonale is right-sided failure that results from lung disease.

110. a. Around the clock, NSAIDs are key to the pain management in pericarditis.

111. d. Nonsteroidal anti-inflammatory drugs (NSAIDs) are routinely used. Fluid intake should be at least 2500 mL/day and recurrence is a possibility that should be discussed with the client.

112. f   113. e   114. a   115. d

116. b   117. c   118. g   119. h

▪ ▪ ▪ **Chapter 29**

1. (a) arteries, (b) arterioles, (c) capillaries, (d) venules, (e) veins, (f) vena cava

2. c. The alternate expansion and contraction of an artery constitutes a pulse.

3. Answers include: blood viscosity, length of a vessel, diameter of a vessel

4. d

5. (a) hypertensive, (b) normotensive, (c) hypertensive, (d) hypotensive

6. a   7. b   8. a   9. b

10. b   11. a   12. b

13. Answers include: lymph nodes, thymus, tonsils, spleen, Peyer's patches

14. Answers may include: activity habits and tolerance, alcohol consumption, smoking history and tobacco use, current medications, prior history of vascular or heart problems

15. a. These symptoms are consistent with arterial insufficiency, not venous problems or an aortic aneurysm.

16. a. The use of IV drugs is less likely to cause swollen lymph glands than exposure to radiation or toxic chemicals, a history of swollen glands, or chronic illness.

17. (a) blood pressure; (b) pulse points; (c) skin; (d–e) edema, ulcerations; (f–g) color, temperature

18. 120 is the first Korotkoff's sound, representing the systolic pressure; 72 is the true diastolic pressure, or a muffling of the Korotkoff's sound; 64 represents the second diastolic sound and it is the level at which sounds are no longer heard.

19. Answers include: an improper cuff size, client supports his/her own arm, inadequate inflation, improper deflation or inflation

20. Answers may include: observe for postural color changes, check capillary refill, palpate pulses, assess venous patterns

21. d 22. d 23. i 24. h 25. k

26. a 27. e 28. f 29. b

30. Answers include: systolic hypertension, dependent edema, carotid bruits

31. stasis dermatitis

32. d 33. b 34. e 35. c 36. a

37. Answers may include: size, shape, symmetry, consistency, delineation, mobility, tenderness, sensation, condition of overlying skin

38. metastatic disease from abdominal or thoracic cancer

39. breast cancer

40. e 41. b 42. c 43. a

44. g 45. d 46. f

47. b. A positive Homans' sign is consistent with calf pain on dorsiflexion. It may or may not indicate thrombophlebitis.

48. b. The nurse should assess circulation, sensation, and motion. The other actions are inappropriate.

49. c

50. Answers include: cardiac tamponade, constrictive pericarditis, severe chronic lung disease

51. True 52. False 53. True

54. False 55. True

56. subjective findings: denies pain and discomfort, forgets to test his blood sugar regularly

57. objective findings: cyanotic right foot; ulcerated area on right great toe; weak pedal pulse in left foot; no palpable pulse right foot; blood sugar, 298 mg; B/P, 138/98

58. His personal and family medical history should be assessed. The onset, characteristics, and course should be more specifically assessed. He should be asked about associated symptoms such as burning, numbness, tingling, leg fatigue or cramps, changes in skin color or temperature, and edema. His nutritional history should be assessed. His current medications should be documented. Socioeconomic factors should be assessed including occupational and psychosocial factors. A full diabetic assessment should be completed.

Physical assessment of the peripheral vascular system should be completed.

■ ■ ■ Chapter 30

1. Answers include: constriction, obstruction, inflammation, vasospasm

2. b

3. c. This elevation in blood pressure should be re-checked and evaluated by a physician. However, there is no need to do it immediately.

4. a 5. b

6. b. One glass of wine is equal to one ounce of alcohol, which is the limit set by the Joint National Committee on Detection, Evaluation, and Treatment of High Blood Pressure.

7. a. Diuretic therapy and antihypertensives are not conservative treatment. Conservative treatment is quitting smoking, not changing brands of cigarettes.

8. Answers may include: decrease sodium, maintain adequate potassium, decrease fat, limit alcohol, maintain adequate dietary calcium and magnesium

9. d. Regular aerobic exercise promotes weight loss and helps lower blood pressure.

10. f 11. d 12. b

13. c 14. e 15. a

16. Answers may include: monitor and record daily weights, balance periods of activity with rest, monitor and record level of consciousness, monitor intake and output, decrease workload of heart

17. c. Mutually set goals are imperative to the client adhering to the treatment plan.

18. c. Oral contraceptives place clients at the highest risk for high blood pressure. Race, gender, weight, and job stress may be co-factors in hypertension.

19. Answers include: estrogen use, renal disease, endocrine disorders, coarctation of the aorta, pregnancy

20. pheochromocytoma

21. c. This blood pressure must be reported and treated promptly to prevent serious complications and death. The other interventions are inappropriate in this emergent situation.

22. (a) Osler's maneuver, (b) pseudo
23. b. The other conditions would not be relieved by rest.
24. c. The other symptoms would not be present in peripheral arterial occlusion.
25. a. The Doppler ultrasound helps the nurse assess pulses.
26. b. Aspirin inhibits platelet aggregation.
27. d. Walking is an appropriate intervention, whereas the other interventions are not appropriate for this condition.
28. a
29. b. The dependent position is appropriate for clients with arterial disorders, as it promotes blood flow.
30. c. The circulation, sensation, and motion should be carefully assessed. Pain is an indication of arterial insufficiency.
31. c. The dependent position promotes arterial flow. The other interventions would reduce arterial flow.
32. c. Heat should not be applied, as it may result in tissue injury. The other interventions are appropriate.
33. a. These symptoms are consistent with arterial insufficiency.
34. b. Calcium channel blockers may reduce postoperative vasospasm.
35. d. Elevating the foot of bed less than 30 degrees will promote venous return without markedly slowing arterial flow.
36. Answers may include: inflammation, polycythemia, dehydration, repeated arterial punctures, atherosclerotic changes, damaged blood vessels
37. c. The client should wear cotton stockings. All the other interventions are appropriate.
38. Answers include: excessive bloody drainage from the incision site; continuous oozing from injection sites; bleeding from the gums; bleeding from the nose; hematuria; petechiae, purpura, ecchymoses
39. c. Smoking cessation will eliminate the vasoconstricting effects of nicotine.
40. (a) raising, (b) lowering, (c) five, (d) 2, (e) elevate the legs from a horizontal position to a 45-degree angle and then lower them to a dependent position
41. b

42. (a) Blue is caused by diminished arterial circulation due to vasospasm. (b) White occurs as circulation becomes more severely diminished. (c) Red occurs as the fingers are warmed and the spasm resolves.
43. swing the arms back and forth to increase perfusion in the small arteries by centrifugal force.
44. d. A history of hypertension contributes to the development of aneurysm.
45. b. A true aneurysm is the result of the long-term, eroding effects of atherosclerosis and hypertension. False aneurysms are caused by a traumatic break in the vessel wall.
46. b. A dissecting thoracic aneurysm is a likely cause of this type of pain. The other problems are much less likely.
47. a. The pain may indicate the severity.
48. b. Lowering the systolic pressure to less than 100 is the goal of therapy.
49. Answers may include: increasing fluid and fiber in the diet, postponing sexual activity and other strenuous activity for 6 to 9 weeks, monitoring wound for signs of infection or bleeding, compliance with medication regimen, reducing stress.
50. c. The other three medications are important: Colace (docusate sodium) to soften stool and prevent Valsalva maneuver, Inderal (propranolol) to lower blood pressure, and morphine to reduce the pain.
51. Answers include: stasis of blood, increased blood coagulability, injury to the vessel wall
52. b. Absent peripheral pulses would indicate arterial, not venous problems. The other symptoms would be present in DVT.
53. c
54. Answers may include: anti-inflammatory medication, applying a moist warm compress to the affected extremity, antibiotic therapy
55. b. The client would remain on bed rest. The leg would be elevated, not massaged, and passive/active range of motion would be performed.
56. b. This intervention is for the treatment of DVT, not its prevention.
57. d. The client's value is twice the control or within therapeutic range.

58. Answers may include: regular follow-up is necessary to be sure that the prothrombin time remains within the desired range; most clients require 2–4 months of oral anticoagulation therapy; report side effects such as bleeding or bruising immediately; dose, purpose, frequency, side effects, dietary and medication interactions

59. b. Life-threatening complications can occur if the client does not adhere to bed rest.

60. b. Compression devices should be removed as directed so the skin can be assessed.

61. Answers include: assess pain, measure the diameter of the affected extremity, apply warm, moist heat to the affected extremity, maintain bed rest

62. b. Congestion of blood in the affected extremity results in chronic venous insufficiency.

63. Answers include: lower leg edema, discoloration of the skin of the lower leg and foot, hardness of the subcutaneous tissues, stasis ulcers

64. b. Walking will promote venous return. The other interventions are appropriate.

65. a. Varicosities can be prevented with regular exercise such as walking.

66. Answers may include: severe aching pain in the leg; leg fatigue; leg heaviness, itching over the affected leg; feelings of heat in the leg; visibly dilated veins; thin, discolored skin above the ankles; stasis ulcers

67. Answers may include: wearing antiembolism stockings, walking, elevating legs for specific periods of time, avoid prolonged sitting or standing

68. d. Disability occurs with lymphedema.

69. a. Respiratory status is evaluated as the dyes used during the procedure can result in respiratory problems.

70. Answers include: elevation, elastic stockings, meticulous skin hygiene, bed rest, restricting dietary sodium

71. Answers may include: restrict dietary intake of sodium, measure the girth of the extremity daily, keep the client's skin clean and dry, elevate the extremites while the client is seated and at bedtime.

72. d. Encourage the client to express her feelings. The other responses are inappropriate.

73. (a) secondary lymphedema, or swelling in the lymph system; filaria, a nematode worm

▪ ▪ ▪ Chapter 31

1. Answers include: bone marrow (myeloid) tissue, lymphatic tissue

2. c   3. a

4. d. Hypoxia is a stimulate to erythropoiesis.

5. b

6. (a) 120, (b) hemolysis

7. (a) jaundice, (b) yellow-appearing skin and sclera

8. (a) erythrocytopenia, microcytic, hypochromic; (b) answers may include: spoon-shaped nails, cheilosis, smooth and sore tongue, pica; (c) administer oral or parenteral iron preparations

9. (a) macrocytic, thin membranes, oval-shaped (rather than concave); (b) answers may include: smooth, sore, beefy, red tongue; diarrhea; paresthesias; (c) parenteral administration of vitamin B_{12}

10. (a) fragile, megoblastic; (b) answers may include: fatigue, SOB, palpitations, glossitis, cheilosis, and diarrhea; (c) folic acid supplements

11. (a) crescent-shaped, (b) answers may include: severe pain during sickling episodes, seizures, congestive heart failure, hematuria, skin ulcers, retinal detachment;(c) none—supportive care such as rest, oxygen, analgesics, and hydration

12. (a) fragile, hypochromic, microcytic with "bull's eye" appearance; (b) answers may include: hepatomegaly, splenomegaly, jaundice, shortness of breath, congestive heart failure; (c) transfusion

13. (a) normochromic, normocytic; (b) answers may include: jaundice, pallor, hemoglobinuria; (c) treatment is dependent on the causative agent

14. (a) normochromic, normocytic; (b) answers may include: fatigue, pallor, weakness, dyspnea, headache; (c) none—remove the offending agent

15. (a) normochromic, normocytic; (b) answers may include: tachycardia, CHF; (c) removal of causative agents

16. c   17. c   18. a   19. a   20. d

21. c   22. a   23. d   24. e   25. b

26. Answers may include: encourage fluids following ingestion of oral iron preparation, stagger the administration of tetracycline, offer the

client a straw to drink the iron preparation, mix the iron preparation with orange juice, monitor laboratory work, monitor for toxic effects of iron, assess for drug interactions

27. a

28. c. Leafy green vegetables are sources of folic acid. The other foods are not.

29. d. Alcohol-based solutions are irritating to the mucous membranes. The other solutions can be used.

30. b. Bland foods should be consumed, not spiced foods or citrus fruit.

31. (a) the heart pumps harder or more rapidly in an attempt to compensate for the decrease in tissue oxygenation; (b) the blood vessels in the skin constrict, allowing blood to be shunted to vital organs; (c) there is a decreased level of oxygen in circulation secondary to below-normal hemoglobin levels.

32. Answers include: chronic, occult blood loss; inadequate dietary intake of iron

33. a. These are findings in iron-deficiency anemia. Hematuria and jaundice are found in sickle-cell anemia. Paresthesias and problems with proprioception are found in B_{12} deficiency. Pancytopenia and infections are found in aplastic anemia.

34. d. Parenteral administration of B_{12} is required when intrinsic factor is absent.

35. b. Priority interventions are providing oxygen and pain relief. Fluids and rest are also important. Folic acid supplements, electrophoresis, and dialysis are not part of the treatment plan for sickle cell anemia. Transfusions may be given, but are not generally a high priority.

36. d. The client may experience discomfort at the puncture site for about 2 days after the procedure.

37. Answers may include: beef, chicken, egg yolk, turkey, bran flakes, brown rice, whole grain breads, dried fruits, and beans

38. Answers may include: leafy green vegetables, broccoli, organ meat, eggs, wheat germ, liver, milk, yeast

39. Answers may include: liver, fresh shrimp and oysters, eggs, milk, kidney, meats, cheese

40. d. He should assess his pulse. Shortness of breath may indicate cardiac decompensation. If his pulse does not return to normal in 4 minutes, he should call his health care provider.

41. c

42. Answers may include: cyanosis, plethora, headaches, dizziness, tinnitus, blurred vision, hypertension, bruising, gastrointestinal bleeding

43. Answers may include: maintaining adequate hydration, preventing blood stasis, using support stockings, following and complying with medical therapy, quitting smoking or avoiding secondhand smoke, reporting bleeding

44. c   45. a

46. d. Thrombocytopenia is a platelet count below 100,000 platelets per milliliter of blood.

47. c   48. b

49. (a) ecchymosis, (b) petechiae, (c) purpura

50. (a) blood clotting, (b) hemorrhaging

51. increased; this test measures the integrity of the platelet plug. In DIC, plasminogen breaks down fibrin before a stable clot is formed.

52. decreased; because of the systemic bleeding that occurs, platelets are used up faster than they can be produced

53. decreased; in an attempt to clot, serum fibrinogen gets used up

54. increased; when fibrin is broken down, FDP products are released into circulation

55. b. Acute pain may be signs of arterial insufficiency and further assessment is required. The other statements are false.

56. d. This finding may indicate impending respiratory failure and further complications of DIC. The doctor should be notified.

57. male

58. d. Cryoprecipitate does not contain factor IX, which is given in hemophilia B.

59. a. IM injections may cause tissue trauma and bleeding.

60. b. Aspirin should not be taken, as it may lead to bleeding. The other statements are true.

61. (a) neutrophils; (b–c) band, stab; (d) 10

62. (a) neutropenia, (b) lymphocytopenia, (c) agranulocytosis

63. c

64. False   65. True

66. False   67. False

68. d   69. a   70. b

71. b. Fruits and vegetables may have a number of pathogens contributing to infection.

72. c. Bence-Jones protein is characteristic of multiple myeloma.

73. b. Protective isolation should be instituted with this low neutrophil count. The other interventions are not appropriate.
74. Explain to the client that freshly cut flowers and plants may have insects that carry infection and should not be placed in the room.
75. c   76. b   77. c
78. Answers include: drug resistance is reduced, toxicity from high doses of a single agent is reduced, cell growth is interrupted at various stages of the cell cycle
79. c. When the WBC is the lowest, the client should be protected from infection.
80. a. Infection is the major risk for individuals with leukemia.
81. d. These findings suggest herpes; they are not consistent with the other problems.
82. d. Oral medications are less invasive and are the preferred route.
83. (a) donor, (b) client
84. (a) invasive
85. Answers include: eat dry foods on arising; eat salty foods if permitted; avoid very sweet, rich, or greasy foods; eat small amounts frequently
86. False   87. False   88. False
89. True   90. False
91. c. The underlying principle should be to minimize exposure to infections. Adults may be as likely to expose her to infections as school-age children.
92. c. All the other statements are true. Immunizations are avoided in leukemia.
93. d. Tampons should not be used. All other statements are correct.
94. Interventions include assessing the roles of the client and the family members and assessing how they have managed stressful situations in the past, assessing coping strategies and their effectiveness, determining sources of strength, using therapeutic communication skills to allow open discussion of losses and permission to grieve, and identifying resources such as self-help groups and making appropriate referrals.
95. b
96. d. This statement provides the client with the facts related to hair loss.
97. c. This statement gives the realistic prognosis for early Hodgkin's disease.

98. refer him for evaluation. A lymph node that has been present this long, with or without pain or other symptoms, should be referred for evaluation.
99. d
100. Answers include: assess factors that precipitate nausea and/or vomiting, use ordered antiemetics, provide teaching to prevent or relieve nausea and vomiting
101. Answers include: nitrogen mustard, vincristine, procarbazine, prednisone

▪ ▪ ▪ **Chapter 32**

1. (a) pulmonary ventilation during which air moves into and out of the lungs, (b) external respiration during which oxygen and carbon dioxide are exchanged between alveoli and blood, (c) gas transport, (d) internal respiration during which oxygen and carbon dioxide are exchanged between blood and cells
2. The upper respiratory system serves as a passageway for air to move into the lungs and carbon dioxide to move out into the external environment; air is cleaned, humidified, and warmed by the upper respiratory passages.
3. Surfactant-containing fluid is necessary for maintaining a moist surface. It reduces surface tension of alveolar fluid and helps prevent collapse of the lungs.
4. simple diffusion
5. Answers include: produces a lubricating fluid that allows the lungs to move easily over the thoracic wall during breathing; holds the lungs to the thoracic wall and creates slightly negative pressure necessary for lung function
6. a
7. (a) alveolar surface tension, (b) lung compliance, (c) lung elasticity
8. g   9. e   10. l   11. h   12. j
13. k   14. p   15. c   16. i   17. m
18. r   19. o   20. n   21. d   22. q
23. f   24. a   25. b
26. f   27. c   28. a
29. d   30. b   31. e
32. Since oxygen is not very soluble in water, it must bind with hemoglobin to be carried to the cells of the body.
33. Answers may include: difficulty breathing, hoarseness, changes in voice quality,

coughing, pausing for breath in the middle of a sentence

34. Answers include: loss of elastic recoil, stiffening of the chest wall, changes in gas exchange

35. Answers include: sedentary lifestyle, obesity

36. c   37. d   38. allergy

39. inspect nose and nasal cavity; assess sense of smell; assess respiratory rate; measure anteroposterior diameter of chest; inspect for intercostal retraction; inspect and palpate for excursion; palpate trachea; palpate tactile fremitus; percuss lungs; percuss posterior chest; auscultate lungs; auscultate voice sounds

40. a   41. b

42. c. These symptoms are consistent with pneumonia. Dyspnea, shortness of breath, fever, persistent coughing, and rusty sputum are consistent with some type of respiratory infection. Crackles and increased voice sounds are also consistent with the presence of foreign matter or exudate in the lower lobe of the right lung. Laboratory and other diagnostic tests are necessary to confirm this suspicion.

43. b   44. d   45. a   46. c

47. Kyphosis is the increased curvature in the spine that occurs in older adults. This may increase the anteroposterior diameter of the thorax, causing a barrel chest. The lungs experience a loss of elastic recoil, stiffening of the chest wall, and changes in gas exchange, decreases in vital capacity and increases in residual volumes. These changes decrease cough effectiveness.

48. The nurse should interview Mr. Chan using the interview questions presented in this chapter. A complete physical examination of the respiratory system should also be performed. Assessing his general health and vital signs would also be appropriate. A more detailed assessment should be conducted if indicated by history or physical examination.

49. Mr. Chan should avoid individuals with respiratory infections and get his flu shots as directed. He also should keep his other immunizations current. He should avoid environmental or respiratory irritants such as smoke. He should eat a well-balanced, nutritious diet. He should see a health care provider on a regular basis and any time he experiences respiratory infections.

50. This change in smell sensation is related to age. He needs to eat a great variety of foods that are appealing to either his taste or smell. Not eating alone is a good strategy for increasing appetite. He needs to be sure to include foods that are rich in calories, nutrients, and minerals. He might find it helpful to consult with a dietician to increase his caloric intake.

▪ ▪ ▪ Chapter 33

1. c. The most important teaching topic for the client with acute or chronic rhinitis is education. Care should be taken to avoid spreading pathogens to others. Increasing fluid intake thins secretions, hastening recovery.

2. b. These medications stimulate the sympathetic nervous system, increasing peripheral vascular resistance, blood pressure, and heart rate.

3. d. Most clients can use over-the-counter preparations for symptomatic relief and to enhance feelings of wellness. Aspirin and acetaminophen do not prevent progression of acute viral rhinitis.

4. a. Teaching clients and families about influenza focuses on prevention.

5. c. Yearly outbreaks of influenza affect about 48 million Americans each winter, accounting for about 3.9 million hospitalizations and 20,000 deaths.

6. b. Tachypnea and/or rapid, shallow respirations may result from fever and muscle ache.

7. d. Fever and decreased oral intake of fluids may cause dehydration and increased viscosity of secretions, which make it more difficult to expectorate. Increasing the water content of inhaled air helps loosen thick secretions and soothe mucous membranes.

8. obstruction

9. b   10. d

11. c   12. a

13. c. Complications of sinusitis involve the local spread of infection. Sinusitis can be an acute or chronic condition and is common in clients who have AIDS.

14. b. Mild analgesics are adequate for pain control. The client should have the head of the bed elevated and ice packs may be

applied to the nose. Nasal packing, which does contribute to the client's discomfort, is not routinely changed.

15. group A beta-hemolytic streptococcus

16. b. Viral infections are communicable for 2–3 days.

17. a. Taking a full course of antibiotics is essential. Penicillin is the drug of choice. If the client is allergic, erythromycin or tetracycline may be used. Clients are not considered contagious once they have taken antibiotics for a 24-hour period. Drugs such as aspirin or acetaminophen are useful in providing symptomatic relief for clients with pharyngitis or tonsillitis.

18. c

19. b. These symptoms are consistent with a peritonsillar abscess and require emergency care. Failure to obtain appropriate medical care could result in respiratory obstruction.

20. (a) airway, (b) breathing, (c) circulation (monitor for hemorrhage)

21. monitoring and maintaining airway patency

22. Answers include: nasal flaring, restlessness, stridor, use of accessory muscles for breathing, and decreased oxygen saturation measurements

23. change in the voice

24. b. *Impaired Verbal Communication* is the priority nursing diagnosis for clients with laryngitis. The other answers listed are also appropriate for the client with epistaxis.

25. pseudomembrane

26. a. The diphtheria antitoxin is derived from horses and a skin test for sensitivity to horse serum should precede immunization.

27. (a) trauma, (b) systemic bleeding

28. Answers may include: elevate the head of the bed; apply cold compresses to the nose; encourage deep, slow breathing through the mouth; monitor for hematemesis; monitor vital signs and respiratory rate; monitor the position of the packing; monitor for bleeding in the posterior pharynx; provide for rest; encourage oral fluids; provide frequent oral hygiene

29. c. These activities could increase pressure and initiate bleeding. The client is advised to avoid strenuous exercise for several days or weeks, to avoid blowing the nose, and to sneeze with the mouth open.

30. c. Direct pressure provided through pinching may control or stop the bleeding. The other actions are appropriate, but not the priority in acute bleeding.

31. a. Placing the client in an upright position with her head forward will minimize the amount of blood draining down the nasopharynx and reduce the risks of aspiration. The other interventions are not the highest priority.

32. c. CSF rhinorrhea occurs in some fractures of the nasoethmoidal or frontal region, but is not a typical clinical manifestation of nasal fracture.

33. *Staphylococcus*   34. glucose

35. Answers include: edema, bleeding

36. maintain a patent airway.

37. c. Swelling may subside in several days, though bruising may persist for several weeks.

38. b

39. b. To prevent bleeding, the client is instructed not to blow the nose for 48 hours after the packing is removed. Breathing exercises are to be done gently. Cold, not warm, compresses may be used. Frequent oral care is encouraged.

40. ingested meat that lodges in the airway.

41. four back blows followed by four abdominal thrusts, repeated until the obstruction is relieved

42. a. The priority of nursing care for the client with a laryngeal obstruction is restoring a patent airway to prevent cerebral anoxia and death. This is a medical emergency requiring immediate intervention.

43. Answers may include: subcutaneous emphysema, voice changes, dysphagia, stridor, coughing (with hemoptysis), crepitus, pain with swallowing

44. soft tissue   45. airway maintenance

46. 10 seconds   47. obstructive

48. c   49. d

50. b. Alcohol is likely to contribute to the occurrence of sleep apnea.

51. a

52. (a) elevating the head of the bed will decrease swelling and maximize lung excursion, (b) pace activities to provide for periods of rest as fatigue can further compromise breathing, (c) apply warm packs to the nose to enhance comfort after surgery

53. c. If posterior bleeding occurs, the client may swallow frequently and note blood at the back of the throat. Swallowed blood may cause nausea and vomiting.
54. Answers include: papillomas, nodules, polyps
55. d. Yelling and screaming will contribute to the severity of the condition.
56. b. A speech therapist can help teach less-damaging use of the voice.
57. (a) 1 to 3, (b–c) alcohol, tobacco
58. (a) leukoplakia, (b) erythroplakia
59. a. Lesions of the true vocal cords, or glottis, occur more frequently than cancers of other regions of the larynx.
60. d. Hoarseness or changes in the voice occur because the tumor prevents a complete closure of the glottis during speech. Choices (a), (b), and (c) are manifestations of supraglottic cancer.
61. a
62. b. Radiation therapy is often the treatment of choice for early laryngeal cancer. Chemotherapy may be used as adjunctive therapy for laryngeal cancer, but it is not the treatment of choice.
63. c. The speech therapist is a vital part of the care team for all total laryngectomy clients; the others may be useful for certain clients, but not essential for all.
64. inform the client that the surgery will affect eating during the postoperative period, and that nutritional and fluid needs will be met with intravenous or enteral feedings. The client should be prepared for the effect of surgery on taste and smell.
65. d. The client who is unable to speak or call out needs the reassurance that help is within reach at all times.
66. Answers may include: assess the client's nutritional status using height and weight charts and reported weight loss; monitor the client's fluid intake and output and food consumption; weigh the client at least once a day; evaluate the client's current and preferred food and eating habits; refer to a dietician; encourage the client to experiment with foods of different textures and temperatures; encourage frequent, small meals; provide mouth care; offer dietary supplements
67. True   68. True

69. False   70. True
71. Answers may include: use of humidity, stoma care, clean technique for tracheostomy care, avoiding water sports, strategies to prevent infection, follow-up care and treatment, alternate communication techniques
72. a. The priority intervention is to encourage the client to express her feelings. Responses (b) and (c) dismiss her feelings and experience. Referring her to a cancer support group may be appropriate, but is not the priority intervention.
73. c. Assessing the patency of the airway is the priority intervention. The other assessments should follow assessment of the airway.
74. Prior to surgery, the nurse should discuss alternative methods of communication, both short- and long-term. The nurse should provide the client with nonverbal means of communication such as pencil and paper, magic slate, or alphabet board. The client should be referred to a speech therapist prior to surgery. The client should always have a call bell within reach and all personnel should know that the client can not respond verbally.

▪ ▪ ▪ Chapter 34

1. (a) teaching (b) smoking cessation
2. b   3. a   4. e   5. d   6. c
7. b. The gag or cough reflex is one of the major defenses against the entry of foreign substances into the lungs.
8. d. Pneumococcal pneumonia vaccine gives lifetime immunity whereas influenza vaccine needs to be given annually.
9. c   10. b   11. c   12. a   13. d   14. b
15. b. *Ineffective Airway Clearance* results in tachypnea.
16. a. Fluid intake of 3000 mL/day is important. Discharge goals should be established on the first day of hospitalization. It is important to provide adequate rest periods for the client and increase activity levels gradually. Small, frequent, nutritious feedings are important for this client.
17. a
18. False   19. True   20. False
21. *Mycobacterium tuberculosis*

22. c
23. Answers include: coughing, weight loss, anorexia, periodic fevers
24. cover the mouth when coughing or sneezing, and dispose of sputum appropriately
25. b   26. c   27. a
28. b. People with AIDS, the homeless, and members of lower socioeconomic groups, which represent the population at highest risk for developing active TB, are also most at risk for being unable to manage the complex treatment regime.
29. Groups include those with HIV infections, those who have had close contact with TB, individuals with medical risk factors, those born in countries with high prevalence of TB, low-income individuals who are medically underserved, alcoholics, IV drug users, residents and staff of long-term residential facilities.
30. 0.1 ml of PPD is injected intradermally into the dorsal aspect of the forearm. This test is read within 48 to 72 hours and recorded as the diameter of induration (raised area, not erythema).
31. b. This is the correct procedure for collecting the sputums. All other responses are incorrect.
32. d. Although this diameter of induration is considered negative, the client still may be infected.
33. False   34. True   35. False
36. False   37. False   38. False
39. False   40. True
41. Answers include: early detection, accurate diagnosis, effective treatment of the disease, prevention of the spread of the disease to others
42. c. In the United States, many fungal lung diseases demonstrate a geographic distribution. Blastomycosis is found throughout North America.
43. histoplasmosis   44. education
45. b   46. a   47. c
48. Answers may include: chest tightness, dyspnea, wheezing, cough, tachypnea, tachycardia, anxiety, apprehension
49. c. The other choices are triggers that represent intrinsic asthma.
50. d. Bronchodilator agents act as sympathomimetics. They would be contraindicated or used with great caution for persons with hypertension, cardiovascular disease, dysrhythmias, or diabetes.
51. b. Choices (a), (c), and (d) may be appropriate, but they do not greatly enhance trust in a relationship. Active listening promotes trust and helps the client express concerns.
52. (a) controlling symptoms and preventing acute asthma
    (b) restoring airway patency and alveolar ventilation
53. Eosinophilia is an elevation of the eosinophil count. It indicates inflammation and is a common finding in asthma.
54. b. Decreasing breath sounds and reduced wheezing may be indicative of impending respiratory therapy. Increased breath sounds and diminished wheezing may be an indication of improvement.
55. a. The mouth should be rinsed after using the inhaler, not before. All the other statements are correct.
56. Four implications include: monitoring the therapeutic blood level, monitoring for signs of toxicity, administering medications with meals or a full glass of water or milk, monitoring the client for therapeutic and adverse effects
57. Teaching should include the importance of taking the medication on an empty stomach, monitoring for a change in the color of stools or urine, or monitoring for jaundice.
58. c. The therapeutic level is 10 to 20 µg/mL.
59. (a) chronic asthma, (b) chronic bronchitis, and (c) emphysema
60. b. Cigarette smoke is the major factor implicated in the development of chronic bronchitis.
61. b. The canister is held upside down, the breath is held for as long as possible after the inhalation, and the client should wait 30 seconds to 2 minutes before taking the second dose.
62. c. The other choices are true for chronic bronchitis.
63. c   64. a   65. d   66. b
67. relatively immune to hypercapnia and use hypoxia as their primary respiratory stimulus
68. d. The influenza immunization is given yearly. Fluid is usually increased to 2000–2500 mL/day; clients should be encouraged to follow a prescribed exercise program and to

maintain activities as tolerated, balancing activity with periods of rest.

69. a,c 70. b 71. c 72. c 73. a 74. a

75. The nurse should assess the client's knowledge and understanding of choices involved and consequences for each. The client's concerns, values, and beliefs should be assessed. The nurse should encourage the client to express his feelings and assist the client to develop a plan or course of action for quitting. Resources to assist the client quit smoking should be identified and the client should be provided with practical information regarding quitting and managing withdrawal symptoms.

76. b. CF is transmitted by an autosomal-recessive gene.

77. False   78. False
79. True   80. False

81. b. The client should be positioned on the unaffected side, putting the affected side in a superior position to enhance drainage.

82. prevention

83. True   84. True
85. True   86. False

87. a. Although choices (b), (c), and (d) apply, the most common problem with occupational lung diseases is activity intolerance. With severe dyspnea, the client's ability to carry out ADLs may be significantly impaired.

88. b 89. a 90. d 91. c

92. often resolves spontaneously

93. Symptoms include anorexia, fatigue, weight loss, fever, dyspnea, arthralgias, and myalgias. Skin lesions, uveitis, lymphadenopathy, and hepatomegaly may be noted.

94. deep veins

95. Answers may include: stasis of blood flow, damage to vein wall, altered coagulation, prolonged immobility, trauma (especially to the hip and femur), surgery (especially orthopedic, pelvic, or gynecologic), obesity, advanced age, myocardial infarction

96. d. Tachycardia and tachypnea are common clinical manifestations of pulmonary embolism.

97. d. Anticoagulant therapy is often given prophylactically. The low doses of heparin affect the PTT very little and carry only a small risk of bleeding. Heparin will not act on a formed clot, but prevents further clotting and embolization.

98. c. The client should be placed in a Fowler's or high-Fowler's position, which facilitates maximal lung expansion and reduces the venous return to the right side of the heart.

99. cor pulmonale

100. True   101. False   102. True

103. cigarette smoking

104. b. Smoke paralyzes the cilia, reducing their ability to remove tars from contact with the respiratory epithelium.

105. c. Dull, aching chest pain occurs as the tumor spreads to the mediastinum.

106. Answers include: the disease, the expected prognosis, the planned treatment strategies

107. True

108. Answers may include: manage pain relief by administering prescribed medication, assist the client with comfort measures (massage, positioning), engage the client and family in activities that distract from the pain, spend as much time with the client as possible, assess pain, spend time with client

109. c. Questions should be answered honestly. The client and family should be encouraged to discuss treatment decisions and prognosis. The loss must be processed.

110. d

111. removing fluid from the pleural space with a needle

112. d. Assessments should be performed at least every 4 hours; the apparatus is not changed unless it is damaged; the apparatus is to be kept below the level of the chest.

113. Answers include: alveolar ventilation, gas exchange

114. (a) blood in the pleural space, (b–c) thoracic trauma, surgery

115. (a) flail chest, (b) paradoxic

116. a. Splinting the chest is not adequate for pain relief, but it should be taught in conjunction with analgesics. Rib fractures are often managed on an outpatient basis. The nurse should emphasize reporting complications to the physician and avoiding respiratory irritants such as cigarette smoke.

117. Answers include: thermal damage to the airways leading to impaired ventilation, carbon monoxide or cyanide poisoning resulting in tissue hypoxia, chemical damage to the lungs from noxious gases that can impair gas exchange

118. cherry-red
119. Answers may include: altered level of consiousness, vomiting, headache, chest pain, restlessness, cyanosis, tachypnea
120. (a) 50–60, (b) 50
121. Neuromuscular blockers provide no sedation or pain relief; muscle paralysis produces extreme anxiety in the client.
122. c. With continued high levels of oxygen delivery, surfactant synthesis is impaired and the lungs become less compliant (more "stiff").
123. a. To maintain positive pressure ventilation, the tube is cuffed with an air-filled or foam sac just above the end of the tube. When the cuff is inflated, it obstructs the upper airway, preventing air from escaping back into the nose or mouth.
124. a
125. a. Clients who are in respiratory failure should not be sedated (this can further depress the respiratory drive); high levels of oxygen may inhibit the respiratory drive; activities and energy expenditures should be minimized—rest is vital to reduce oxygen and energy demands.
126. d. Clients who receive neuromuscular blockers are totally alert unless sedated, so they need analgesia, usually morphine; the agents are given by slow injection or infusion; the alarms should never be turned off because the client is unable to move or communicate distress. Neostigmine is the antidote for the neuromuscular blockers.
127. d
128. a
129. c. Dyspnea and tachypnea are the initial manifestations. Choices (a), (b), and (d) occur later as the disease progresses.
130. a. The mainstay of ARDS management is endotracheal intubation and mechanical ventilation. This takes priority over the other therapies.
131. c. Choices (a), (b), and (d) would indicate that the cardiac output is improving.
132. a. ARDS is not the result of lifestyle, but a consequence of serious illness. Clients who survive the initial insult of ARDS generally recover with significant long-term adverse effects. If the client has been a smoker, the importance of completely avoiding cigarette smoking in the future should be stressed.

▪ ▪ ▪ **Chapter 35**

1. e   2. c   3. f   4. g   5. i
6. b   7. a   8. j   9. h   10. d

11. Answers may include: provide support for soft tissue, serve as a storage site for fat and minerals, serve as a site for blood cell formation, protect vital organs from injury, serve to move body parts
12. Answers include: secretion of parathyroid hormone stimulates calcium release from the bone, increasing serum calcium levels; secretion of calcitonin stimulates calcium salt deposit in the bone matrix; bones that are in use and therefore subject to stress respond by increasing osteoblastic activity to increase ossification
13. Answers include: excitability—the cell's ability to receive and respond to stimulus; contractibility—the cell's ability to respond to a stimulus by forcibly shortening; extensibility—the ability of muscle to respond to a stimulus by extending and relaxing; elasticity—the cell's ability to resume its resting length after it has shortened or lengthened
14. (a) strenuous exercise eventually results in the buildup of lactic acid and reduced energy in the muscle, or muscle fatigue; (b) regular exercise increases the size and strength of muscles and maintains muscle tone; (c) inactivity, or lack of use, causes a decrease in muscle tone and strength known as atrophy
15. (a) acetylcholine, (b) Sodium ions
16. b
17. The nurse's questions should focus on the chief complaint of pain. The questions should address onset, characteristics, course, severity, location, precipitating and relieving factors, and any associated manifestations. Past injuries and measures to self-treat the problem should also be addressed. Appropriate questions include: Describe the pain in your leg. When did it start? How long has it lasted? Where exactly is the pain located? How severe is your pain and has it gotten worse? What relieves or aggravates the pain? What medications are you taking for the pain? Have you noticed any redness, swelling, or limited mobility? Have you ever injured your leg before?

18. Answers may include: range-of-motion, inspection, palpation, measurement of muscle mass
19. c
20. assess gait and posture; inspect and palpate bones for obvious deformities, changes in size or shape, and pain; measure length and circumference of extremities with client in supine position; assess muscle mass; assess joints for swelling, pain, redness, warmth, crepitus and ROM.
21. j   22. b   23. h   24. i   25. g
26. a   27. e   28. c   29. d   30. f
31. A previous history of back problems makes Ms. Destone more likely to incur future problems because repeated injuries alter the strength and tone of muscle. Ms. Destone's job as a home health aide requires her to be able to assist clients with a variety of basic skills, such as ADLs and mobility issues. This type of work will be likely to place additional strain on Ms. Destone's back; she may need to reconsider her career choice dependent on the nature and severity of her current problem. Ms. Destone's weight is excessive for her height, which also contributes to muscle strain in her back. Her leg-length discrepancy most likely causes her to limp, although her weight is also a contributing factor; special shoes and/or shoe inserts may be needed to equalize leg length and possibly eliminate her limping. Ms. Destone's inability to touch her toes is probably associated with changes in the flexion and extension capabilities of her lumbar spine secondary to lumbar muscle injury (such as strain, sprain, and spasm). Additional diagnostic tests and focused assessments are necessary to evaluate the extent of injury and the nature of treatment.
32. c   33. d
34. True   35. False   36. False
37. False   38. True

▪ ▪ ▪ **Chapter 36**

1. (a) growth, (b) maintenance
2. 80%
3. a
4. d. Exercise helps with bone remodeling.

5. Answers may include: low back pain, progressive curvature of spine, loss of height, fractures of forearm, spine, or hip
6. 30
7. c. Estrogen helps prevent bone mass loss.
8. b. Withdrawal of estrogen may result in breakthrough bleeding.
9. a. Estrogen may affect glucose tolerance, leading to a possible change in dose in the oral hypoglycemic medication.
10. Answers may include: yogurt or low-fat cheeses, broccoli or beans, leafy green vegetables, calcium-fortified orange juice, sardines, salmon
11. False. A 35-year-old client who still is menstruating is not a candidate for estrogen-replacement therapy.
12. dietary sources of calcium are absorbed better than pills
13. vitamin D
14. bone density
15. (a) 1000, (b) 1500
16. The absorbency of a calcium supplement may be tested by placing a tablet in vinegar; if it dissolves in 30–45 minutes, it will be absorbed in the stomach.
17. *Risk for Injury*
18. a. Nutritional deficiencies contribute to osteomalacia.
19. Answers include: insufficient calcium absorption from the intestine, increased loss of phosphorous in the urine
20. d. Chronic renal failure leads to inadequate metabolism of vitamin D.
21. c. Bone pain is a common symptom of osteomalacia.
22. a. An elevated calcium level can occur with vitamin D therapy.
23. Answers may include: evaluate home setting for hazards and protect from injury, provide adequate lighting, teach safety measures, consult with physical therapist about use of assistive devices, evaluate vision
24. Answers may include: ice cream, yogurt, cheese
25. c
26. (a) increase, (b) minimal, (c) absent
27. c. This medication should not be taken within 2 hours of the ingestion of foods high in calcium or with antacids.

28. a. Heartburn and tingling around the mouth are adverse effects and the response to these medications is slow.
29. Key components include providing an appropriate assistive device, teaching the client about good body mechanics, planning exercise protocols and activity regimens and instructing the client about them.
30. a
31. b. Alkaline phosphatase levels increase in untreated Paget's disease.
32. b   33. a   34. a
35. c   36. b   37. a
38. a. Warmth at the site may occur early in osteomyelitis.
39. d. A bone scan or gallium scan are the most sensitive tests for early osteomyelitis.
40. c. Change in cognitive status is an early symptom of infection in older adults.
41. d
42. b. The client should be encouraged to drink fluids to reduce excessive radiation to the bladder and gonads.
43. Answers include: shoulder, hip, scapula
44. c. The client with Paget's disease is at risk for kyphosis.
45. b. Corrective shoes may relieve pain and discomfort.
46. a
47. c. Morton's neuroma occurs as the result of tight, confining shoes.
48. d. Numbness may indicate more serious neurologic complications that may require hospitalization.
49. b. An activity not usually pursued may lead to acute pain.
50. b. Exercises assist the client to restore mobility.
51. c
52. Answers may include: depression, chronic anxiety, psychiatric syndromes
53. c. Providing the client with knowledge about the benefits of surgery will help the client understand the benefits of conservative treatment.
54. a. This position will relieve compression of the spinal nerves.
55. d. Avoiding prolonged heat or cold prevents rebound phenomenon, which is a reverse effect.

56. Answers may include: using proper body mechanics; modifying the workplace to minimize stress to the back; achieving and maintaining ideal body weight, stopping smoking; avoiding prolonged sitting, standing, lying prone, or wearing high heels
57. d
58. d. Often the type of bone tumor cannot be determined until it and the surrounding tissue are removed.
59. Answers may include: worsening bony pain, pain at night or during rest, muscular weakness, soft tissue mass, fever, change in ability to perform activities of daily living
60. elevated
61. a
62. c. To date, there is no way to detect the genetic defect.
63. Answers include: promote independence, promote mobility, provide psychological support to the client and family

▪ ▪ ▪ **Chapter 37**

1. b
2. Answers include: blunt force distributes energy over a large area and does not disrupt the skin, penetrating force directly causes a break in the skin integrity
3. d. For older adults, falls often result in musculoskeletal trauma.
4. d. Restoring homeostasis is the focus of nursing interventions. The other components of care are part of restoring homeostasis.
5. c   6. f   7. b   8. a
9. e   10. d   11. c
12. Answers include: straight (skin) traction, balanced traction, skeletal traction
13. d   14. b
15. a. neurovascular assessment is a priority after reduction of a fracture, as nerve function and blood flow may be interrupted following this procedure.
16. b. in compartment syndrome, there is decreasing arterial blood flow. Assessing the pulse helps determine the presence or absence of arterial flow in the larger vessels.
17. (a) within 48 hours, (b) edema
18. prevention

19. c. Petechiae are classic findings in fat embolism.
20. Answers include: pain, pulses, paresthesias, pallor, paralysis
21. Answers may include: deformity, pain, swelling, numbness, guarding, crepitus, muscle spasms, ecchymosis
22. b
23. c. A plaster cast should not become wet.
24. d. Worsening pain often occurs before other symptoms occur.
25. Answers may include: home safety measures; exercises to improve strength, gait, and balance; correct use of assistive devices; use of proper footwear; uses of corrective glasses and hearing aids; side effects of medication; methods to prevent dizziness when changing position
26. Answers may include: decreased blood flow, injury to vessel wall, coagulopathy
27. False   28. True   29. False
30. False   31. True   32. True
33. a. A fracture of the clavicle could not be immobilized in a cast—it is usually immobilized through use of a splint. The other fractures could be immobilized in a cast.
34. d
35. a. Deep breathing will ensure full expansion of the lungs and prevent atelectasis.
36. c. All the other assessments are important, but airway assessment is the priority.
37. The most appropriate action is to not move this victim and to immobilize the head and neck until further help arrives.
38. This individual's extremities should be assessed for sensation, movement, and circulation.
39. It may be treated with a cervical collar fastened shut with plaster, a halo immobilizer brace, a thoracic brace, or a body cast.
40. Assess the vital signs, circulation, and sensation of the lower extremities. Assess for pain and provide reassurance and support.
41. The client needs to understand how to manage her pain and splint her fractures. She needs to understand the importance of deep breathing and using an incentive spirometer. She needs to understand signs and symptoms to report and the importance of follow-up care.

42. Following this type of fracture, most clients can not bear weight for a period of up to 6 weeks. In his work as a hairdresser, he may find it very difficult to modify his work environment. He needs to consult with his physician regarding any physical limitations and how to plan for a return to work.
43. d
44. b. Abduction should be maintained to prevent adduction, which could lead to dislocation.
45. c. Using a high chair will help prevent dislocation. The client should use a walker and exercise legs and knees as directed.
46. c. The pillow prevents adduction and promotes abduction.
47. a
48. a. The client will get out of bed the first day postoperatively. Delaying early activity may lead to complications.
49. a
50. a. This position will prevent contracture.
51. c. Injured nerve endings contribute to phantom pain.
52. b. This position prevents flexion contractures.
53. c. Wrapping distal to proximal promotes venous return.
54. Encourage the client to verbalize his or her feelings, wear clothing from home, look at the stump, and participate in self-care activities and care of the stump. Active involvement in rehabilitation will be helpful, and a visit from a fellow amputee may also be helpful.
55. Monitor the client's vital signs and assess the pain on a regular basis. Splint and support the injured area and elevate the stump on a pillow for 24 hours. Move the client gently and slowly, encourage distraction and administer pain medications as ordered. Also encourage deep breathing and relaxation exercises. Reposition the client every 2 hours and prn.
56. The client should be taught to elevate the stump with the knee extended. All joints should receive either active or passive ROM every 2–4 hours. The client should change position every 2 hours. Prolonged sitting should be avoided.
57. strain   58. sprain

59. contusion
60. R = rest, I = ice, C = compression,
    E = elevation
61. b. Applying heat may help in venous return
    and decrease edema and pain.
62. (a) hip, (b) shoulder
63. a
64. b. Assessing neurovascular status is a priority
    intervention. Usually, the client will return
    with a splint in place. The other interventions
    may be important, but are not a priority.

▪ ▪ ▪ **Chapter 38**

1. d
2. Arthritis is inflammation of a joint.
3. (a) inflammatory, (b) articular cartilage
4. c
5. b. CPM is used after a total knee replacement
   to ensure extension and prevent flexion
   contracture.
6. d. Early activity will promote recovery. The
   other points may be important, but not as
   crucial as early mobility.
7. b. Clients are allowed out of bed the first day
   after surgery.
8. b. An abduction pillow will prevent adduction. Hip flexion should be 90 degrees or less.
9. c. Application of heat may relieve discomfort.
   Prednisone is not indicated in osteoarthritis.
   Cold and vigorous activity may increase pain.
10. a. Weight loss will relieve stress on the joints.
    The other interventions will not prevent
    osteoarthritis.
11. Answers include: dislocation, infection, circu-
    latory impairment, thromboembolism, nerve
    injury, component loosening or wear
12. 90
13. c. Worsening pain may indicate dislocation.
    The other interventions are inappropriate in
    this situation.
14. Answers may include: exercise regularly,
    avoid overuse or stress on affected joints, bal-
    ance exercise with rest, attain and maintain
    ideal body weight, sit in a straight chair, sleep
    on a firm mattress
15. d   16. secondary
17. c. Pain is the most distinct feature of acute
    gout.

18. c. Vigorous activity is not associated with
    acute gout. The typical gout attack occurs in
    the middle of the night, in the metatarsopha-
    langeal joint of the great toe, and after ingest-
    ing a heavy meal.
19. Answers include: uric acid, ESR, white blood
    count
20. e   21. a   22. d   23. a   24. c
25. b   26. c   27. d   28. c
29. rheumatoid factors
30. pannus
31. c
32. d. Cloudy fluid is an indication of infection,
    not inflammation.
33. (a) systemic, (b) extra-articular manifesta-
    tions
34. c. Only 70% of individuals with RA have an
    elevated RF.
35. Answers include: balancing rest with activity,
    prioritizing activities, engaging in regular
    physical activity, receiving support and
    counseling, planning rest periods throughout
    the day
36. False   37. True
38. True   39. False
40. b. A butterfly skin rash is a classic manifesta-
    tion of SLE.
41. b. These antibodies are rarely found in other
    disorders.
42. c. These are the primary concerns related to
    this drug.
43. b. Infection is a high-priority concern.
44. b. Joint pain occurs in 90% of those with SLE.
45. c. These symptoms are consistent with celluli-
    tis and should be assessed by a physician.
46. c. Pregnancy is safe as long as there are no
    other contraindications. Birth control pills
    may be contraindicated.
47. (a) calcinosis, (b) Raynaud's phenomenon,
    (c) esophageal dysfunction, (d) sclerodactyly,
    (e) telangiectasia
48. b. In scleroderma the skin is tight, shiny, and
    hyperpigmented.
49. Answers include: impaired skin integrity,
    impaired physical mobility
50. b   51. c   52. d   53. a
54. f   55. e   56. g   57. d
58. c. These symptoms suggest Lyme disease and
    should be evaluated and treated.

59. The nurse should provide specific recommendations for fibromyalgia such as exercise, relaxation, good nutrition, and trigger-point therapy.

▪ ▪ ▪ **Chapter 39**

1. The central nervous system (CNS) is made up of the brain and spinal cord. The peripheral nervous system is made up of cranial nerves, spinal nerves, and the autonomic nervous system.
2. b
3. myelin sheath
4. Afferent neurons relay impulses from the skin, muscles, and other organs to the central nervous system (CNS), while efferent neurons transmit impulses from the CNS to cause some type of action.
5. Answers include: sodium, potassium
6. c   7. a   8. j   9. i   10. b
11. c   12. g   13. f   14. a   15. e
16. d   17. h   18. k   19. b   20. c
21. a   22. e   23. f   24. d
25. (a) receive, (b) transmit information from and about the external environment, (c) regulate the internal environment of the body
26. b   27. d
28. Glasgow Coma Scale
29. ask family members or significant others
30. Answers include: mental status exam, cranial nerve exam, sensory exam, motor exam, cerebellar exam, reflex exam
31. b
32. inability to understand verbal or written language
33. c   34. h   35. g   36. a   37. e   38. b
39. c   40. i   41. d   42. f   43. a
44. (a) abnormal assessment findings: slurred speech, difficulty pronouncing words with many syllables, homonymous hemianopsia (loss of half of each visual field), ptosis of left eyelid, decreased facial sensation, dysphagia (difficulty swallowing), ataxia (unsteady gait). (b) contributing factors: 82 years old, widow, lives alone (may be less likely to report early abnormal signs and symptoms), children live out-of-state (unavailability of significant others to notice changes in early

stages), full-time customer service work (sedentary), history of smoking, weight excessive for height, B/P = 168/94 (elevated). (Mrs. Larue is probably experiencing residual effects of a right-sided stroke.)
45. Answers may include: lessened ability to taste and smell, a slower and more deliberate gait, vibratory sensation, diminished reflexes and sensations, slight decrease in motor strength, senile tremor, difficulty in performing alternating movements
46. b. When Brudzinski's or Kernig's signs are positive, they may indicate meningeal irritation. A lesion of the pons results in decerebrate posturing, whereas a lesion of the corticospinal tracts results in decorticate posturing. With a ruptured disc there is pain with straight leg raising.
47. b. The nurse should stand close to the client to prevent falling. During this test, the client stands with the feet together and with the eyes closed.
48. c   49. b   50. a
51. The Glasgow Coma Scale assists in assessing level of consciousness. It assigns a certain score to an individual's response to verbal directions, such as "open your eyes" and "move your upper arms," and their responses to questions related to their name, the date, the time, and place. The higher the score, the higher the level of function.
52. True   53. False
54. False   55. True

▪ ▪ ▪ **Chapter 40**

1. e   2. c   3. a   4. d   5. b   6. f
7. (a) arousal, (b) cognition
8. Answers include: responsiveness to stimuli and behavior
9. Answers include: blood, oxygen, glucose
10. b. Apnea does not occur with all seizures. There is decreased sensory input during sleep, not just seizures, and only striated muscle has a refractory period.
11. 1. LOC, 2. pupillary responses, 3. oculomotor responses, 4. motor responses, 5. breathing
12. (a) doll's eyes, (b) brain stem
13. levels of glucose below 40–50 mg/dL may

result in irreversible brain damage; hyper-glycemia may result in fluid and acid-base imbalances that are detrimental to the brain

14. c. Naloxone (Narcan) is the antidote for narcotics.

15. d. Elevation of the head decreases cerebral edema. Turning every 2 hours prevents skin breakdown, and the side-lying position protects from aspiration.

16. d. The other assessments are important, but patency of the airway is the priority.

17. (a) oral-pharyngeal, (b) 15

18. a. Taping the eyelids closed will prevent corneal irritation and abrasions.

19. c   20. cerebral edema   21. b

22. d. Behavior and personality characteristics are functions of the cortex.

23. c. Widening pulse pressure, increasing blood pressure, and decreasing pulse and respira-tions with an elevation in temperature may indicate increased ICP.

24. 48–72

25. herniation

26. b. The most commonly used drugs are manni-tol and dexamethasone.

27. a. The elevated head with the neck in a neutral plane enhances venous blood flow, thus decreasing cerebral edema.

28. a, d

29. c. Vision problems are an early sign of increased ICP.

30. c   31. b   32. d   33. a

34. Responsibilites include monitoring vital signs and electrolyte values closely, fluid status, blood pressure and pulse before and during administration, renal laboratory studies, and using an infusing pump to ensure accurate dosage.

35. c. Hypoosmolar fluids are generally not administered when ICP is suspected as it can result in further cerebral edema. The order should be verified before proceeding.

36. b

37. (a) seizure, (b) epilepsy

38. b. Complex seizures are characterized by an altered consciousness, often with nonpur-poseful activities.

39. d. The clonic phase consists of alternating contractions and relaxation of muscles.

40. c. Options (a) and (b) are sometimes used, but (c) is the drug of choice.

41. b. Washing the hair prior to the test removes oils that might interfere with the placements of electrodes.

42. d

43. b. Nothing should be forced or placed in the mouth when the client is actively seizing, as it may result in airway obstruction.

44. a. Alcohol should be avoided completely, as consumption of alcohol may lower the seizure threshold.

45. c. State and local laws determine whether or not he can drive. Driving is usually prohibited for 6 months to 2 years. The physician will have this information.

46. c. Migraine headaches have a familial charac-teristic and are associated with the menstrual cycle.

47. b. Cluster headaches are more common in males. Options (c) and (d) are both related to tension headaches.

48. d. the drug should be taken only when the first symptom occurs; if there is an aura, it should be taken at that time.

49. Three stages of a migraine headache include: (a) the aura stage—characterized by sensory manifestations lasting 5 to 50 minutes, (b) the headache stage—characterized by a throbbing headache, nausea, vomiting, tender scalp, and may last for hours or 1–2 days, (c) the postheadache stage—characterized by a sensitive headache area and a deep aching with exhaustion

50. Trigger factors for migraine headaches include rapid changes in blood glucose, stress, emo-tional excitement, fatigue, hormonal changes related to menstruation, bright lights, and food high in tyramine. Hypertension and febrile states can make the condition worse.

51. a. This is the only incorrect statement. Beta-blockers like atenolol are taken on a regular basis in an effort to prevent migraines.

52. Two nursing responsibilities include assessing the client for a history of peripheral vascular disease, renal or hepatic problems, and preg-nancy, and evaluating relief of migraine headaches.

53. The client should be taught not to take more than 2 injections in a 24-hour period; to allow at least 1 hour between injections; to use the autoinjector to administer the medication; how to administer the injection; how to dis-

pose of the syringe; and to report wheezing, heart palpitations, skin rash, swelling of the eyelids or face, or chest pain.

54. d

55. a. A leakage of spinal fluid indicates there is a direct route for infective agents to enter the CNS.

56. b. Edema from a brain contusion is most likely to peak 12–24 hours after the injury.

57. motor vehicle accident (MVA)

58. False   59. True   60. False

61. True   62. True

63. c   64. b   65. a   66. a   67. c

68. b   69. c   70. c   71. a

72. c. The other answers are true for intracerebral bleeds.

73. d. This case history is classic for a chronic subdural hematoma: it occurred at the time of injury and has now become a chronic condition, causing symptoms.

74. a. Alcohol abusers and older adults are at greatest risk for intracerebral hematomas related to falls.

75. c. Airway and ventilation must be the primary focus; the other options are components of the collaborative care and nursing care, but are not the primary focus.

76. (a) direct extension from trauma or invasive procedure, (b) bloodstream

77. d

78. c. Corticosteroids, antipyretics, and anticonvulsant agents may be a part of the therapy used to treat manifestations of meningitis, but they are not given in high doses.

79. a. Viruses are the most common causative organism for encephalitis.

80. c. Middle ear infections can extend into the brain, resulting in an abscess.

81. False   82. True

83. Symptoms include fever, chills, headache, back and abdominal pain, nausea, and vomiting.

84. Brudzinski's sign means that flexion of the neck causes the hip and knee to flex.

85. Kernig's sign relates to an inability to extend the knee while the hip is flexed at a 90-degree angle.

86. c   87. e   88. a

89. d   90. b

91. b. Glioblastoma multiforme is the most highly malignant brain tumor.

92. c. Lung tumors are most likely to metastasize to the brain.

93. d. The basis for cerebral edema resulting from a brain tumor is not known, but is well documented.

94. Answers may include: swollen, bruised eyelids; distorted facial features; an endotracheal tube or a tracheostomy tube will be in place, and client will be unable to speak; there will be a large bulky dressing. Assure them that all of this is usually temporary.

95. Answers may include: safety, comfort, pain, nausea/vomiting, communication, visual disturbances, cosmetic concerns, support groups, community resources, manifestations of complications

96. b. If the fluid tests positive for glucose, it is CSF and indicates a CSF leak. The nose should not be packed or suctioned. The head of bed should be maintained at 20 degrees unless contraindicated.

97. c. Narcotic analgesics may mask changes in eye signs and depress respirations.

■ ■ ■ Chapter 41

1. 20   2. a

3. Answers include: gravity, pressure

4. Answers may include: sneezing, coughing, straining for a bowel movement, vomiting

5. b   6. d   7. a   8. c

9. Answers may include: hypertension, diabetes mellitus, sickle cell disease, substance abuse, atherosclerosis, previous history of CVA, family history, obesity, sedentary lifestyle, hyperlipidemia, cardiac disease, use of oral contraceptives

10. b. A CVA causes deficits in the contralateral side.

11. e   12. c   13. b

14. d   15. a

16. b. Agnosia is the inability to recognize familiar objects.

17. d. the individual with expressive aphasia can understand speech, but has a limited ability to respond verbally.

18. c. The head will be immobilized.

19. b

20. b. Aspirin is used for its antiplatelet effect.

21. d. Heparin would increase bleeding.

22. a. Calcium channel blockers may reduce cerebral vasospasm.

23. b. *Ineffective Airway Clearance* is the highest priority in an unconscious client.

24. c. He should be side-lying to prevent aspiration.

25. c. Complaints of tightness may be an indication of neck swelling and bleeding. The operative site should be assessed.

26. help the client dress the affected extremity first, then allow the client to finish dressing alone. Using the unaffected extremities and participating in self-care promotes functionality and independence.

27. a. Prodromal signs of a cerebral aneurysm can be related to headaches, visual problems, nausea, and vomiting.

28. c. An explosive headache is a common complaint with an aneurysm.

29. d. The client would be in a deep coma. Grade I means no symptoms or slight headache; grade V means deep coma.

30. c. A quiet, restful environment helps prevent an increase in blood pressure.

31. (a) the first 48 hours, (b) 7–10 days

32. encourage passive activities such as watching TV or videos to promote relaxation and help control B/P. Visitors should be limited.

33. b. An AV malformation is a tangled collection of dilated arteries and veins that allows blood to flow directly from the arterial into the venous system.

34. Answers include: radiation therapy, laser therapy

35. c. 60% of individuals with cord injuries are males 16–30.

36. d. Motor vehicle accidents account for 45.5% of cord injuries.

37. c   38. c   39. d   40. b   41. e

42. c   43. a   44. c   45. d

46. d. A spinal cord injury in the cervical level will result in impaired respiratory function.

47. a. Immobilizing the neck will prevent further tissue damage.

48. b. A Halo traction device allows for early mobility.

49. c

50. b. Self-catheterization is a frequently used bladder routine.

51. The nurse should inform the client that erections and ejaculations are still possible and may be used to inseminate his wife.

52. a. The HOB should be elevated and TEDS removed to decrease venous return, thus decreasing B/P. B/P should be frequently assessed.

53. c. The lumbar disks are most frequently herniated.

54. c   55. a   56. b   57. a   58. a   59. b

60. a. Initially a client with an acute ruptured intervertebral disk will be recommended to take a short period of bed rest.

61. b. A myelogram lasts for about 1 hour.

62. b. Unexplained incontinence may be an indication of decreased motor function and/or hematoma formation, and should be reported immediately.

63. c. Shoes should be flat-heeled and provide good support.

64. c

65. (a–b) rapidly, slowly; (c–d) hard, soft

66. False   67. True

68. True   69. False

70. Important assessments include monitoring neurologic function and any changes and assessing pain and pain control.

▪ ▪ ▪ **Chapter 42**

1. b

2. Answers include: neurofibrillary tangles, neuritic plaques

3. c. Echolalia is the term used when one repeats words over and over.

4. d   5. b

6. a. These findings are consistent with stage 2. Option (b) describes stage 1, and options (c) and (d) describe stage 3.

7. d. Increased monitoring and assessment is appropriate.

8. b. This diagnosis is only made after other causes have been ruled out. A brain biopsy would only be performed postmortem in this situation.

9. b. A score below 24 indicates possible dementia, depression, delirium, or schizophrenia.

10. Answers include: assess for fatigue and agitation, maintain a consistent daily environment,

remove client from situations causing increased anxiety, schedule rest periods or quiet time

11. c. If the client smokes, serum levels may decrease and the dose may need to be increased.

12. a. Weakness after a warm bath is Uhthoff's sign and may indicate MS.

13. c. Visual signs are often a first sign of MS.

14. d

15. the worsening of the client's condition may be due to an autoimmune response. Removing inflammatory agents is the purpose of plasmapheresis.

16. demyelination

17. d. An MRI detects lesions in the white matter.

18. c. Jaundice should be reported immediately, as this medication can induce hepatitis.

19. Answers include: nonintention tremor, bradykinesia, muscle rigidity

20. a. Insufficient dopamine in the basal ganglia best describes Parkinson's disease.

21. a. Resting tremor is characteristic of Parkinson's disease.

22. d. There are no laboratory or diagnostic tests for Parkinson's disease.

23. Monoamine oxidase (MAO) inhibitor works by *inhibiting* the enzyme that *inactivates* dopamine. Example: Eldepryl (selegiline)

24. Dopaminergics cross the blood-brain barrier to be converted to dopamine. Example: carbidopa-levodopa

25. Dopamine agonist directly activates dopamine receptors in the brain. Example: Parlodel (bromocriptine)

26. Anticholinergics block the action of acetylcholine. Example: Cogentin (benztropine)

27. Phenothiazines

28. b   29. e   30. d   31. a   32. c   33. f

34. a. This medication may not take effect for weeks or months.

35. d. This drug can cause urinary retention. A client with benign prostatic hypertrophy may develop urinary retention.

36. Answers include: dementia, chorea

37. b

38. c. Decreasing stimuli may be helpful when caring for the client with Huntington's chorea.

39. a. Aspiration is the most common cause of death.

40. a. The client may have the genetic marker. Although carriers can be identified, there is no cure. Symptoms of the disease may occur as late as age 30–40, when the gene has already been passed on to the next generation.

41. b

42. (a–b) answers include: weakness, paresis; (c) one muscle group

43. focal twitching of involved muscles

44. a. A decreasing O_2 saturation may indicate increasing respiratory difficulty. The HOB should be elevated at least 30 degrees, and the client should be turned every 2 hours. Clear lung sounds are a normal finding.

45. a   46. c

47. d. Improved muscle strength after administration of an anticholinesterase drug is diagnostic of myasthenia gravis.

48. a   49. b

50. Answers include: planning meals to promote medication effectiveness, providing prompts to chew food thoroughly, teaching caregivers the Heimlich maneuver, matching food consistency with ability to swallow, schedule meals when client is well-rested

51. a

52. a. Plasmapheresis is most helpful in the earliest stages of Guillain-Barré syndrome.

53. c. Applying heat or cold to the affected area may relieve pain.

54. c. This vital capacity may indicate a need for ventilatory support. The physician should be notified.

55. d. Facial pain is the primary symptom of trigeminal neuralgia.

56. Answers may include: use artificial tears 4 times per day, do not rub eyes, wear protective sunglasses when indicated, schedule regular eye exams, blink frequently, wear an eye patch at night, check eye for redness and swelling daily

57. a. Pain behind the ear or along the jaw may precede the paralysis.

58. b   59. c

60. Answers may include: massage the affected side of the face TID, manually close the eyelid BID, practice wrinkling the forehead, practice closing the eyes, practice blowing air out of a puckered mouth, whistle for 5 minutes TID or QID

61. c

62. b. A darkened, quiet room decreases stimulation.
63. a. Active immunization prevents tetanus.
64. 50
65. (a) 10, (b) 5
66. d. Botulism occurs from eating improperly canned or cooked foods.
67. 12 to 36
68. respiratory paralysis causing death
69. True   70. False
71. True   72. True
73. Points to include: processing home-canned food in a pressure cooker rather than boiling water; not eating home-processed foods that are soft, contain air bubbles, or have a bad odor; heating home-processed foods and commercial foods at temperatures over 248F; discarding home-processed or commercially canned or bottled foods with defective seals; discarding commercially prepared canned foods that are damaged or have bulging sides or leaking contents
74. False   75. True   76. True
77. (a) transmissible, (b) progressively fatal, (c) 55 and 74
78. The most appropriate response is that the disease is diagnosed with a thorough neurologic examination, an EEG, and CT scan. The final diagnosis is made on postmortem examination.
79. The most appropriate response is that in the early stages it is hard to distinguish CJD from AD. It progresses faster and usually is fatal within 3 to 12 months.

■ ■ ■ **Chapter 43**

1. Answers include: to encode the patterns of light from the environment through photoreceptors, to carry coded information from the eyes to the brain
2. Answers include: intraocular, extraocular
3. (a) Extraocular or accessory structures, (b) Intraocular structures
4. optic chiasma
5. a
6. (a) light rays bend as they pass from one medium to another medium of different optical density, (b) refracted light rays are bent at the lens so they come together at a single point on the retina. Focusing of this image is known as accommodation.

7. Answers include: hearing, maintaining equilibrium
8. Answers include: trapping foreign bodies, protecting tympanic membrane and middle ear from infections
9. d   10. k   11. g   12. q   13. t
14. b   15. u   16. l   17. m   18. f
19. s   20. c   21. e   22. h   23. v
24. n   25. a   26. o   27. r   28. j
29. p   30. i   31. b   32. f   33. d
34. g   35. a   36. h   37. e   38. c
39. (a) static balance, (b) dynamic balance
40. (a) squinting, (b) abnormal eye movements
41. ringing in the ears
42. d. The Rosenbaum chart is used for testing near vision.
43. strabismus
44. b
45. Unequal pupillary size may indicate severe neurologic problems, such as increased intracranial pressure.
46. by shining a light obliquely into one eye at a time as the client looks straight ahead, and observing constriction of the pupil in the opposite eye.
47. c
48. ophthalmoscope
49. cataract
50. a. The ears and hearing are assessed primarily through inspection of external structures, the external auditory canal, and the tympanic membrane.
51. tuning fork
52. d
53. Answers include: pearly gray, shiny, semi-transparent
54. b. These symptoms are descriptive of age-related changes in the older adult.
55. less cerumen production is an age-related change in the older adult that results in a dry auditory canal and increased risk for impaction of cerumen.
56. Presbycusis is an age-related loss of the ability to hear high frequency sounds.
57. high frequency sounds such as normal speech
58. Arcus senilis is an accumulation of calcium and cholesterol salts around the limbus that creates a gray halo around the outer edge of the cornea. It should not affect Mr. Ramos or

his vision. He might notice the gray halo when he looks at his eyes closely.

■ ■ ■ **Chapter 44**

1. c. Decreased corneal sensitivity increases the potential for damage due to a foreign body or trauma and is a common age-related change in the eye.
2. c. Tear secretion is decreased with age. This condition increases the potential for infection or damage due to environmental pollution.
3. b
4. a. Hordeolum is a staphylococcal abscess that may occur on either the external or internal margin of the lid.
5. Trachoma
6. d. Because there is no blood supply, immune defenses have difficulty fending off infections of the cornea.
7. c. A frequent cause of corneal ulcer is bacterial infection following trauma or contact lens overuse.
8. c. The client should avoid activities that increase intraocular pressure, such as bending over or lifting heavy objects.
9. a. This position reduces intraocular pressure.
10. Answers may include: instructing the client to call for help before getting up or ambulating after surgery, administering prescribed analgesics and antiemetics postoperatively, instructing the client not to rub or scratch the eye, reinforcing the importance of using eye protection during hazardous activities, teaching client to apply a night shield, helping client deep breathe
11. b. The client should avoid wearing contact lenses until the cornea has healed completely.
12. (a) explosions, (b) flash burn injuries
13. In a penetrating injury, the layers of the eye spontaneously reapproximate after entry of a sharp-pointed object or small missile into the globe. In a perforating injury, the layers of the eye do not spontaneously reapproximate, resulting in rupture of the globe and potential loss of ocular contents.
14. Answers include: educating people about the prevention of eye injuries, providing direct care to clients with eye injuries

15. Causes include: contact lenses, eyelashes, small foreign bodies, and fingernails
16. (a) Chemical burns are treated initially with irrigation with copious amounts of fluids, preferably normal saline.
    (b) Immediate care for penetrating wounds focuses on pain relief and protecting the eyes from further injury.
    (c) Emergency treatment for blunt trauma includes bed rest in semi-Fowler's position and protecting the eyes from further injury with an eye shield.
17. b
18. Answers may include: avoid reading, lifting, or strenuous activity; leave the eye dressing in place; take prescribed medications; avoid sleeping on operative side; schedule a follow-up appointment
19. True   20. False
21. True   22. True
23. Glaucoma is a condition characterized by increased intraocular pressure of the eye and a gradual loss of vision.
24. d. Normal intraocular pressure is 12–20 mm Hg.
25. b   26. b   27. a   28. b
29. c. The angle of the anterior chamber of the eye is assessed with gonioscopy.
30. d. Timoptic (timolol) and other beta-adrenergic blockers have the advantage of a longer duration of activity than the miotics, allowing fewer doses per day.
31. c. Dorzolamide (Trusopt) is a diuretic in the carbonic anhydrase inhibitor group.
32. False. Surgical management includes improving the drainage of aqueous humor from the anterior chamber of the eye.
33. True
34. b. Clients need to understand the importance of lifetime therapy.
35. d. Floaters—irregular dark lines or spots in the field of vision—represent an important clinical manifestation of retinal detachment.
36. c. Correct positioning allows the contents of the posterior portion of the eye to place pressure on the detached area, bringing the retina in closer contact with the choroid.
37. Teaching points include signs and symptoms to report, the risk of future retinal detachment, the importance of seeking immediate treatment if recurrent symptoms occur, the

need to maintain regular follow-up care, and positioning.

38. a. When the macula is damaged, central vision becomes blurred and distorted, but peripheral vision remains intact.

39. b. Large-print books and magazines, the use of a magnifying glass, and high-intensity lighting can help the client to cope with the reduced vision of macular degeneration.

40. b. The initial manifestation of retinitis pigmentosa—difficulty with night vision—is often noted during childhood.

41. a. In the client with diabetes, the extent of retinopathy is reflective of the length of time the client has had the disease and the degree of control that has been maintained.

42. c. Yearly retinal examination is recommended for all adults with diabetes.

43. False   44. False   45. True

46. d. CMV retinitis develops in 10–15% of people with AIDS.

47. Answers may include: trauma, infection, glaucoma, intractable pain, malignancy

48. True. The person who has been blind from birth has developed numerous adaptive strategies that the newly blind person has yet to learn.

49. True   50. False

51. True   52. False

53. Causes include: cataracts, trachoma, glaucoma, onchocerciasis, nutritional deficits, trauma

54. c. Disruption of the normal environment within the external auditory canal typically precedes the inflammatory process. The removal of cerumen leaves the skin of the ear canal vulnerable to invasion and infection.

55. a. The pain of otitis externa can be differentiated from that associated with otitis media by manipulation of the auricle or tragus. In external otitis, this maneuver increases the pain. The client with otitis media experiences no change in pain perception.

56. b

57. d. Inform clients that ear canals rarely need cleansing beyond washing of the external meatus with soap and water.

58. a. When an organic foreign body is suspected, water should not be instilled into the ear canal because it may cause the object to swell, making its removal more difficult.

59. Clients should be taught that their ears rarely need cleaning and that they should never insert anything smaller than a finger wrapped with a washcloth into the ear canal.

60. c. On examination, the tympanic membrane demonstrates decreased mobility and may appear retracted or bulging.

61. d. A pneumatic otoscope allows a puff of air to be instilled into the ear canal so that the examiner can evaluate the mobility of the tympanic membrane.

62. b. A rapid change in barometric pressure can increase the client's pain significantly.

63. a. As soon as the pressure is released, pain subsides and hearing improves.

64. b. Pain that subsides abruptly may indicate spontaneous perforation of the tympanic membrane with relief of pressure within the middle ear.

65. prevention

66. True   67. False   68. True

69. Signs and symptoms include: recurrent earache, hearing loss, persistent pain, throbbing, tenderness over the mastoid process, redness, inflammation, swelling, fever, tinnitus, headache

70. Cholesteatomas

71. Yes. Otosclerosis is a hereditary disorder with an autosomal dominant pattern of inheritance.

72. False   73. True

74. True   75. True

76. c. A fast-acting diuretic, such as intravenous furosemide (Lasix), may be administered to the client to decrease fluid pressure in the inner ear. An acute temporary hearing improvement is considered diagnostic for Ménière's disease. An oral diuretic, such as oral furosemide, helps maintain a lower labyrinthine pressure.

77. True   78. False   79. False

80. b   81. b   82. a

83. b   84. a

85. b. These assistive devices do nothing to prevent, minimize, or treat the hearing loss, but they amplify the sound presented to the hearing apparatus of the ear.

86. The nurse should explain to the client that the cochlear prostheses will provide the perception of sound, but normal hearing will not be restored.

▪ ▪ ▪ Chapter 45

1. Answers include: provide for sexual pleasure, produce children, produce hormones for biological development and sexual behavior
2. e   3. a   4. h   5. c
6. k   7. g   8. b   9. j
10 f   11. i   12. d
13. (a) nourishes the sperm, (b) provides bulk, (c) increases alkalinity
14. Spermatogenesis
15. (a) androgens, (b) testosterone
16. g   17. c   18. d   19. i
20. k   21. a   22. e   23. j
24. f   25. h   26. b
27. Estrogen
28. Progesterone
29. Androgens
30. d   31. a
32. (a) menstrual, (b) proliferative, (c) secretory
33. b
34. b. Use of clinically correct terms for anatomical parts can be embarassing or intimidating for the client.
35. c
36. Answers include: chronic disease, medication use, stress
37. a   38. d
39. subjective: 52 years old, divorced, difficulty starting urination, dribbling, nocturia, no history of STDs, sexually active, wears condoms, multiple partners, no changes in urine appearance
    objective: uncircumcised penis, slight phimosis, normal testicles and scrotum, small inguinal bulge on right, enlarged prostate without tenderness
    abnormal assessment findings and possible etiologies: tight foreskin related to uncircumcised penis; small bulge in right inguinal area, possible right inguinal hernia; enlarged nontender prostate, probable benign prostatic hypertrophy
40. breasts
41. lithotomy
42. vaginal speculum
43. bimanual pelvic exam

▪ ▪ ▪ Chapter 46

1. c
2. (a) nocturia, (b) reflux of urine into the ureters
3. d. Hypertonic fluids may lead to fluid volume excess.
4. c. This problem should be evaluated by a physician. They are not age-related changes and a catheter is not the appropriate treatment. These symptoms indicate BPH, not prostatic cancer. A PSA may be performed, but evaluation by a physician is most important.
5. False   6. True
7. False   8. True
9. d. Disturbances in urine flow are the most common manifestation.
10. bowel
11. a. PSA is the specific test for detecting prostatic cancer.
12. b. In advanced cancer, surgery is only palliative.
13. a. Kegel exercises can eliminate or lessen stress incontinence.
14. b. An orchiectomy can result in permanent erectile dysfunction.
15. a. Blood clots are an indication of excessive bleeding and should be reported.
16. (a) 40
17. Answers may include: assess the client's and family's knowledge about surgery, inform the client he will have a catheter postoperatively, address concerns and anxieties regarding the surgery, obtain a signed consent, provide bowel preparation if ordered, ask about receiving blood transfusions
18. c. Movement should not be discouraged, but encouraged.
19. c. Some bleeding may be expected; excessive bleeding should be reported.
20. True   21. False   22. False
23. (a) incisional pain, (b) bladder spasm, (c) abdominal cramps related to intestinal gas
24. b. The tape is applied to the catheter tubing and applied tightly to help prevent bleeding.
25. b
26. d. Belladonna and opium suppositories provide relief of bladder spasms more effectively than the other measures.

27. (a) fluid volume deficit, (b) hyponatremia
28. (a) hyponatremia, (b) decreased hematocrit,
    (c) hypertension, (d) bradycardia,
    (e) nausea and confusion
29. a. Depending on the type of prostatectomy,
    the client may be able to resume his sexual
    activities 6 weeks after surgery.
30. Key elements include avoiding strenuous
    activity and heavy lifting, not driving for 2
    weeks, not taking long walks, taking stairs
    slowly and carefully, continuing dorsiflexion
    exercises, taking showers, and avoiding tub
    baths.
31. d. Sexual intercourse may relieve some con-
    gestion in the prostate.
32. c. Sitz baths and soaking may relieve
    congestion.
33. c. A painless nodule is the most common
    symptom.
34. a. An orchiectomy is always performed.
35. b. The testicles should be gently rolled, not
    squeezed.
36. d. In some forms of testicular cancer, sperm
    banking may be indicated. However, an
    orchiectomy for testicular cancer may not
    always change reproductive status.
37. True   38. False
39. False   40. False
41. e   42. c   43. a   44 b   45. d   46. a
47. Answers include: inguinal nodes, bones,
    lungs, liver
48. c   49. b
50. c. Physiologic reasons are the most common
    cause of erectile dysfunction.
51. Answers include: revascularization, penile
    implant
52 revascularization
53. a
54. c. Sildenafil can only be taken once a day.
55. False   56. True   57. False   58. False

Chapter 47

1. (a) estrogen, (b) progesterone,
   (c) aldosterone
2. b
3. Answers may include: abdominal pain,
   headache, diarrhea, breast tenderness, fatigue,
   nausea, vomiting
4. False   5. True   6. False

7. c   8. a   9 d   10. b   11 a
12. d. Resting and avoiding straining is an appro-
    priate intervention.
13. c. Heavy bleeding is not expected and should
    be reported.
14. c
15. Answers include: heart disease, osteoporosis,
    breast cancer
16. b. She should have a mammogram before
    starting the medication. The medication does
    have side effects and should be taken regu-
    larly as prescribed.
17. Answers may include: keep track of symp-
    toms, continue normal activities while hot
    flash is occurring, stay calm, keep moving,
    avoid hot-flash triggers, keep cool, keep learn-
    ing, keep involved, keep talking
18. True   19. False   20. False   21. True
22. (a) reduced risk of coronary artery disease,
    (b) reduced risk of Alzheimer's disease,
    (c) reduced risk of osteoporosis
23. b. This is the calcium requirement. All the
    other statements are correct.
24. c. Water-soluble lubricants will prevent vagi-
    nal irritation. All the other statements are
    false.
25. Answers include: uterine prolapse, cystocele,
    rectocele
26. c
27. Answers include: the possible benefits of hor-
    mone-replacement therapy, proper perineal
    care, decreasing caffeine intake, how to per-
    form Kegel exercises, use of perineal pads
28. False   29. True
30. e   31. d   32. f   33. b   34. a
35. True   36. False   37. False
38. True   39. False
40. estrogen
41. (a) lungs, (b) liver, (c) bone
42. (a) endometrial biopsy, (b) D and C
43. surgery
44. c
45. c. Abdominal bloating and constipation
    should be evaluated.
46. approximately 75%
47. d. A 40–60 watt light bulb should be used.
48. Risk factors include: early sexual experience,
    multiple sex partners, multiple pregnancies,
    human papilloma virus infections, genital
    herpes infections, cigarette smoking

49. b. Sexual intercourse can be resumed when vaginal discharge ceases (approximately one week).

50. because it is often asymptomatic until it is quite advanced

51. c   52. d   53. b   54. a

55. Answers include: client education, personal hygiene practices, safer sex

56. a. Diabetes is often associated with recurrent vaginal infections.

57. False   58. True

59. False   60. False

61. c. Super-absorbent tampons have been associated with TSS and should not be used. If tampons are used, they should be low absorbency and changed every 4 hours, with a tampon-free period each day.

62. Answers include: menopause is the death of a woman's sexuality, hysterectomy results in the loss of sexual function

63. a

64. False   65. True

■ ■ ■ **Chapter 48**

1. True   2. False   3. False

4. True   5. False

6. Noninvasive breast cancer represents the proliferation of malignant cells within the ducts and lobules of the breast without the invasion of surrounding tissues.
Invasive breast cancer refers to the penetration of the tumor into the surrounding tissues.

7. Answers include: female gender, age

8. nipple epithelium

9. Answers include: bloodstream, lymphatic system

10. d   11. e   12. a   13. b   14. c

15. Answers include: tumor size, lymph node involvement, metastasis to distant sites

16. a

17. Answers include: mammography, breast self-exam, breast clinical examination

18. a. Culturally sensitive material will increase compliance.

19. Answers include: arms relaxed at sides, arms lifted overhead, hands pressed against hips and together at waist level, leaning forward

20. c. This is the recommended approach to BSE.

21. d   22. b   23. a

24. e   25. c

26. Answers include: lumpectomy, radiation therapy

27. d. An estrogen-positive breast cancer in a postmenopausal woman means that tamoxifen can be used to prevent recurrences.

28. b. Breast cancer is not a local disease; it is treated as a systemic illness. The nurse should be able to answer this question without referring her to the doctor. Chemotherapy is not always part of the standard therapy; it reduces, but does not eliminate, the risks of metastasis.

29. a. Radiation in this instance is palliative and will assist in controlling pain and preventing fractures; it will not destroy cancer cells. Surgery in these regions is not indicated.

30. d. Massage will prevent development of a fibrous capsule.

31. c. Weight gain is a common side effect of this drug.

32. a. The nonaffected arm should be used to assess blood pressure and for venipunctures.

33. c. The client should avoid heavy lifting such as carrying grocery bags.

34. b. The client should avoid abduction and not raise the elbow above shoulder height. Holding the arm still will lead to contractures. Pain and discomfort may be late signs of excessive movement. Activity should be gradually increased once the drain is removed.

35. b. Research suggests that older women have less emotional distress than younger women. Older women have greater needs for personal and home care services. They may not have higher pain thresholds.

36. False   37. True

38. True   39. False

40. Answers include: aging, hormonal changes

41. c. Eliminating caffeine is recommended in fibrocystic breast changes.

42. d   43. e   44. b   45. a   46. c

■ ■ ■ **Chapter 49**

1. Answers may include: a more permissive attitude towards sexuality, the use of oral contraceptives instead of condoms, emergence of HIV/AIDS

2. Answers include: people of color in urban populations of lower socioeconomic status, those with less education

3. b. Latex condoms help control the spread of infection.

4. 25

5. state and federal agencies

6. Answers may include: blood, saliva, open lesions, body fluids

7. c. A genital chancre would be present in the early stages of syphilis.

8. b. This is a confirmatory test for syphilis.

9. c

10. Answers may include: referring all sexual partners for evaluation and treatment, abstaining from all sexual contact for 1 month after treatment, using a condom to avoid transmitting or contracting infections in the future, attending follow-up evaluations at 3- and 6-month intervals, taking any and all precribed medications, understanding signs and symptoms of re-infection

11. d

12. d. Painful papules below the trunk are consistent with genital herpes.

13. d. Antivirals such as acyclovir would be prescribed.

14. Answers include: water, soap, hydrogen peroxide

15. (a) cervical cancer, (b) infection of neonate during delivery

16. b

17. Answers include: take medications as ordered and keep follow-up appointments, abstain from sex until cured of infection

18. False   19. True

20. False   21. True

22. c

23. Answers include: PID, endometritis, chronic pelvic pain, salpingitis

24. a. A Pap smear will be helpful in detecting cervical cancer, which may occur as a result of genital warts.

25. False   26. False   27. False

28. True   29. False   30. True